THE DISSECTION OF
A DEGENERATIVE DISEASE

THE DISSECTION OF
A DEGENERATIVE DISEASE

Proceedings of Four Round-Table Conferences on the Pathogenesis of Batten's Disease (Neuronal Ceroid-Lipofuscinosis)

Editors:

WOLFGANG ZEMAN
Indiana University, Indianapolis, U.S.A.

and

J. ALFRED RIDER
President, Children's Brain Diseases Foundation, San Francisco, U.S.A.

 1975

EXCERPTA MEDICA – AMSTERDAM · OXFORD
AMERICAN ELSEVIER PUBLISHING CO. – NEW YORK

ISBN Excerpta Medica 90 219 2100 6
ISBN American Elsevier 0 444 16715 3

Sole distributors for the U.S.A. and Canada:

American Elsevier Publishing Company, Inc.
52 Vanderbilt Avenue
New York, N.Y. 10017

Printed in The Netherlands

Dedicated to

Charles Alfred Rider

our inspiration

PREFACE

Medicine in the United States is becoming increasingly government oriented. Electrorate, trade unions, and politicians alike demand and successfully obtain more and more government control. Today the government directs the major part of scientific inquiry into diseases and their treatment. Consequently, enormous amounts of tax funds are spent on such major disabling and killing diseases as cancer, respiratory disorders and cardiovascular illnesses; but the political pressure of minority groups has also succeeded in making substantial funds available to the study of less common diseases, for example sickle cell anemia and multiple sclerosis.

The potential rewards offered by productive research on major health problems are high, both with respect to financial return and to scientific glory. This promise, however, tends to obscure and neglect the possibility that exceedingly rare but equally disabling diseases may yield to scientific inquiry and thus become amenable to prevention and perhaps cure. These diseases also result in loss of manpower and in enormous costs for medical care, frequently borne by society but often by the individuals and families so affected. As regards these "minor" health problems, one notes with relief that currently a large number of heredodegenerative diseases can be diagnosed prenatally, by demonstrating the genetically controlled enzyme defect on the amniotic contents. This enables the parents to obtain a therapeutic abortion, eliminating the threat of prolonged heartbreak and of financial disaster. In many instances, the investigations which led to these beneficial developments were spurred by the initiative of individuals. Consequently, these efforts were more often supported by private rather than fiscal funds.

Against this background, we, the editors decided in 1968 to generate private funds in support of furthering the knowledge on a then little known disease, "Juvenile Amaurotic Idiocy", with the aim to develop data upon which rational treatment could be designed. This decision was made because one of us (J.A.R.) after years of futile medical consultations had been apprised that his firstborn son suffered from this disease. At that time, little was known about the pathogenesis of this recessively inherited brain degeneration except for the fact that it definitely was not related to the "Amaurotic Familial Idiocy" of the Tay-Sachs type, a lysosomal disorder due to

i

a deficiency of β-N-hexosaminidase.

Our task appeared formidable and our situation unique;
how does one approach the solution to a practically undefined
medical problem? The present volume partly answers the question
in providing the transcripts of four round table conferences
solely devoted to the pathogenesis and the possible treatment
of Juvenile Amaurotic Idiocy which subsequently became recognized
as one of several disorders which make up the group of Neuronal
Ceroid-Lipofuscinoses.

In contrast to the typical biomedical symposia which
have proliferated during the past two decades, the conferences
did not primarily attempt to gather medical investigators
who had already made contributions to the understanding of
the disease under question; rather, from the beginning our
aim was to have a major emphasis from scientists whose ideas
would be unencumbered by preconceived opinions. One guiding
principle helped us shape these conferences and that was the
observation that the disorder, which we as a form of laboratory
jargon call "Batten's Disease", is characterized by the massive
accumulation of autofluorescent lipopigments which result
from the peroxidation of unsaturated fatty acids. Therefore,
lipid peroxidation seemed to be a prime suspect for the pathogenesis and the editors made every attempt to secure the cooperation of researchers active in this field.

The present volume is not a monograph devoted to Batten's
disease or neuronal ceroid-lipofuscinosis. Although it does
contain information on the clinical, genetic, morphological
and biochemical aspects of this group of diseases, the clinician
or neuropathologist who has to deal with the problem will
search in vain for complete, let alone exhaustive information.

In a sense, this book is a guide into the uncharted terra
incognita of a specific human disease but it may very well
serve as a map for the inquiry into the pathogenesis of other
unknown or little understood diseases. It is a lively account
as to how scientists with radically different backgrounds
confer and discuss, propose hypotheses, and dissect the thoughts
and proposals of others. It uncovers some autistic thinking,
particularly of the scientifically trained physician, but
it also shows how the physician can gain immeasurably from
scientific intercourse with the pure scientist.

Much information on lipid peroxidation, its chain-breaking
prevention, the role of free radicals on enzymatic and chemical
protection against lipid peroxidation, and on monitoring of
peroxidase activity will be found in this volume. Some search-
ing thoughts on the biochemical expression of genetic defects
are recorded. Extended passages deal with the role of vitamin
E, not only as a chain-breaker in lipid peroxidation, but
also as a co-factor for the enzymes operative in heme synthesis.

General discussions probe into the possibilities of studying fatty acid and lipid turnover in monolayer cultures and explants and into the promise of enzyme replacement therapy. Most important are the repeated references to lipid peroxidation as a factor in aging, and the presentation of promising data on the extension of the mean life span by the use of antioxidants.

Much of this information has been previously published; some of it is entirely new. The most fascinating aspect of these discussions however is to see how a particular concept, shaped after many experiments and observations, becomes refined and more sophisticated under the impact of discussion and dissection by scientists representing different fields. It is obvious that this book does not address itself to a medical specialty; rather, it cuts across the barriers which separate specialists and therefore appeals to the biomedical community in general.

Needless to say, the approach on which the present volume is based has some drawbacks. In the first place, there is some repetition because of the changing composition of the participants in the four conferences. Furthermore, it is intriguing to note how some of the participants go off on a tangent, completely missing the problem under discussion. The editors felt that these parts of the transcript should not be deleted for the same reason that they exercised great care in leaving the spoken word intact rather than transform the recorded and transcribed proceedings into a more stereotyped text. This decision has preserved the enlivened style and makes for smooth reading even of those parts in which the discussion degenerates into some meaningless and irrelevant talk.

Owing to financial risk envisioned by the publisher, the editors decided to produce the volume by making negatives for offset printing available to the publisher. Therefore all the copy editing had to be done by us and only we are responsible for errors, omissions, and garbled phraseology. We felt, however, that we should proceed with this venture and make this unique volume available to the scientific community as an exercise in scientific methodology and progress.

W.Z.
J.A.R.
July, 1975

FOREWORD

Those who now make up the Board of Trustees of the Children's
Brain Diseases Foundation, having close personal knowledge of
the tremendous battle for survival which my wife and I were
waging on behalf of our son, Charles, were as distressed as we
were that there was no practical way to diagnose, let
alone treat, an unknown cerebral degenerative disease. Consequently, the concept of the foundation for children's brain
diseases was developed and in 1968 the Children's Brain Diseases
Foundation was created as a non-profit, tax exempt, charitable
organization to determine the cause and cure of various progressively deteriorating brain diseases occurring in infancy
and childhood. After many years, Charles' condition had finally
been diagnosed as Spielmeyer-Vogt Batten's disease by Doctor
Wallace Tourtellotte and confirmed by Doctor Wolfgang Zeman.
The first goal of the Foundation, therefore, because of the
stimulus provided by Charles' plight, was to study this disease.
We elected to shorten the term to Batten's disease for historical
and pragmatic reasons and it is the feeling of the Foundation
that this term should be retained. To the Foundation Board
of Trustees it became immediately and painfully apparent that,
contrary to what was available for cancer, heart disease,
diabetes, etc., there was a lack of public or private funds
available to study brain diseases. To this end, the Foundation
has managed to raise money and as a result has sponsored six
Round Table Conferences, four of which make up this publication.
These were conducted as "think tank" sessions without prepared
presentations, wherein each participant was encouraged to
have a free-flow of ideas concerning the etiology and treatment
of Batten's disease. As a direct result of these conferences,
various research projects were sponsored by the Foundation.
It is hoped that this publication will provide a wealth of
material concerning specifically Batten's disease as well
as other cerebral degenerative diseases and including the
so-called "normal" aging brain.

Over the last seven years a much better understanding
of Batten's disease has evolved and it has become clear that
it is not as rare as previously supposed, and that there are
families in which as many as four children are affected.

The brain lesion has been more precisely identified and
has been shown to consist of an accumulation of two specific

iv

classes of pigment, the yellow ceroid and the brown lipofuscin. It is probable however, that this accumulation is the end product of the disease and not its cause. With the recent work of Dr. Armstrong, confirmed by Dr. Zeman, it is apparent that there is a measurable lack of peroxidase enzyme in children with Batten's disease. Knowledge of this enzyme defect has now reinforced and strengthened earlier concepts suggested by Dr. Tappel and Dr. Zeman that the defect in Batten's disease must be somehow related to defective peroxidation in the brain cells. Thus, a study of enzymes responsible for these reactions and treatment directed toward influencing these reactions by antioxidants has been instituted.

The thrust of the 6th conference was to report on additional studies involving whole families who have children with Batten's disease. It is now clear that every child with Batten's disease has a low peroxidase enzyme level. However, some of the brothers and sisters also have a low enzyme level and either the father or mother have a low level and yet all of these subjects do not have the disease. Therefore, it is now apparent that it is just as important to investigate why the relatives with low enzyme levels do not have the disease as why certain children do have the disease. In other words, there must be protective mechanisms or enzymes that are making up or compensating for this lack. The healthy have this, the sick do not.

At the 6th conference the next steps for investigation were defined. These include the following:

1. Study of companion enzymes (iso-enzymes or co-enzymes) in the sick children and their healthy relatives.

2. Study of possible activation factors which would make the lesser amount of enzyme more effective.

3. Study of the possibility of the presence of an activator of the peroxidase enzyme in the healthy children and adults who have a low level.

4. Study of a theory that two defects may be necessary for the disease. One of these is the lack of peroxidase which the subject inherits from one of his parents and the other a second unknown factor which he inherits from the other parent or a lack of a protective factor which he did not inherit from either parent.

5. Finding an inhibitor for the increased peroxide which results from a deficiency in peroxidase.

6. Finding a way to enhance and increase the utility of the deficient peroxidase.

7. Finding a replacement for the deficient peroxidase.

Since we have on our hands a group of children with a disease which is slowly progressing and at present is eventually fatal, we feel it most important to continue treating these subjects with the broad spectrum approach while the pure research and scientific programs are going on. Thus, from this conference--on theoretical grounds--the suggestion was again made to use antioxidants or activators of peroxidase. Drugs such as nicotinic acid, p-chlorophenoxy acetate of tocopherol, methionine, glutathione, thiazolidin carboxylic acid, benzoic acid and imidazole will be utilized, in addition to continuing previous treatment with vitamin E, vitamin C, L-Dopa, synthetic antioxidants used as food preservatives such as butylated hydroxytoluene, and peroxidase (both crystalline and natural forms, such as horseradish and avocado). Further progress will be reported and a follow-up conference will be held next year, or sooner if warranted.

Hopefully, this publication will prove to be of benefit to the neurologist, pediatrician, neurosurgeon, neuropathologist, biochemist, enzyme chemist, clinician and all physicians in general. Furthermore, we hope that the background of the Foundation and the results obtained to date will act as encouragement for other similar organizations to raise funds and sponsor medical research. From this may there be light from darkness, order out of chaos, hope where there was despair, encouragement where there was discouragement, a future where there was a past; and may the physician be able and allowed to think freely, clearly and creatively, unencumbered by administrative red tape, rules and regulations.

J.A.R.

ACKNOWLEDGEMENTS

We wish to express appreciation and thanks to the following members of the Board of Trustees of the Children's Brain Diseases Foundation--Charles I. Kramer, James Martin MacInnis, Graclynn L. Rider, Richard D. Rider, M.D., Robert B. Sutherland and Jay W. Walsh, Jr.; to the Women's Auxillary of the Children's Brain Diseases Foundation, especially the officers, Mrs. J. Alfred Rider, Mrs. Richard D. Rider, Mrs. Barry F. Regan, Mrs. Raymond Vuksich, Mrs. Francis J. Keane and to the committee chairmen, Mrs. Milton Romey and Mrs. Jack Kennedy; to the participants of these round table conferences; to Dr. Vimal Patel for editorial help; to our secretarial assistants, Nilda Greene, Marilyn Kampsnider, Joyce Swader and Vivian Eldridge; and most deeply to the numerous financial contributors to the Foundation.

Our publisher most graciously accepted the risk of producing this volume, despite its novel and untried approach. In this connection, specific thanks are directed to Dr. P. Vinken, Dr. G. W. Bruyn, and Dr. J. Franklin for their generous help and understanding attitude.

INTRODUCTION

Sometime in 1956, Charles Rider, a vivacious, attractive
and intelligent boy of 8 years began to experience occasional
slight difficulty in maintaining his equilibrium and in performing complex movements. His parents noticed that he would
fall while playing more frequently than the circumstances
would explain and certainly more often than would be expected
for a normally active child. His father, a physician, immediately realized that something was wrong with the boy's motor
function, but expert medical consultation did not uncover
any neurological abnormalities. In fact, the parents were
told not to worry about these changes in the development of
their son. Consequently they took comfort in the realization
that the child's scholastic abilities were exceptional and
immensely rewarding and tried to overlook the motor disturbance.
However, within the next several months Charles had a generalized
seizure, his scholastic performance declined and what had
been considered a mere clumsiness developed into overt motor
incapacitation. Having easy access to the best trained medical
colleagues in the country, his parents spared no effort to
arrive at a diagnosis. However, these pains eventually terminated in the office of a psychiatrist who told the parents
that the symptoms and signs of the child were the reflection
of their emotional problems and that the child therefore would
benefit from a psychotherapeutic effort brought to bear on
patient and parents as well. Only after an illness of 10
years, when Charles had become practically blind and was
dysarthric and ataxic, did a neurologist diagnose "juvenile
amaurotic idiocy."

Parenthetically one may remark that it is not unusual
for a variety of degenerative brain diseases in children to
cause such persistent diagnostic difficulties. In the first
place these conditions are exceedingly rare and therefore
are observed only in a few instances, even by the busiest
pediatric neurologist. Furthermore, only recently has sufficiently detailed information been disseminated in medical
journals for the practioner to arrive at a correct diagnosis.

Finally, whenever the opinions of parents and physicians
differ about symptoms in a child, the parents' concern is
often interpreted as proof of their emotional instability,
especially if objective neurological signs of the disease
are minimal or missing. This occurs in spite of the fact

1

that an intelligent parent, with the advantages of continuous observation of the child in a variety of circumstances and the comparison with normal siblings, is often a better and more objective observer than a physician.

Dr. Rider, being a highly successful researcher of his own right, and a pragmatist, immediately consulted the literature on juvenile amaurotic idiocy, but to his disappointment found little tangible information. Instead of resigning himself to the fact that his son suffered from a rare, little known intractable disease, Dr. Rider wrote to and obtained from the then National Institute of Neurological Disease and Blindness, a list of investigators engaged in what we now call lysosomal diseases. Dr. Rider sent personal letters to each of them, inquiring about the latest information on juvenile amaurotic idiocy. In this way he got in touch with me in 1967 and although we had done a considerable number of studies on this particular disorder, I was not able to tell him the etiology of the disease. I could only point out that the term "juvenile amaurotic idiocy" was misleading, because it alluded to an etiopathogenetic relationship to Tay-Sachs disease, or infantile amaurotic idiocy, whereas our research had clearly proven that no disturbance of ganglioside or even sphingolipid metabolism was demonstrable in juvenile amaurotic idiocy. I could also tell him that this disease, together with a few others, was characterized by the accumulation of autofluorescent lipopigments, a process which was invariably associated with loss of neurons. Since this particular clinicopathological correlation had first been described by F. E. Batten in 1903, we had come to call the condition Batten's disease, following the British who spoke of the Batten type of amaurotic idiocy.

The term Batten's disease proved to be a poor choice. In the first place many colleagues objected to abandoning the names of other investigators who also had made contributions to the knowledge of these conditions. They pointed out that one of the critical papers was published by Mayou in 1904 and that Batten and Mayou had combined their forces in 1914 in order to more precisely define the condition in terms of clinical and pathomorphologic findings. It was also remarked that H. Vogt and Spielmeyer in Germany had done much to clarify the nature of this disease. In the German-speaking countries juvenile amaurotic idiocy thus became known as Spielmeyer-Vogt disease whereas in Great Britain apparently the same condition was designated as Batten-Mayou disease. Subsequently, however, these terms took on different meanings and ophthalmologists used the eponym Batten-Mayou to designate certain fundic changes such as macular degeneration whereas the Spielmeyer-Vogt type was supposed to designate a retinitis pigmentosa-like picture.

Our justification for using the term Batten's disease was predicated on the fact that Batten described not only instances of the juvenile type of the disease but also of the so-called late infantile type later defined by Bielschowsky (1913). In this context it must be mentioned that in 1908 the Czech psychiatrist Jansky had already delineated a late infantile type of amaurotic idiocy which he considered different from the infantile type of amaurotic idiocy or Tay-Sachs disease. Since the "juvenile" and the "late infantile" types are indeed quite similar with respect to histopathology, it seemed appropriate to retain the name Batten, to which we added that of Vogt, who like Batten, had also considered both types to be closely related. Thus we began to use the term Batten-Vogt syndrome.

The almost arbitrary use of eponyms for the age-dependent subtypes of amaurotic familial idiocy, to which Seitelberger (1961) added a "myoclonic variant", made it mandatory to devise a new terminology based on morphological features. The emphasis on morphologic criteria became a necessity, since the clinical features of amaurosis and dementia turned out not to be invariant signs of the disorder, whereas the accumulation of autofluorescent lipopigments and the loss of cerebral nerve cells represented consistent and pathognomonic findings. Accordingly, we chose the term "neuronal ceroid-lipofuscinoses" for all disorders with evidence of primary excessive formation of autofluorescent pigments which were retained in the nerve cells. Those cases conforming to the Jansky and Bielschowsky definition--a pernicious, rapidly progressive degenerative brain disease, highlighted by intractable convulsions and rapid loss of mental functions--were termed the Jansky-Bielschowsky type of the neuronal ceroid-lipofuscinoses. Similarly, the cases of amaurotic idiocy originally described by Spielmeyer and later confirmed as a separate entity by Sjögren were designated the Spielmeyer-Sjögren type of neuronal ceroid-lipofuscinoses. The scattered observations of cases clinically manifested during adulthood were called the Kufs type of neuronal ceroid-lipofuscinoses, named for the author of the casus princeps (1925). In 1971 Dr. Koppang applied the term to a disease in dogs when he realized that a degenerative brain disease in English Setters, inherited as an autosomal recessive, had all the hallmarks of what we defined as neuronal ceroid-lipofuscinoses. In 1973 Santavuori and Haltia, with other Finnish pediatricians and neuropathologists, proved conclusively that the neuronal ceroid-lipofuscinoses also include a disease which becomes manifest during the first year of life (originally described by Hagberg, Sourander and Svennerholm in 1968). We had included similar cases with the Jansky-Bielschowsky type but Santavuori and Haltia demonstrated the faulty nature of this classification.

Currently we consider the neuronal ceroid-lipofuscinoses to consist of four distinguishable human disorders and a well-defined disease in English Setters as shown in Table 1.

	Clinical Highlights	Gross Neuropathology	Ultrastructure of Residual Bodies	Deficiency of PPD-peroxidase
Santavuori-Haltia type	Onset during infancy; rapid deterioration of cerebral functions. Rare seizures. Prolonged state of decortication.	Extreme atrophy of brain, 250-500 gram. Extensive loss of myelinated fibers.	Predominantly with granular matrix.	Unknown
Jansky-Bielschowsky type	Onset during early childhood or adolence. Rapid deterioration of cerebral function. Frequent intractable seizures, Relatively short survival.	Severe atrophy of brain, 500 to 800 grams.	Curvilinear profiles, fingerprint pattern and granular matrix.	Yes
Spielmeyer-Sjögren type	Onset with visual failure during childhood. Slowly progressive deterioration of cerebral functions. Seizures as late manifestation.	Moderate atrophy of brain, 800-1400 grams.	Fingerprint pattern, curvilinear profiles and granular matrix.	Yes
Kufs type	Onset during adulthood usually with motor disturbances. No visual problems. Dementia mild to absent.	Moderate atrophy of brain, 1000-1400 grams.	Granular matrix, often with lipid vacuoles (lipofuscin?)	Yes
Canine NCL (Koppang)	Stereotyped picture with onset around age 15 months. Loss of orientation, incoordination and weakness. Death at age 25 months.	Atrophy of brain about 70% of normal weight.	Pleomorphic inclusions, fingerprint pattern, curvilinear profiles and others	Yes

Table 1. Current classification of the Neuronal Ceroid-Lipofuscinoses.

It must be pointed out that not all observations fit into this rigid scheme and that certain cases must be called transitional forms.

Unfortunately, the term neuronal ceroid-lipofuscinosis is clumsy and does not lend itself to being used easily in conversation. It is presumably for this reason that other designations are still being used, and we who coined the new term are no exception. Thus, it has become customary in our daily laboratory jargon to speak of Batten's disease with the understanding that a) this terminology is inadequate and b) that the word "disease" is wrongly used because we are really dealing with a syndrome, and possibly a variety of diseases. Nevertheless this term is almost exclusively employed in the discussions which are recorded in this book.

Although terminology was only a peripheral issue in relation to Dr. Rider's probing questions, it was obviously necessary to clarify what diseases we were considering because even today many physicians and even investigators in the field of degenerative brain diseases in children hold the opinion that the diseases now called the neuronal ceroid-lipofuscinoses are all due to specific disturbances in ganglioside metabolism, as has been proven for Tay-Sachs disease and therefore implied by the now abandoned term, "amaurotic idiocy."

After the diagnosis of Charles Rider's disease had been made and confirmed, Dr. Rider was understandably determined to have his son treated. He pointed out correctly that Steinberg, by having uncovered the pathogenesis of Refsum's disease, had found a way of treating patients with this condition dietetically by withholding any type of food that would result in the intermediary production of phytanic acid and it was Dr. Rider's hope that a similar approach might prove successful in "Batten's disease." Unfortunately, I had to admit that nothing was known about the pathogenesis of Batten's disease, although it was my opinion that the basic defect was the formation of lipopigment, possibly the result of polyunsaturated fatty acid peroxidation. However this view was not shared by any of my colleagues, neither did I have the means or the knowledge and training to prove my hypothesis. To Dr. Rider this professed inability was no serious obstacle but rather a challenge.

He raised a substantial amount of money with which to establish a laboratory by the end of 1968. In this laboratory Dr. Siakotos performed his classical studies on the isolation and purification of lipopigments. At the same time we felt that a critical evaluation of our hypothesis was needed and that we had to develop a mechanism by which this hypothesis could be expertly evaluated. We felt that such experts need not be knowledgeable about the neuronal ceroid-lipofuscinoses nor did we think it necessary that they be physicians. The question of polyunsaturated fatty acid peroxidation and pigment formation was deemed to be the most important subject for a critical evaluation.

This is the historical background of the events which led to a series of round table conferences, all sponsored by the Children's Brain Diseases Foundation, an organization created by Dr. Rider. The conferences were conceived with the idea of providing a forum for discussion, criticism, and the mapping of projective studies exclusively concerned with the pathogenesis and the possible treatment of Batten's disease. From the beginning it was determined that the number of participants would be limited to 12 or 15 active discussants. Furthermore, the participants should be assured that submission or even preparation of a manuscript was actually undesirable

5

and that the discussions should be moderated only slightly
by somebody who had a general overview of the problem. Thus
the conferences would take a direction largely determined
by the selection of participants. As a final criterion the
duration of the discussions was restricted to 8 hours, divided
into 2 sessions.

The first round table conference was held in December,
1969. The hypothesis that all types of Batten's disease were
due to an unchecked rate of peroxidation of polyunsaturated
fatty acids found reasonable support from studies by A. L.
Tappel on in vitro peroxidation. However an unduly large
amount of time was wasted by repetitious efforts to document
to the participants the pigmentary nature of the deposits
and to properly delineate the neuronal ceroid-lipofuscinoses
from superficially similar lysosomal diseases. In other
words, the thinking of many of the participants turned out
to be directed towards the presumed close relationship of
the gangliosidoses, an obstacle which had to be overcome
before meaningful discussions could ensue. Nevertheless,
the first symposium lead to the important result that the
very carefully executed studies of Tappel and his co-workers
proved the working hypothesis to be reasonable. More important,
however, these experiments provided an explanation for the
entire pathomorphological syndrome in Batten's disease: accumulation of lipopigments, the damage to nerve cells leading
to a slow death via atrophy and the complete lack of evidence
for a specific lipid accumulating in the diseased brain tissue
such as is the case for the various lysosomal diseases. Of
utmost significance was Dr. Tappel's demonstration that polyunsaturated fatty acid peroxidation not only destroys fatty
acids, but results in a chain reaction with the formation
of cross-linked polymers at the expense of biological species
such as proteins, i.e., enzymes, and of subcellular organelles,
in particular their lipoprotein membranes. Since the unraveling
of the chemical pathogenesis of lipopigment formation does
not reveal the causation of the increased rate of polyunsaturated
fatty acid peroxidation, the participants of the first symposium
agreed that Dr. Siakotos should be encouraged to produce
preparations of highly purified pigments for analytical studies,
with the hope that such analysis would provide the data from
which could be developed clues to the mechanisms by which
polyunsaturated fatty acid peroxidation is enhanced. As it
turned out this was not an easy task and several years went
by before these projected analyses became a reality. Even
then, and this is reflected by the transcriptions of the 3rd
and 4th conferences available here, analytical data on composition of the lipopigments did not reveal their pathogenesis.

Following the recommendations made by the participants
of the first conference, the 2nd conference was almost exclusively concerned with discussions on the isolation and purifi-

cation of the pigments, an effort which led to the physico-chemical differentiation of ceroid from lipofuscin. This terminology was introduced in order to express the following correlations: Ceroid was isolated from the brain of a patient clinically diagnosed as "ceroid storage disease" who on post-mortem studies turned out to have suffered from the Santavouri-Haltia type of neuronal ceroid-lipofuscinosis. Ceroid pigment is bright yellow in the purified state and contrary to expectations turned out to be extremely unstable to salt solutions and ion exchange. Its density is from 1.27 to 1.33. Lipofuscin on the other hand is the characteristic age pigment of brain, heart and muscles. It is dark brown to black in the purified state and its density ranges from 1.10 to 1.25, depending upon the amount of admixed neutral fats. Lipofuscin is stable to all types of manipulations, especially to those procedures which cause disintegration of ceroid pigments. Aside from these important results which are repeatedly presented and discussed in the subsequent conferences, the transactions of the 2nd conference are of limited interest.

Substantial progress towards a better understanding of the pathogenesis of the neuronal ceroid-lipofuscinoses was made during the 3rd, 4th, 5th and 6th round table conferences, held at yearly intervals. Therefore, the transactions are presented here in the form of a monograph. The transcript clearly proves the value of the round table concept and of the request to bring along an open mind rather than a prepared manuscript. The nature of the problem has been clarified to the extent that a testable working hypothesis could be developed. Only time will show its validity. Consequently, this monograph, though containing many definitive statements, remains a fragment. Its purpose, however, to give an unabridged account of the thinking and the deliberations of a number of assembled scientists has been fulfilled.

The evidence which had been developed during the 1st conference already warranted an experimental therapeutic approach for the neuronal ceroid-lipofuscinoses. Following a suggestion by A. L. Tappel, treatment was instituted in the form of daily doses of 200 mg of butylated hydroxytoluene as an antioxidant, 2 gms of Vitamin E also an antioxidant, 500 mg of Vitamin C as a hydrogen donor and 1 gm of DL-methionine as a scavenger for free radicals. This treatment has produced encouraging results by retarding the progression of the disease in a number of patients but it did not provide any cure. In the English Setters this same treatment causes the manifestations of the disease to be retarded by several months, but to date no extension of the life span has been observed.

The 3rd conference provided a detailed definition of the clinical features and the pathology of Batten's disease. Dr. Siakotos presented his observations on the isolation and

the characterization of lipopigments which he had purified
by highly intricate gradient ultracentrifugation. The major
part of the discussions turned around various aspects of the
peroxidation of polyunsaturated fatty acids, the results of
this reaction and the interaction with antioxidants such as
Vitamin E. Methods of measuring the fluorescent Schiff-base
product from the interaction of the products of polyunsaturated
fatty acid peroxidation with biological species was covered
in great detail as were the protection afforded by α-tocopherol
and the effect of free radicals upon biological species.
In these discussions the ever present question of primary
metabolic effect versus epiphenomenon cropped up repeatedly
and the reader will be impressed by the sincerity of the participants in their efforts to arrive at a logically satisfactory
answer. It turned out that the formation of malonaldehyde
by the peroxidation of polyunsaturated fatty acids is an easily
detected indication that this process is taking place in the
tissues. However, the yield of this reaction is relatively
minor and therefore cannot be considered to account for the
entire phenomenon of autofluorescent lipopigment formation.

    Much speculation went into the presumed metabolic distur-
bance, whether it be a primary loss of protection against
oxidants or an enzymatic defect. The possibility that the
different types of Batten's disease which become manifest
at various ages may be an expression of the age-dependent
change in the translatability of the degenerate genetic code
was considered, as were other feasible mechanisms which could
express a mutated gene. However, the participants did not
develop any testable hypothesis on the pathogenesis of the
neuronal ceroid-lipofuscinoses. Instead, a forum for ventilating
ideas for constructive criticism had been provided. Although
repeated calls were made for collaborative studies, little
or no collaboration ensued, a fact perhaps explained by preoccupation of the participants with their own work and also
by the lack of research funds which began to be felt quite
seriously around the time of this conference.

    The 4th conference brought a wealth of new information
and it was therefore decided to include in the transcripts
references and illustrative material in the form of tables
and pictures. Again, the physicochemical characterization
of the lipopigment occupied a relatively large part of the
discussions, because the participants still felt that precise
chemical analysis might lead to an indication as to how the
increased rate of polyunsaturated fatty acid peroxidation,
the existence of which was now fully accepted, is triggered.
Barber raised the possibility that genetically controlled
conformational changes in the protein moieties of lipoprotein
micelles might account for the increased rate of peroxidation
by way of an exposure of the hydrophobic chains to oxidants.
The hydrophobic chains are normally protected by the protein

envelope. However, other participants pointed out that such conformational changes would be expressed as a dominant mutant, rather than a recessive. The recent findings of repetitive changes in leukocytic and liver hydrolases, not as the genetic basis of the disease but rather as a possible diagnostic tool, were thoroughly discussed.

The pharmacological role of vitamin E as a cofactor for hemesynthesis received major attention after Dr. Nair had documented this particular function. It was speculated that a faulty hemesynthesis, due to a decreased activity of δ-amino-levulinic acid (ALA) synthesase and dehydratase may eventually lead to the excessive accumulation of ferrous iron, a known oxidant. These speculations are supported by the very high iron content of ceroid, which has 1500 parts per million in comparison to 300 parts per million of ferrous iron in lipofuscin. Although the participants felt that the determination of vitamin E in the serum and in tissues of patients with the Batten's syndrome and heterozygous carriers should be vigorously pursued, it became clear in the discussion that current techniques are tricky and possibly unreliable. Furthermore, determinations of ALA synthesase and dehydratase are currently performed only in the laboratory of Dr. Nair and some doubt was expressed as to the significance and reproducibility of these determinations. These criticisms were elicited by the report that in several blind studies, these two enzymes, the substrate of which is δ-amino-levulinic acid, were markedly depressed in three patients with the Batten's syndrome, but they did not show the expected correlated anemia.

At the preceeding conference, the accumulation of enormous amounts of ceroid in the aging drosophiliae had been discussed. It again became a topic of major interest when Dr. Miquel reported his relevant studies and showed that a vitamin E supplement to the diet of these fruit flies extended the life span significantly. No comparable observations have been made in mammals.

Reports from Italy that the fatty acid moiety of gangliosides is markedly altered in Batten's syndrome received considerable attention. However, it was felt that the changes were such that they could not possibly express the effects of a mutated gene and that they might therefore be epiphenomena. Likewise, the hypothesis was rejected that malonaldehyde oxidase might be genetically deficient, thus leading to the accumulation and lack of detoxification of malonaldehyde, which is a known cross-linking agent that develops as a by-product of polyunsaturated fatty peroxidation, but with a yield of 1:300, only.

Dr. Philippart reported his studies on the half-lives

of various fatty acids from tissue cultures obtained by explants
of brain tissue from patients with Batten's disease. Practically all fatty acids showed an increased half-life up to
29 days in the explants from brains with Batten's disease,
in comparison to 17 days for stearic acid in normal controls.
Similar findings were obtained on explants from puppies of
English Setters homozygous for the trait.

Since this wealth of new observations did not produce
direct insight into the nature of the disease, it was suggested
that co-cultivation according to the Neufeld principle should
be seriously considered. By co-cultivating fibroblasts from
patients with the Hunter and Hurler type of mucopolysaccharidoses, Neufeld could demonstrate that the enzymatic defect
in the two conditions, which are very similar, must be different,
for co-cultivation prevented the accumulation of tertiary
lysosomes containing mucopolysaccharides. Since fibroblasts
from patients with Batten's disease do not produce lipopigment,
the co-cultivation experiments would have to be performed
with pigment producing cells such as thyroid or brain tissue,
systems which have a notoriously short life in culture.

The importance of early diagnosis of Batten's disease
received much attention. This was predicated on the fact
that treatment with the antioxidant-free radical scavenger
mixture had shown best results in patients and in affected
dogs when instituted early during the course of the disease
or even before the manifestation of clinical signs. Dr. Desnick
reviewed the possibilities of enzyme replacement therapy and
called for experiments in which crosstransplantation of kidneys
as a possible source of enzyme therapy was envisioned. It
may be pointed out in this context that these experiments
were indeed performed but did not produce tangible results.
That is to say that a homozygous affected donor of a kidney
from a closely matched heterozygous sibling developed the
disease with its natural course whereas the heterozygous normal
donor did not show any ill effect from the graft. Transplant
studies were performed also with lymphatic stem cells injected
intravenously and into the bone marrow at the time of birth
into four homozygous affected animals. Again, these recipients
did not show any deviation from the natural evolution of the
disease.

Obviously these studies were instituted because the enzyme
defect was not known at the time of this symposium and therefore purified enzyme preparations could not be selected for
direct application.

The 4th conference did produce a limited collaboration
among participants, for example Dr. Desnick received English
Setters from us for the kidney transplant studies and Dr.
Philippart obtained viable brain cell cultures from ascertained

homozygous affected canine puppies and fetuses.

Shortly after the 4th conference, Dr. James Austin and Donald Armstrong reported that they had observed a significant reduction of a leukocytic peroxidase in patients with the Spielmeyer-Sjögren type of Batten's disease. They had used the procedure of Lück (1965) which calls for p-phenylene diamine as a hydrogen donor whereas we had been using methoxybenzidine and in particular guiacol as hydrogen donor because these compounds are many times more efficient than p-phenylenediamine. Using p-phenylenediamine however, we also found in some of our patients a reduction in enzyme activity to approximately 20% of normal and it was therefore felt that Austin and Armstrong should present their data at another conference attended predominantly by enzymologists and neurochemists.

Consequently, the 5th conference was almost exclusively concerned with enzymological studies in Batten's disease. Three investigators reported detailed studies on the activity of various peroxidases in tissues and leukocytes of patients with the disease and in heterozygous carriers. The discovery by A. L. Tappel of the glutathione oxidase-reductase system as a detoxifying mechanism for fatty acid peroxides had given rise to a number of carefully detailed studies. This enzyme system was an a priori suspect of being deficient; however, none of the three laboratories engaged in testing this hypothesis could produce the slightest indication of such a presumed defect. Likewise, true peroxidase and catalase had come under scrutiny. With respect to catalase, the case was made that this enzyme is apparently organspecific and therefore determinations should be done on only those tissues which suffer pathologic evidence of pigment accumulation. The determination of catalase activity in approximately one dozen brain specimens from patients and from dogs with neuronal ceroid-lipofuscinosis, carefully matched for age and anatomical structure, produced absolutely no differences in comparison to controls. The same was observed for glutathione peroxidase, although it appeared that the activity of this enzyme was actually increased in some of the pathological specimens, suggesting perhaps a compensatory derepression of the enzyme on account of the accumulated peroxides.

The highlight of this conference was Armstrong's report on the peroxidase deficiency determined by assay of leukocytes. It became quite clear that only p-phenylenediamine as a hydrogen donor would reveal the defect which amounts to approximately 90% and, if his technique was carefully followed, that the enzyme defect was actually a reproducible observation. Armstrong's data were confirmed by at least three other laboratories at this occasion which left little doubt as to their validity.

At this time the p-phenylenediamine-mediated peroxidase defect was shown to occur in both the Spielmeyer-Sjögren and the Jansky-Bielschowsky type, a fact which was not bothersome to the participants because it is well known that these two conditions are closely related to each other and connected by the relatively common occurence of transitional forms. Thus, there was a strong feeling that the basic enzyme defect had been discovered. On account of the normal values for glutathione peroxidase, true peroxidase, and catalase, it was concluded that the PPD-mediated peroxidase must catalize a highly specific organic peroxide, which a priori would not be an aliphatic fatty acid peroxide because these are all catabolized by glutathione peroxidase. Several ingenious proposals were made as to how to discover and identify the presumed specific peroxide and it was felt that cholesterol hydroperoxide and perhaps other sterol-hydroperoxides could possibly be the as yet unknown specific substrate.

The results of the 5th conference left everyone in an elated mood, because it appeared that the etiopathogenesis of this puzzling disease had finally been resolved. Subsequently, however, it turned out that the dogs with Batten's disease as well as patients with the dominantly inherited Kufs type have the same enzyme defect. These observations cast some doubt on the validity of the concept that the PPD-mediated peroxidase is indeed the primary expression of the genetic mutation, although a number of theoretical possibilities seem to exist which would permit retention of this concept.

Despite determined efforts by several laboratories to come to grips with the problem, little progress had been made and the question still remained as to whether the deficiency of PPD-mediated peroxidase activity represents an expression of the genetic defect. Obviously this impasse called for a different kind of expertise than needed previously and it was decided to submit the problem to a panel of experts convened at the 6th round table conference, the proceedings of which conclude this monograph.

THIRD ROUND TABLE CONFERENCE ON BATTEN'S DISEASE
SAN FRANCISCO, CALIFORNIA
January 23-24, 1971

Dr. Albert A. Barber
Department of Zoology
University of California
Los Angeles, California

Dr. Denham Harman
University of Nebraska
College of Medicine
Omaha, Nebraska

Dr. Ralph T. Holman
Hormel Institute
University of Minnesota
Austin, Minnesota

Dr. Robert Horvat
U.S. Department of Agriculture
Richard Russell Research Center
Athens, Georgia

Dr. K. U. Ingold
Division of Chemistry
National Research Council of Canada
Ottawa, Ontario, Canada

Dr. Paul McCay
Oklahoma Medical Research Foundation
Oklahoma City, Oklahoma

Dr. Michael J. Malone
Department of Neurology
U.C.L.A. School of Medicine
Los Angeles, California

Dr. Jaime Miquel
Experimental Pathology Branch
NASA, Ames Research Center
Moffett Field, California

Dr. J. Alfred Rider
Children's Brain Diseases Foundation
Franklin Hospital
San Francisco, California

Dr. A. N. Siakotos
Department of Pathology
Indiana University Medical Center
Indianapolis, Indiana

Dr. Bernard Strehler
Department of Biological Sciences
University of Southern California

Dr. A. L. Tappel
Division of Food Science & Technology
University of California
Davis, California

Dr. Lloyd A. Witting
Illinois Department of Mental Health
Elgin State Hospital
Elgin, Illinois

Dr. Wolfgang Zeman
Department of Pathology
Indiana University Medical Center
Indianaplis, Indiana

THIRD ROUND TABLE CONFERENCE ON BATTEN'S DISEASE

Dr. Rider: I want to thank every one present for being
here. I suppose about half of you have been here before and
about half of you have not. We have a copy of the previous
symposiums held on December 13 and 14, 1968 and July 26 and
27, 1969 available for those of you who so desire. The whole
purpose of the symposium is to bring everyone together with
your ideas and see if we can push along our research on Batten's
disease, which is what we are primarily interested in. Dr.
Zeman will be the moderator and start the ball rolling.

Dr. Zeman: I would like to give a very brief rundown
on Batten's disease and on previous discussions which we have
held in this group. I have made an effort to reach all of
you and make literature available to you which delineates
the problem. However, I will briefly refresh your memory
and try to put the problem into perspective.

There is a group of human diseases that is generically
referred to as amaurotic idiocy. This condition was first
described exactly 90 years ago in England by an ophthalmologist,
Waren Tay (1881), and later on studied more extensively in
the United States by Bernie Sachs. Sachs was not aware that
he was concerned with the same disease as Tay, a fact not
demonstrated until many years later. Sachs undoubtedly made
the more profound clinical studies and pathological observations.
He coined the term amaurotic family idiocy, pointing out that
he had discovered a disease which was presumably controlled
by hereditary factors, that led to blindness and idiocy.
He felt that this was possibly due to a maldevelopment of
the brain.

For many years this disease has occupied the mind of
clinicians and of neuropathologists. In 1901 a Hungarian
neuropathologist, Schaffer, performed the first meaningful
pathological studies. He discovered that there was a rather
ubiquitous distension of the nerve cell bodies throughout
the brain and that these nerve cells did contain lipid matter.
Following this lead, a number of human diseases have been
discovered in which very similar findings were made, namely
a distension of the nerve cell bodies by lipid matter.

In a relatively short period of time, no more than 10
years, the term amaurotic idiocy, a clinical term, had been

15

attached to all diseases with nerve cell changes which showed
this peculiar pathomorphologic change--the "Schaffer cell
process."

What was originally a clinical concept, namely idiocy
and blindness, was now employed as "amaurotic nerve cell change"
to designate a pathogenetic alteration. It was this usurpation
of clinical observations by pathologists which has completely
confused the issue of this group of diseases. We can say
today that what Tay and Sachs described 90 years ago is a
lysosomal disease in which a genetically controlled deficiency
and in some cases a complete absence of N-acetylhexosaminidase
leads to the accumulation of ganglioside GM_2. As the specific
lysosomal hexosaminidase is absent, the cell cannot rid itself
catabolically of GM_2 ganglioside, which, especially during
early infancy and childhood, is subject to a rather massive
turnover. With the discovery of this biochemical defect,
Tay-Sachs disease or GM_2-gangliosidosis Type A, is now included
among the well-defined lysosomal diseases with known hydrolytic
enzyme defects.

About 50 to 60 different lysosomal hydrolases are known.
If one of them is defective, the substrate which it normally
catabolizes will accumulate, producing cytoplasmic distention.
If the missing hydrolase happens to catabolize a lipid, then
lipids will preferentially accumulate; however many complex
lipids will trap other biological species, including proteins,
which results in the accumulation of a complex mixture. If
the lysosomal hydrolase acid maltase is deficient or absent,
glycogen accumulates, which, being chemically rather inert,
does not trap other compounds to any extent. In every instance,
the accumulation follows a stereotyped pattern; in the course
of programmed focal cell lysis, autophagic vacuoles are formed
and their contents digested by way of fusion with primary
lysosomes which supply the hydrolytic enzymes. The non-catabolizable substrate and the trapped compounds remain undigested,
the autophagic vacuole does not dissolve but contracts and
remains in the cytosol as a tertiary lysosome or a residual
body.

Basically, all lysosomal diseases follow a similar pattern,
but they are different with respect to the focal point of
manifestation in the metazoic body. Since gangliosides are
rapidly turned over in the developing brain the deficiency
of any enzyme that catabolizes gangliosides will result in
a disorder of cerebral function and structure, predominantly
in infants. Vice versa, in glycogenosis type II or Pompe's
disease, the major lesions and abnormalities of function are
encountered in the liver and the striated muscles, tissues
that normally contain large quantities of glycogen.

16

After these facts had become understood, it developed that residual bodies or tertiary lysosomes can accumulate under conditions which apparently do not involve the deficiency of an enzyme, although like in the lysosomal diseases, the affected cells, for reasons unknown, cannot rid themselves of the residual bodies. This process has even been observed in protozoa and appears to be due to the formation of chemicals which cannot be broken down by the physiologically present hydrolases. Examples of this type of accumulation of residual bodies are poisoning with tellurium and quinine derivatives.

Finally, we know a third group of conditions with accumulation of residual bodies, which in this case contain auto-fluorescent lipopigments. These substances are generally considered to be insoluble in polar and non-polar solvents and remain in the cells, even after extraction with xylene. Lipopigments accumulate preferentially in nerve cells, liver and heart as a function of time, similar to the accumulation process in the lysosomal diseases. The rate of progression is, however, much slower, perhaps by 2 orders of magnitude, and cellular distention is therefore minimal.

The problem of characterizing lipopigments has met with considerable difficulty for several reasons. In the first place lipopigments, as has been known for about 100 years, are found in a variety of tissues of absolutely healthy people. Thus, very little attention was accorded to them. Secondly, while the staining reaction and even the histological and ultrastructural features of these pigments received considerable attention and were studied quite extensively, it was almost impossible to do meaningful biochemical studies on them for it proved most difficult to isolate them. Several procedures have now been developed for the isolation of those pigments, especially in Sweden by Börkerud. However, the isolation procedures were generally damaging and were performed at a time when little knowledge about lysosomes was extant. So the early studies of Heidenreich and Siebert, for example, established that these pigments had some hydrolase activity. They demonstrated activity of cathepsin type C but they never thought of studying acid phosphatase which we have come to recognize as a much better marker for lysosomes. By putting various observations together, by discussing the problem with several investigators and by studying whatever could be studied with available techniques, the following picture has emerged.

There is indeed a group of diseases which has formerly been identified with the amaurotic idiocies in which there is no proven accumulation of any major lipid. There is, however, a progressive and rather rapid accumulation of lipopigments. These lipopigments become incorporated in lysosomes to form residual bodies, very much the same as in the better known and better understood lysosomal disorders due to lysosomal

17

enzyme deficiencies. Furthermore, it has transpired that the pigments which accumulate in this group of diseases are similar to the naturally occurring age pigment or lipofuscin. Apparently age pigment and the pigment in Batten's disease develop along different lines, for the rate of accumulation of pigments in Batten's disease must be very high indeed, perhaps 100 times higher than the rate of age pigment accumulation under physiological conditions. In other words, Dr. Siakotos has been able to isolate up to 5% (on a wet weight basis) of pigments from the brains of children, aged 6 to 10, whereas the normal mature individual in the age group between 30 and 50 years yields no more than about 35 milligrams of pigment per brain which is 3/100 of 1%. We are really talking in terms of a hundredfold difference in the rate of accumulation and perhaps more. It is therefore of great interest--and this has been part of our previous discussions-- to really pin down the factors which are rate-determining for the process of lipid peroxidation and of polymerization by cross-linkage, presumably due to carbonyls and similar compounds. This is the present state of knowledge with respect to Batten's disease.

Batten's disease as I define here is not a disease or a nosological entity. Rather, it appears that a variety of mutations can, in the homozygous state, lead to the same end product, namely the accumulation of residual bodies which contain autofluorescent insoluble lipopigments. The etiopathogenesis of Batten's disease is therefore multifold. Firstly, we can delineate at least three clinically different conditions in which the common denominator with respect to morphological findings is the massive accumulation of lipopigments in the brain and in other parts of the body. The clinical differences are of major magnitude. We know of one group of conditions, the Jansky Bielschowsky type, in which the disease is fatal within 1 to 5 years, that usually begins in infancy or early childhood. The children die at ages 4 to 12 years with an enormous wasting of the brain, the brain weights being reduced to 25% of normal. We know a second clinical syndrome, the Spielmeyer-Sjögren type, in which the disease takes a much slower and more benign course, the median duration being 11 years. The onset of the disease is anywhere between 2 and 8 years of age. The presenting clinical signs which persist for many years are almost exclusively restricted to visual disturbance and only the final phase of the disease answers the general description of blindness and idiocy. This condition seems to be particularly prevalent in the Scandinavian countries and in Germany where this type was first described. Yet another form, the Kufs type, affects adults, people with an entirely normal development until age 20, 30 and even 40 years, who then undergo a relatively rapid mental, intellectual and physical degeneration and whose brain also shows an enormous accumulation of lipopigments. Here are three clinically different syndromes which have the common denominator of lipopigment accumulation.

There are other nosologic differences. In the vast majority of the patients who have been described in the literature or who have been observed by some of us, the disease appears to be inherited as an autosomal recessive. That is to say that the patients are homozygous for the mutated gene; they must carry two mutated alleles in order to express the disease. There is, however, one family which has been very well documented both by chemical and electron microscopic studies, as well as by genetic investigations in which the disease begins around age 30 years and leads to death within 7 years that is inherited as a Mendelian dominant with 100% penetrance and without variability of expressivity. In other words, and this is characteristic for the entire group of the Batten syndrome, the condition is extremely homotypic and homochronic. By this we mean that the disease within one and the same family has a tendency to develop around the same year of age in the various affected members and that it will run a very similar course with an almost identical and repetitive pattern of the evolution of the disease. It is from this type of observation and a consideration of homotypism and homochromism that we have come to question whether these conditions may not be the expression of a variety of mutated genes with modifier genes that determine homotypism and homochronism in one and the same family.

Biochemically the present information suggests that the formation of lipopigments may very well be an autocatalytic reaction which does not require a specific enzyme and which is solely governed by thermodynamic principles. As some of the possible catalytic factors, we may consider that relatively high focal concentrations of polyunsaturated fatty acids may drive forward the reaction of lipid peroxidation as does the presence of relatively high concentrations of oxidants such as bivalent metal ions, heme and certain radicals. In this respect, it is perhaps of interest to note that in at least one patient, a child that developed the characteristic picture of the so-called Jansky-Bielschowsky type, the concentration of free fatty acids was profoundly altered as determined by Hagberg, Sourander and Svennerholm (1968).[1] They suggested a specific inability of the brain and of other tissues to perform chain-lengthening reactions for ω:3 fatty acids which leads to the accumulation of linoleic acid and, as assumed by Svennerholm, initiates the autocatalytic reaction of lipid peroxidation. This is the only, and rather tenuous, information which is available on the biochemical pathogenesis of those pigments. Considering that we are dealing with a relatively

---

[1] This case is now classified as Haltia-Santavuori type.

19

specific mechanism which does recur in a variety of themes, presumably catalyzed by different enzymes, there is reason to assume that we are talking about a general pathogenetic principle which can be the expression of genetic heterogeneity, or of epistasis, or of both. We assembled here to examine this concept with critical eyes to find ways as to how to proceed further in order to unravel some of the spurious facts which have emerged from these observations.

In closing, I should stress that the assumption that lipid peroxidation represents the major pathogenic factor for the Batten syndrome as proposed by Dr. Tappel, must appeal to the neuropathologist, for this concept simultaneously explains two almost invariant findings, namely: the accumulation of autofluorescent lipopigments and the breakdown of tissue, or perhaps we should say, the damage to nerve cells. As Dr. Tappel has shown, lipid peroxidation can be exceedingly damaging because it does inactivate not only biological molecules but it can fix and inactivate subcellular organelles. The yields are very high and the per mole inactivation by lipid peroxidation compares favorably with the per mole inactivation by ionizing radiation. Assuming, however, that lipid peroxidation is continuously going on in our body and that we have a rather efficient mechanism of molecular repair in most of our cells, it does appear that the rate at which this damage does occur is the limiting factor. If the rate of peroxidation is well below the rate of synthetic capability of the affected cell, we would expect that this peroxidation-induced cellular damage is easily compensated for because we are subject to contin- uous damage in our body and in our systems and life itself is a continuous struggle. The built-in factors of safety and the margin of biological compensation suggest that con- siderable damage can be inflicted upon the body before it is rendered unfunctional.

We have now reached the real crux of the problem--namely the hypothesis that an enhanced rate of lipid peroxidation spells the difference between health and disease. With this, I would like to turn over the discussion to other participants with the intent to clarify certain questions. Also, let me re-emphasize that the picture I have given here is actually a hypothesis that has not received the attention we ultimately hope for, but we believe it is a reasonable working hypothesis and you should, if you wish, consider it as a straw man which you would like to knock down. For the next half hour, however, we restrict our discussion to an amplification of this concept.

Dr. Harman: Could I begin with a few questions: What do we know about the diet of these individuals? In particular, the amount and degree of unsaturation of the fat they eat and their intake (for example, how much copper or iron). What is the distribution of the lipofuscin or age pigment

in their tissues--is it just in the brain or is it in the
same locations that we see under normal aging conditions?
In regard to treatment, has anyone tried treating these children
with vitamin E or some other antioxidant? Are there any other
diseases associated with it, particularly in the older age
groups? For instance, do you see any increased incidence of
cancer? Do you see an increased incidence of atherosclerosis
in the people who develop this in middle age?

Dr. Zeman: In response to your questions, Dr. Harman,
the distribution of the disease is such that we have no reason
to assume that food and mineral intake play a major role in
its pathogenesis. However, this does not rule out that these
patients may have a genetically controlled disturbance in
the utilization or detoxification of certain foodstuffs and
minerals. Minerals, that is bivalent metals are indeed very
important because in the isolated pigments we find up to 400
parts per million of zinc, up to 1500 parts per million of
iron and also markedly increased amounts of copper and calcium.

The distribution of the pigment is favoring the brain.
That is to say the pigment can be demonstrated in obviously
increased amounts in a variety of tissues including striated
muscle, thyroid gland, intestines, liver and kidneys but the
largest accumulation is undoubtedly in the nerve cells of
the brain and in the peripheral nerve cells such as the sym-
pathetic neurons of Auerbach's and Meissner's plexus. These
patients do indeed show an increased incidence of arteriosclero-
sis and it is particularly noteworthy that patients dying
in their twenties show or may show advanced arteriosclersis
of the aorta. Also it is noteworthy that such patients do
show cholelithiasis and other concretions in the bile system.

Now to the question about antioxidants. We are treating
approximately 25 patients with antioxidants, following Dr.
Tappel's suggestions. These patients receive 100 mg of butylated
hydroxytoluene (BHT), 1 gram of vitamin E, 500 mg of vitamin
C and 1 gram of DL methionine per day. No patients have been
treated for a long enough period that would permit an evaluation
of the efficacy of the treatment. What is perhaps noteworthy
is that two patients that I have been treating for 10 months
in Indianapolis have not only been stable during this period
of time but the parents, perhaps wishfully, noted that the
children became brighter and participated more actively in
the family life. However, I don't believe that these two
individuals represent good subjects for this type of study
because we put them on this treatment when both were in a
fairly advanced stage of the disease. Both were blind, severely
demented, and the only definite change--and this might be
coincidental--is that the older of these two siblings, a girl
aged 18, was unable to walk when she was put on the experimental
regimen and she is now able to walk erect. However, the disease

21

proceeds at such a slow pace that we cannot be certain at this time whether the subjective improvement is due to the treatment. We are now treating 20 patients in Helsinki and 2 patients in Copenhagen with antioxidants. These patients are in relatively early stages of the disease, much earlier than we get to see them here in the United States because, as Dr. Rider can tell you from his own experience, the Batten syndrome is so little known in the United States that unless a patient is lucky and is seen by one of the few physicians familiar with the condition, the diagnosis is not made. It took approximately ten years for Charles' condition to be diagnosed. In Sweden, Finland, Norway and Denmark the disease is very well known and the diagnosis is usually made during the initial stages when the children show the first signs of visual disturbances. Patients in this country should be put on this treatment but we just do not have access to them.

Dr. Harman: I would like to ask two more questions. Firstly, you didn't answer my first question in regard to cancer incidence in these individuals particularly among the older members, or leukemia in the younger patients. Secondly, is there any geographic distribution in regard to this disorder?

Dr. Zeman: There is no information with respect to cancer. I am not aware of a single instance in the literature. There are perhaps 250 cases recorded in the literature and my own experience is restricted to some 40 or 50 patients whom I have personally examined. I have never seen leukemia nor have I observed other malignancies in these patients. Of course, many of them are still alive; thus what I have said is applicable only to those that have died and have come to autops

As far as geographic distribution is concerned, the incidence of the disease in the United States is practically unknown and no pertinent studies have been made. On account of our interest we do get referrals from out of state. I would say that during the past 10 years we have seen about 20 patients with these disorders in the state of Indiana with a population of about 5,000,000. Were the general practitioners better informed, we would presumably find a relatively even distribution throughout the United States. The disease is definitely more common in the Scandinavian countries, presumably due to ancestral loss. I don't know whether you are familiar with the concept that in relatively closely knit ethnic groups the number of theoretical ancestors, which as you know grows by powers of two with each generation, is reduced so that 10 generations back when the total number of ancestors should be 1,024, these people have an actual number of ancestors of as few as a few hundred. Genetic studies are done with great ease in all Scandinavian countries because of the excellent church records and because these countries have not been subject to the less desirable achievements of modern civilization, namely war. Thus, this data is rather firm. It so happens that in a country like Sweden the distribution of the disease is very uneven. In the population of southern Sweden which is about 2 million there are perhaps as many as 150 documented cases, whereas in central Sweden with a population of about 3 million the incidence of disease is markedly less, perhaps by as much as a factor of ten. The gene distribution is uneven, is determined by ethnic factors and the cancer incidence is at least zero from what I know.

Dr. Miquel: In relation to Dr. Zeman's comments that this disease is very hard to find in early stages, I would like to comment on two cases that have been studied at Stanford University School of Medicine by Dr. Mary M. Herman. One of the patients was 3 and the other 4 years of age when they were diagnosed. I believe one of these children is still alive, in a mental institution of the State of California. He is blind and cannot stand, and might possibly benefit from antioxidant therapy.

I would also like to ask Dr. Zeman about the influence of racial factors, because I have read that this disease is prevalent in Jewish families of German, French and Russian background. From the two cases which I have mentioned, one is an American and the other is Mexican.

I would also like to ask Dr. Zeman about the sex factor. Is this disease more prevalent in male or in female children?

I think it would also be of interest to consider what is going on in the brain development at age 3 to 4 years. How is the myelinization proceeding? Is there anything that makes the brain more sensitive to this disease at this particular age?

Dr. Zeman: The data on the ethnic prevalence of the disease in what you probably refer to as Ashkenazi Jews is erroneous. It is very definitely true for GM_2 gangliosidosis or Tay-Sachs disease and also for a variety of other lysosomal disorders such as Gaucher's and Niemann-Pick disease, a sphing-omyelinase deficiency. However, in Batten's disease or to use a more descriptive term, neuronal ceroid-lipofuscinosis, we find no racial or ethnic prevalence. That might simply be accidental because the prevalence for true lysosomal disorders among the Ashkenazi Jews can be traced back to the presumed occurrence of the first mutation in the 17th century. Again, due to ancestral loss, the mutated gene has been preserved in this ethnic group and, as shown by Myrianthopoulos (1966), the gene for both Gaucher's disease and Tay-Sachs disease does have some usefulness with respect to the heterozygote, perhaps also in dystonia musculorum deformans, we don't know.

23

It seems that with these disorders there is an increased intelligence in the heterozygous carrier. Neuronal ceroid-lipofuscinosis or Batten's disease does occur in Jews and I have examined three or four cases which were sent to me by Dr. Wolman from Israel. They concerned Yemenites but neither Ashkenazi nor Sephardic Jews. We can assume a worldwide distribution of the mutant gene with definite ethnic enrichment on the basis of simple population dynamics.

As far as sex is concerned, nobody has ever demonstrated any difference. Of course, this has supported the assumption that it is an autosomal recessive.

As far as diagnosis is concerned, were you making reference to the fact that the diagnosis has been made clinically or had been made by biopsy?

Dr. Miquel: Biopsy.

Dr. Zeman: Well, this is the usual state of affairs. However, in Scandinavia where state-directed medicine has reached a much wider segment of the population than in this country, the diagnosis is usually made when the first symptoms of visual failure occur and there is not a single ophthalmologist in Scandinavia who would not almost automatically consider this diagnosis in a child that displays visual disturbances at the time of school enrollment.

Dr. Miquel: But what about the brain? How advanced is the myelinization?

Dr. Zeman: You weren't here when I gave my little talk. The point is that from all we can infer there are the following possibilities; all the diseases in which the only pathologic finding is the excessive accumulation of lipopigments in the neuronal perikaryon and other parts of the body, associated with a profound destruction of nerve cells and a loss of parenchyma, are the expression of different mutated genes. In other words we are dealing with genetic heterogeneity, presumably under the influence of modifier genes; or we deal with a combination of these two situations. Now there is only one case which has been relatively but by no means conclusively well documented and shown to result from a disturbance in the chain-lengthening mechanism of ω:3 fatty acids. If we take this singular instance as a point of departure, and I hope that Dr. Malone will enlighten us here, then there should be several periods during the development where specific or relatively specific biochemical situations exist which would engender a thermodynamic situation that facilitates pigment formation. Perhaps Dr. Malone you can speak about this.

Dr. Malone: We have been interested for some time now

in brain development, particularly from the standpoint of
molecular development or chemical architectonics. The amount
of information in this area is fairly good right now and seems
to be getting a bit better each day. Of course one of the
reasons for looking at this is the hope that one may be able
to tie together specific biochemical molecular deficits with
evolving clinical pictures. The problem that has struck me
is the fact that as a neurologist, one rarely sees these
cases over a sufficient time span. The evolution of a clinical
course through a series of well-defined clinical stages has
been presented by Hagberg in metachromatic leukodystrophy.
These clinical entities evolve. If you happen to see the
patient, for example, at stage one, it may not be clinically
possible to make the diagnosis at that point. Stage two would
be a little easier. Stage three would be, perhaps, obvious.
In terms of development we have been interested among other
things in myelinization as a developmental index with obvious
application to clinical problems in pediatric neurology.
Several years ago studies were begun by Folch and his collabor-
ators. They measured changes of lipid entities in evolving
rat brain and they defined the "critical period" of development.
This critical period was thought to be characterized by myelinization and in the rat brain which they studied it was
found that the quantitative appearance of specific lipid and
lipid protein complexes appeared as an S curve in development.
These entities were present in minimal quantities during the
first two weeks of life; the curve rose over a 3-5 day period
and approximated adult levels by weeks 3-4. Since the increase
of these specific lipids corresponded to the morphologic process
of myelinization, the term "myelin lipids" was applied to
sulfatides, cerebrosides and proteolipids. In the human an
analogous period may occur around the second year of life.
The situation is complicated by species difference and the
increase in myelin lipids is more protracted and less dramatic.
One may speculate that a specific enzyme deficit, involved
in the synthesis or degradation of a molecule or molecular
species, might not show a clinical effect at all until the
point in development was reached where you really needed to
fit this particular entity into the structure that you are
building. If such a defect in synthesis of myelin "building
blocks" were present, one might see a perfectly normal course
of early development up to this critical period. Beyond this
period the organism would no longer be able to function normally;
this is to say no longer able to develop normally.

Dr. Zeman: Thank you very much Dr. Malone. Are there
any further questions?

Dr. Holman: How did Svennerholm determine that chain
elongation was not taking place normally?

Dr. Zeman: That was a rather circumstantial argument.

He found an increase of linoleic acid and a decrease of all other ω:3 fatty acids.

Dr. Holman: Well, if polymerization and autooxidation were going on, the same acids would have been removed by those processes.

Dr. Zeman: Perhaps so; that is, of course, a moot point. We have never been able to really find out what becomes polymerized into these lipopigments. Perhaps Dr. Siakotos could show us a slide and Dr. Tappel and Dr. Barber who have studied this process under more critical conditions in the test tube could enlighten us on this situation.

Dr. Tappel: It might be more appropriate to hear from Dr. Siakotos first as he has worked on the disease pigments.

Dr. Zeman: This is a real problem and we hope to make progress towards its solution or at least find a promising approach.

Dr. Siakotos: First I will go through what we have found to date, what pigments are involved, what they look like, etc.

Basically when we started out in this area the problem was really the fact that pathologists and physicians had called these pigments all sorts of names interchangably without making any distinctions between one pigment and another; for example, lipofuscin was used quite widely, lipoprotein pigment, fat pigment, lipochrome, wear and tear pigment. The pigment of vitamin E deficiency was really used for the first time to distinguish ceroid. Then ceroid was referred to as the pigment accumulating in alcoholic livers and the pigment that accumulated in ceroid storage disease, or what we call Batten's disease and what Dr. Zeman has recently termed neuronal ceroid-lipofuscinosis. Now our approach to this problem was essentially to try to make some sense out of what was known as far as the pathologists were concerned. This slide summarizes the basic differences that Hartroft (1965) and others have used to distinguish ceroid, interceroid and lipofuscin from each other and that is their respective solubilities, whether or not they contain iron and similar properties. What we did was to go in and try to isolate these particulates starting about 2 years ago. What we show here is a generalized scheme for fractionating brain. In our system we use beef brain as a model system for human brain but when one does the same thing with fresh human brain, one gets similar results. The basic difference that we found early in the game was that lipofuscin was a very light material, as recovered from brain, and ceroid, found in Batten's disease or ceroid storage disease, is a very dense material with a density equivalent to nuclei.

On specific gravity alone these two pigments could be distinguished, at least in brain.

Starting with that, we developed a procedure for isolating lipofuscin from brain. This procedure essentially capitalizes on the fact that lipofuscin is a very light pigment. The lipofuscin will concentrate as a layer of material floating on the surface of a 0.4M sucrose solution. When we treat this with dextran sulfate and pass it through a gradient of sodium chloride, this material becomes very, very light and even floats on water. This is the basic procedure that we use to isolate and purify lipofuscin from brain. Now if we had a mixture of ceroid and lipofuscin, these two pigments could be resolved. In normal human brain there is about 35 mg of lipofuscin per 1.2 kg of brain. In the brain of an alcoholic this is about 5 times greater, but it's the same brown lipofuscin pigment that one sees in the aged brain.

Dr. Zeman: That's low density pigment.

Dr. Siakotos: It's very light density pigment. This is an electron micrograph of lipofuscin from brain. You can see it is a very heterogeneous mixture of pigments. There are about six morphological types. We have tried to classify these with Dr. Watanabe who is a member of Dr. Zeman's electron microscopy group. As you can see they are actually very heterogenous; for example in this large particle here there are structures such as mitochondria.

Let's take a look at the lipofuscin one isolates from normal human liver. You can see that this pigment is very homogeneous, unlike the brain pigment.

Dr. Menkes: Coming back to that last slide, you said there were 6 different morphologic types. Did you see any that looked like curvilinear bodies?

Dr. Siakotos: No. Not in normal brain. This is normal liver lipofuscin from human liver. It behaves in the same manner as the brain pigment in that it changes it's density in sodium chloride. This is apparently because the pigment has enough phospholipid in it that it will pick up water and swell and approach the density of water.

Now this is the lipofuscin one obtains from normal human heart. You can see it is quite different. It doesn't have these large lipid-like vesicles, but the density of this material is also altered by salt. It is a dark brown pigment and it is heavier than the normal human brain lipofuscin that we find in normal aged individuals.

We have put together the lipofuscins that we find in

brain, heart and liver.

Dr. Malone: Was there seen at any time any suggestion of membranous element components to either the light or heavy material that you have been showing?

Dr. Siakotos: Yes, in the liver and in the normal human brain there is generally a membrane involved.

We are satisfied that these represent the general types of lipofuscins that we find in human organs. We then started to look at ceroid. The distinguishing feature of the isolation procedure for ceroid is that we collect the very dense fraction, the heavy fraction which contains mitochondria, nerve endings and nuclei and this is the fraction that we isolate ceroid from. There is a large difference in density. We are talking of a density difference of at least 1.5 to 2 molar sucrose. In the brain the major problem is to resolve the nuclei from this pigment. The other thing you have to remember is that this ceroid has the dendritic elements interwoven among the ceroid granules. We have used an enzyme called Nagarse, a very strong proteolytic enzyme, which digests away everything except nucleic acid. Under these conditions the nucleic acid is filtered off on glass wool. The pigment will go right through and we can make a 95% isolation of the nucleic acid and discard it. Then we take the filtrate, the pigment rich fraction, and purify it on cesium chloride because sucrose cannot be made up in a dense enough solution conveniently to isolate the ceroid. We go up to about 50% cesium chloride to isolate this pigment. You must have the nucleic acid removed or else in cesium chloride or other salt solutions the nucleic acid clumps and causes an aggregation of nucleic acid and ceroid, making the separation very difficult.

Dr. Barber: What is the density of the cesium chloride you're using?

Dr. Siakotos: It's about 1.30 specific gravity. The surprising thing is that when ceroid is isolated under these conditions, it shows the normal complement of lysosomal enzymes, thus we are not destroying the enzymes in the pigment.

Let's now take a look at one of the ceroid fractions. This was isolated from an 11-year-old patient. 5% of the total wet weight of the brain was this material here--a yellow pigment unlike lipofuscin.

Dr. Menkes: Did you say 5%?

Dr. Siakotos: Five per cent by wet weight.

Dr. Zeman: I think we should emphasize one point, Dr.

Siakotos, namely that the terminology which we use is entirely
arbitrary. When we speak of ceroid then we mean those pigments
that have been first isolated from a patient with Batten's
disease that came to autopsy at the University of Minnesota
and was described in the literature as a degenerative brain
disease with the storage of "ceroid" in the bone marrow.
When we speak of lipofuscin we talk about those pigments that
in the neuropathological literature are identified as constituents of normal nerve cells in normal individuals which show
an age dependent increase and are therefore also called "age
pigments." This terminology is simply arbitrary. It is,
however, remarkable that these two pigments share insolubility
and a relatively specific autofluorescence. They also exhibit
a pigmentary nature--that is to say they appear as colored
particles in unstained histologic preparations and they also
share certain tinctorial properties. They stain with oil red
0, Sudan black B with an indophenol reaction, are acid fast
and PAS positive.

Dr. Menkes: Five per cent of wet weight of brain means
50% of lipids. Is that right?

Dr. Siakotos: Well, this brain at 11 years of age weighed
254 grams at autopsy. Of that 5% was pigment.

Dr. Zeman: I should mention that this brain was severely
atrophic weighing less than 25% of what you would expect for
a girl in this age group. It was not only severely atrophic
but it was completely demyelinated. Most of the nerve cell
bodies had been lost. Histologically the pigment was almost
exclusively found in astrocytic processes and the child had
been in a state of decerebration for at least 6 years prior
to death. Perhaps this does explain the situation.

Dr. Siakotos: This is the major pigment fraction in
this patient. There was another very minor fraction. This
second fraction was more dense and could be resolved from
the previous fraction.

Now this is another case of Batten's disease and these
are the so-called curvilinear bodies. This pigment has exactly
the same specific gravity, the same fluorescence, the same
enzymes as the previous pigment did.

This pigment was isolated from a strain of English setters
which have the same disease. These English setters are found
in Norway and are raised by Dr. Koppang. This is the pigment
as we isolated it in a preparation by the same exact procedure,
has the same density, the same fluorescent properties, the
same color--but what we saw in this pigment were all of these
black dots and this very indistinct pattern. We thought this
was cesium chloride at first so we treated this pigment with

29

Dowex 50 to see if we could get a cleaner picture and this is the picture we got. The strange thing that happens though is that this pigment falls apart when it is treated with Dowex 50 or a chelator such as EDTA.

Dr. Zeman: Which pigment?

Dr. Siakotos: Ceroid.

Dr. Zeman: All ceroid?

Dr. Siakotos: All ceroid falls apart when you treat it with an ion exchanger or a chelator. That's quite different from lipofuscin. This pigment is apparently held together by bivalent ions. One of the problems of working with neuronal ceroid-lipofuscinosis or Batten's disease in this country is the rarity of specimens from which to isolate pigment to work with. Thus, we began to look at cirrhotic livers. Since this pigment is classified as ceroid, we tried recently to isolate this and I think we have a procedure which is now successful, a working procedure to isolate gram quantities of this material so that we can work out many of the parameters that are necessary to characterize these pigments. Then we can isolate ceroid from Batten's disease with what we know from ceroid from cirrhotic liver.

This is a preliminary electron micrograph from one of our preparations and here is the ceroid surrounded by a pencil mark, this is not a membrane, from a cirrhotic liver. This pigment can be isolated in the order of 5 grams per hundred grams of liver, depending upon the degree of cirrhosis. These patients for the most part have an alcoholic cirrhosis unlike a drug cirrhosis. These structures were bacteria--this liver was frozen and thawed about six times. It took us about six runs to get a successful preparation. The preparations which we now have are very clean. This pigment behaves exactly the same way to chelators in density and color as does the pigment isolated from Batten's disease. We now have a number of pigments which are similar in many properties and we put this scheme together as to how we would characterize them and how we separate them. What are the unique features of each of these classes of pigments: (1) the specific gravity, and whether this specific gravity changes with the addition of sodium chloride; (2) does this pigment dissociate in the presence of chelators or ion exchange resins; (3) morphology, but this is often very confusing as we found out in the case of a pigment that was isolated, that we tried to isolate from Drosophilae, which from the electron micrographs of Dr. Miquel's work we had assumed that this was a lipofuscin, but much to our surprise it turns out to be a ceroid, since it completely disappeared in the presence of EDTA. The enzymes are not good characteristics because ceroid and lipofuscin have essentially the same specific activities as far as we can tell in so far as the general lysosomal enzymes. One of our surprises, at least to date, has been that pure lipofuscin, for example, has very little native lipid in it, but is very rich in lipid polymers. The other thing is that these pigments appear to be distinguished from each other on the basis of metal composition. The amino acid composition is something that is under way but we have no information on that at the present time. Just to give you an idea of the types of enzymes that we have found, these pigments are very rich in acid phosphatase, they are very rich in alpha glucosidase, and they have a general distribution of normal lysosomal enzymes. I don't know whether Dr. Zeman mentioned this to you but the proposed pathway of synthesis of these pigments is supposed to be through a lysosomal mechanism.

Here are the cations that are found in these pigments (see Table 3 page 124). These are just two samples that we subjected to neutron activation. You can see some distinguishing features; (1) ceroid is much richer in calcium, as we have previously shown this pigment falls apart in the presence of chelators, (2) it is much richer in iron, (3) it has less zinc than normal lipofuscin. On the basis of these metals, at least these pigments can be distinguished.

This is a two-dimensional thin layer chromatogram of a pure preparation of brain lipofuscin (see Figure 2 page 123). The material has been passed through a Sephadex G_{25} column in a partition system which removes all of the sugars, salts and amino acids. From those of you who are familiar with the Folch procedure, this is like washing with your salt solutions to remove these materials. The material is applied here and in this particular chromatogram this was 800 micrograms of material and we ran up on this solvent system here with chloroform/methanol/ammonia, dry the plate, turn it 90 degrees, run in this solvent in this direction within an acetic acid solvent system, cholesterol for example is in this region here, but that may not be cholesterol. The strange things that we see here are a number of compounds or a number of spots which do not match exactly those of any known phospholipids. In particular is this very large spot here. This is a lipid-like compound and we are assuming that these materials here represent polymers.

Dr. Zeman: Ceroid or lipofuscin?

Dr. Siakotos: This is normal lipofuscin from brain.

Dr. Malone: In the system that you have examined, have you considered the possibility that the material which is close to the origin on TLC plates might be a phosphoinositide or a polyphosphoinositide?

Dr. Siakotos: We've considered that but that is an awful lot of phosphoinositide for any known structure.

Dr. Tappel: Are those pigments, the ones that you now identify as being polymers, are they fluorescent? Also, is the phosphatidyl ethanolamine fluorescent?

Dr. Siakotos: If this is phosphatidal ethanolamine, this is really a trace component. This is less than 5%. This compound here for example is less than 5%. These lipids here make up 90% of the lipid extract.

Dr. Tappel: Are they fluorescent?

Dr. Siakotos: As far as we can tell, yes. We haven't checked this out.

Now we are going to separate these out into a polystyrene column to determine molecular weight ranges to see whether they differ and so on and so forth between the various pigment species.

Dr. Zeman: I should interject here in response to Dr. Tappel's questions that up to the point of application of the sample all these pigments are indeed autofluorescent. We have not looked for fluorescence after the separation.

Dr. Siakotos: Al, you have made extracts in chloroform methanol and they are highly fluorescent, aren't they?

Dr. Tappel: Yes, and I have some of the spectra here which I can show at the appropriate time.

Dr. Siakotos: In summary, these are the lipid fractions that we have isolated from pigments in normal brain, brain from Batten's disease patients, normal heart, normal liver and cirrhotic liver (Table 2). On this column here we have classes on the basis of density. In normal heart we have a very high concentration of a floating lipid layer which is apparently fatty material. No matter how you dissect the excess fat off a normal heart from an aged patient there is still plenty in between the muscle fibers and it comes off in this fraction here. The same thing is true for normal liver from human patients. This is not true for liver, say from a dog. Most humans who die from some cause in a hospital generally go without feeding for sometime, their livers usually become very fatty. Thus the problem of isolating lipofuscin from an animal liver is really quite different than that of isolating lipofuscin from a human liver obtained at postmortem. The same type of fraction is obtained in cirrhotic liver. In normal brain the principal pigment is lipofuscin and it is obtained in the range of 35 to 50 milligrams per 1.2 kilograms.

Density	Brain, Normal	Brain, NCL	Heart, Normal	Liver, Normal	Liver, Cirrhotic
-1.00			Very high "floating lipid"	Very high (human) Very low (animal) "floating lipid"	Low to high "floating lipid"
1.00-1.05	.05 gm/Kg Lipofus-cin	Trace Lipo-fuscin	Trace Lipo-fuscin	5-50 gm/Kg Lipofuscin	Very low to high Lipofuscin
1.10-1.25	Trace Lipofus-cin		1-50 gm/Kg Lipofuscin	Trace Lipofuscin	Very low to high Lipofuscin
1.25-1.30		10-25 gm/Kg Ceroid			1-10 gm/Kg Ceroid

Table 2. Classification of auto fluorescent lipopigments by density.

There is a trace of a heavier lipofuscin but a very small percentage. In brains from patients with Batten's disease there is just a minor component in the normal light lipofuscin fraction. The major pigment is this ceroid, the yellow pigment, unlike the lipofuscin which is brown which has a greater density. This can be obtained in very high concentrations, depending upon how long this patient has lived. In normal heart one has a heavy lipofuscin which can be obtained in very high concentration. In normal liver the principal lipofuscin or lipopigment is the lipofuscin which is very similar in density and in other parameters to the one that we find in normal brain. There is also a trace of this heavier lipofuscin as in the case in brain. In the cirrhotic liver the principal pigment is ceroid as we find in brains from patients with Batten's disease. This ceroid has similar properties. Recently we have had a liver from a cirrhotic patient who had both lipofuscin and ceroid.

Dr. Zeman: Just one question, Dr. Siakotos. When you have lipofuscin from a normal heart, does that really have a density of about 1.12 to 1.13?

Dr. Siakotos: It's about 1.25.

Dr. Zeman: So it is in the range of ceroid.

Dr. Siakotos: It's slightly lighter than ceroid that we normally obtain from Batten's diesease patients.

33

Dr. Zeman: The difference would then be the stability under chelation and what else?

Dr. Siakotos: Color and I would assume fluorescence spectra.

Dr. Rider: Dr. Zeman, at one time didn't we feel that the pigment in Batten's disease was primarily lipofuscin rather than ceroid? Has this changed or is my memory incorrect?

Dr. Zeman: Your memory is quite correct but my assumptions as of a year or two ago were incorrect. We observed in patients with Batten's disease a variety of ultrastructurally different pigment granules, among them what we called granular pigment bodies and curvilinear bodies and bodies with fingerprint pattern. In order to keep the issue open we said these organelles or pigment bodies show characteristics of what has been described as lipofuscin and what has been described as ceroid. We had no means, however, of differentiating those until Dr. Siakotos developed his particulate fractionation procedures. It did indeed come as a surprise to all of us and post hoc perhaps justified our wanton diffuseness in terminology. In Batten's disease the pigments which morphologically and ultrastructurally look like lipofuscin, indeed behave like ceroid.

In all fairness we have to say that, as yet, we have not been able to get hold of a specimen that could be identified as the adult type of neuronal ceroid-lipofuscinosis, these are patients who die in the forties or fifties and who develop the disease during adulthood. It would of course be a wild but educated guess that this pigment might indeed behave like lipofuscin and might be stable under conditions of chelation but we don't know. Even worse, we have not yet had a case that we could without reservation classify as the Spielmeyer-Sjögren type of ceroid-lipofuscinosis, that is to say, a condition which is relatively chronic and slowly progressive. All the present data comes from the more pernicious form of neuronal ceroid-lipofuscinosis that runs a relatively short course of only a few years, and predominates in young children. However, there is at least one case of this disorder, a 25-year-old male whose disease was fatal within two years and whose brain contained ceroid rather than lipofuscin. Whether the same pigment occurs in the Spielmeyer-Sjögren type is unknown because our sampling has been restricted to the more pernicious form of Batten's disease. That is one of the reasons why we have been sending letters to numerous neurologists and neuropathologists, asking their help in making specimens available to us. We have one case from Milan, that is a Spielmeyer-Sjögren type, but we haven't isolated the pigment as yet.

Dr. Holman: Referring back to the previous slide with the two-dimensional chromatography, was that chromatography on a solution of the lipofuscin itself or was it some fraction of it?

Dr. Siakotos: That was a chloroform-methanol extract. We started out with a 2:1 chloroform methanol and went through various dilutions all the way up to absolute alcohol and then went back to 7:1 chloroform-methanol plus ammonia. This material is very thoroughly extracted and it's filtered on a sintered glass filter.

Dr. Holman: Can we assume that the protein components are not there any more?

Dr. Siakotos: We would assume that some of the protein may be extracted; that's presumably extracted out and remains on the Sephadex column.

Dr. Holman: What we are looking at here is then the separation of abnormal lipid soluble material. Has anything been done to study the possible hydrolysis products of these things?

Dr. Siakotos: No. We've concentrated the last year in establishing the purification of the pigments. This is not as easy as it sounds because in normal human brain the lipofuscin fraction is very low in concentration and we have now switched to zonal rotors. We can now process 12 total brains in one 3-day run. What we would like to do is to obtain grams of these materials and ship them around the country to whoever is a specialist in any particular area and have these experts characterize the components that fit into their specialty. This is really what we have been aiming for. Now that we can do this and we have the equipment to isolate very pure fractions of this pigment, the next step is to push the very thorough characterization of all components in these pigments.

Dr. Rider: In the cirrhotic patient, did you check the brain for ceroid to see if it was more...

Dr. Siakotos: No. In an alcoholic, particularly one who has a very severe cirrhotic liver, the brain has up to 5 times the normal concentration of normal lipofuscin. In other words, they don't accumulate ceroid in their brain, they accumulate lipofuscin. This is much higher than in a normal human brain.

Dr. Rider: Clinically, isn't it rather disturbing that you would find high ceroid in the cirrhotic if you are going to say that in Batten's disease they have a high concentration of ceroid? It's hard to see any correlation between these.

35

Dr. Siakotos: No. There are two problems here. One
is to obtain enough ceroid to work with because the brain
samples that we get from patients with Batten's disease, we
may get just a slice. When you are talking about working
and thoroughly characterizing 100 mg of pigment then you have
to know precisely what you are going to do with it. There
is no room for wasting any of this material.

Dr. Rider: In the cirrhotic you find the excess ceroid
in the liver and in Batten's disease you find the excess ceroid
in the brain. From the pathogenic standpoint is the ceroid
really significant in Batten's disease if it's also present
in other disease or other organs...

Dr. Siakotos: What you have to remember is that the
ceroid which is found in the brain of the Batten's disease
patient is found in a very young patient. Most alcoholics
that we normally see, rarely are they under 40 years old.
By normal accounts they have had a chance to accumulate a
fair amount of lipofuscin in the brain anyway. The problem
is that we haven't had any adult patients with Batten's disease.
We've seen ceroid and lipofuscin in the brains of some Batten's
patients.

Dr. Rider: You've said that the ceroid in the brain
of the children with Batten's disease is higher than normal.

Dr. Siakotos: There is no ceroid in a normal brain.

Dr. Rider: You've an abnormal finding in Batten's disease.
In the cirrhotic you have a high ceroid content in the liver...

Dr. Siakotos: That's right. You can say the reason
for having this very high concentration of ceroid in the liver
and this very high concentration of lipofuscin in the brain,
which is an organ somewhat distant from the liver, is that
the metabolism of alcohol produces a large number of free
radicals during the process of turning alcohol to aldehyde
and then to acid and then to its metabolites. This high concentration of free radicals may end up accelerating the same
type of damage in the brain but it doesn't result in ceroid,
it results in lipofuscin.

Dr. Rider: You're not damaging nerve cells in the liver.
Thus, the ceroid is coming from some different source than
nerve cells. If you are going to say that Batten's disease
has a destruction of the neurons and this destruction results
in ceroid or that ceroid destroys the nerve cells, it seems
to me that you have a different mechanism....

Dr. Siakotos: The brain of an alcoholic has a large
destruction of neurons too.

<u>Dr. Rider</u>: But ceroid....

<u>Dr. Zeman</u>: I would like to settle this argument and then continue with a short remark by Dr. Miquel.

Actually, there is no evidence that the destruction of any tissue under otherwise normal conditions does produce lipopigments. Lipopigments can be produced in experimental situations with a variety of damaging procedures; for example, vitamin E deficiency, antioxidant deprivation, or hypoxia and we all know about the epididymal fat pad model of Hartroft where the intimate mixture of heme with relatively neutral triglycerides and cholesterol esters produces large quantities of lipopigments. However, if you look at any brain with evidence of degenerative disease or with destructive lesions for any other reason, there is very little evidence of lipopigment formation. I believe the situation is rather the other way around. The process which accounts for the rapid accumulation and massive formation of lipopigments represents, indeed, the cause for the damage to the neurons and the loss of the neurons in Batten's disease. In this respect what we should be looking for is a similar cell damage to the liver parenchyma under the formation of ceroid in cirrhotic livers. The question here is whether the pigment occurs in the scar or does it occur in the still viable hepatocytes, a question which is not fully resolved. Before we have Dr. Tappel elaborate on some of his observations which really form the connecting link between the observations of Dr. Siakotos and the assumption that we are dealing with products of lipid peroxidation, Dr. Miquel is going to show us a few of his preparations. I might mention that Dr. Miquel may have discovered a very elegant system to study ceroid, namely the aging Drosophila. Dr. Miquel is not only able to show that the aging flies have tissues which are loaded with these pigments but he also has developed a variety of performance tests which permit the correlation between biological aging and pigments on the one hand and functional performance on the other hand. Unfortunately, he didn't bring his movies along, but he will be very happy to receive any one of you in his laboratory and show the movies on the changing pattern of mating behavior of Drosophila which is probably the best yardstick for aging. He is going to show us a few of his observations.

<u>Dr. Miquel</u>: My presentation will be very short. However, I wish to give credit to those who have been interested in the Drosophila model so far, among them Dr. Tappel who has demonstrated in our flies fluorescent pigments similar to mammalian lipofuscin. Also, I am very grateful to the electron microscopy laboratories which are performing a systematic investigation of practically all the tissues of Drosophila. In particular I wish to acknowledge the contributions of Dr. Mary M. Herman and Dr. Klaus Bensch from the Stanford Department of Pathology, of Dr. Delbert E. Philpott from our own laboratory.

I have been very pleased to learn that Dr. Siakotos has isolated ceroid from old Drosophila tissues. I was surprised to hear that ceroid pigment may amount to 2% of the fruit fly's body weight. This is a tremendous amount. However, after looking again at our electron micrographs, I see no cause for surprise in Dr. Siakotos' finding. Here you can see a cell from the midgut of old Drosophila that has about 30% of the cytoplasm filled by ceroid pigment. As you can see, the dense bodies are very similar to those shown by Dr. Siakotos in mammalian tissue.

Regarding the physiological parameters, Drosophila is ideally suited for a study of the decrease in performance with age. Moreover, to investigate behavioral changes we don't need to train the flies as psychologists train rats. All that is required is to house male and female Drosophila together and monitor the mating performance. In this slide we have plotted the "vitality" of the flies as expressed by the mating ability of human males. The slide shows a linear decline for both parameters with the passage of time. It is our opinion that Drosophila is an excellent model to investigate the biological significance of the ceroid accumulation.

Dr. Menkes: When you performed your test, Dr. Siakotos, did you look at testes? There is a peculiar polyunsaturated fatty acid in testes. I was wondering if you looked at that.

Dr. Holman: The polyunsaturated fatty acids in testes of rats are highly unsaturated and long-chained. I don't recall any that are unusual, i.e., the whole family of them seems to occur.

Dr. Witting: I think that what he is referring to is that the $\omega 22:5$ there is in high concentration.

Dr. Holman: Well, the 22:5 acids as a group are rich in testes.

Dr. Witting: We tried feeding nonessential polyunsaturated fatty acids to rats and it's rather hard to get the ω:3s incorporated into the testis' phospholipid. They are resistant to incorporation with ω:3s.

Dr. Zeman: Perhaps along the same line of argument, I understand that the outer segments of the retinal rods also do contain a very high concentration of polyenic fatty acids, according to Svennerholm. This is a part of the human body in which Batten's disease begins and produces a very early destructive lesion. I wonder whether Dr. Holman or Dr. Witting knows any more particulars about these polyenic acids in the retinal rods? No. Well, then Dr. Miquel....

38

Dr. Miquel: We have developed culture conditions for
Drosophila which result in mortality curves of the rectangular
type. This means that our flies are very healthy and most
likely die as a consequence of degenerative processes associated
with normal aging. The longevity curve shows a long plateau
during which practically no flies die, and then a rather abrupt
inflection, with most flies dying between 70 and 120 days.
The flies used for electron microscopy investigations were
from 84 to 120 days old, the age at which we see abundant
pigment accumulation. In our opinion a very interesting feature
of Drosophila morphology and physiology may be responsible
for the intensity of the pigment accumulation, namely that
Drosophila does not rely on blood vessels to transport oxygen
to the tissues, but instead has tracheolae pumping air to
the cells and therefore the intracellular oxygen tension may
be very high.

The most intense accumulation of ceroid occurs in the
oenocytes, which are secretory cells involved in the maintenance
of the exoskeleton. Some mitochondria in the oenocytes of
old flies show intact cristae, but most mitochondria have
a dense core that, in our opinion, is the first stage in a
process of peroxidation. There are also typical dense bodies
that are the product of severe mitochondrial degeneration.
We believe that in this particular tissue the dense bodies
arise from mitochondria because we see transitional forms.
We have not performed histochemical studies and at the present
time we don't know if the lysosomes are involved in this process.

We have found age pigment accumulation in the Drosophila
fat body. This tissue has a very important role in the insect
metabolism since it synthetizes proteins and stores neutral
fat and glycogen. In old flies we see dense bodies that look
like lipofuscin, and also a process of mitochondrial degeneration
with appearance of intramitochondrial crystals.

In the cells of the midgut we have found some dense bodies
with the appearance of autophagic vacuoles and others that
had a hollow core and were similar to dense bodies found in
the mitochondria of mammals, for instance of thallium-intoxicated
rats as shown by Herman and Bensch.

There is also a tremendous accumulation of dense bodies
in the thoracic muscle of old Drosophila. In humans lipofuscin
is predominantly found in those muscles (ocular, cardiac)
which are the most consistently active through life (as shown
by Rubinstein). The activity of these muscles, however, does
not come close to that of insect flight muscle with its high
complement of mitochondria, which may account for approximately
40% of total cell volume. The required oxygen is generously
supplied by tracheolae closely applied to the fiber surface.

These special features of flight muscle structure and metabolism may be responsible for the striking accumulation of age pigment in this tissue.

In conclusion, I believe that Drosophila is an excellent model to study age pigments for the following reasons: (1) The accumulation of ceroid in old flies is not a pathological process, as in mammals, but a consequence of normal aging. This feature of Drosophila aging may be related to the concentration of antioxidants in the tissues or to the oxygen level. In any case, further studies may throw light on the pathogenesis of ceroid accumulation both in insects and in mammals. (2) Since the flies live approximately 3 to 4 months, samples of old tissues are easily obtained. For instance, we have already preserved frozen in liquid nitrogen 50,000 old animals (50 grams) for Dr. Siakotos. (3) In Drosophila we can easily correlate age pigment accumulation with physiological performance.

Dr. Zeman: Thank you very much Dr. Miquel. I might just mention in passing that these observations are very important for the reasons outlined by Dr. Miquel and that is that the metabolism and structural organization of these flies is markedly different from mammals, and yet apparently a very similar process is going on in these animals as a function in time as in men.

Dr. Tappel will now present some of his data.

Dr. Rider: Can you see grossly this pigment or not? Is this all microscopic?

Dr. Zeman: You can see it grossly. Brains from patients with Batten's disease have a bright yellow-brownish cortex in comparison with a normal brain.

Dr. Tappel: I will try to address myself particularly to some of the questions or topics that have come up.

The first one--the question of damage--we hope to bring in the free radical chemists at this point to help the biochemists and biologists with the question of free radical damage.

The second question I would like to address is the origin of the fluorescent pigment because I think the pigment can be used as a tracer to connect what the pathologists see and have seen for a long time with what the biochemist understands about lipid peroxidation.

Thirdly, I would like to address myself particularly to the use of antioxidants in vivo to inhibit the development of the fluorescent pigment.

With the first slide I am showing a fairly conventional presentation of the free radical peroxidation process being initiated. The L stands for the polyunsaturated lipid which reacts avidly with oxygen to form the hydroperoxyl radical. In the middle of the figure is shown the breakdown of the hydroperoxide, usually by a homolytic scission. This is often a chain-branching region in which free radical chain reactions multiply. The circular method of presentation is meant to imply the free radical chain-reaction. I think it will be interesting for this group to discuss what may be the major free radicals that cause the molecular damage because we have the hydroperoxy radical (LOOH), the alkoxyl radical and the hydroxyl radical. Finally, the formation of some lipid peroxides is represented by LOOH and further break down products by the carbonyls.

We will try to put this into some perspective of what is known about mechanisms of damage in terms of the structure of the membrane. If you will, visualize that this figure represents a cross-sectional view of a membrane, that there are proteins on the surface, and these tuning fork-like structures are the polyunsaturated phospholipids. We could visualize that as a peroxidation is initiated, as shown by the LOOH, it might undergo chain branching. This free radical chain reaction might translate to the membrane in the direction shown by the arrows. Each arrow might be a free radical re-action, causing either a peroxidation or hitting a protein to cause free radical chain-polymerization. In this case the oxidation might oxidize the methionine, a very labile amino acid. One product you get--and we'll show that this is one of the fluorescent products--is a Schiff-base, for example from a phosphatidyl ethanolamine. Another possibility is the crosslinking via carbonyl compounds of enzymes or other amines of the body. You also get the Schiff-base products and they fluoresce with the same fluorescence properties as the pigments Dr. Siakotos discussed.

We will describe now some of the methodology that is used to measure peroxidation by the biochemist and the chemist and indicate the type of reaction that forms the fluorescent products. I think we are mostly familiar with the polyunsat-urated lipids forming peroxides. One can measure the oxygen absorption; one can measure carbonyl products; one can measure changes in the polyunsaturated lipids. In small quantities some of these carbonyls--and the only structural requirement they have to have is either to be an unsaturated carbonyl or to be something like dicarbonyl like malonaldehyde--react with the various amines, and they will react with all of them to form fluorescent products. This fluorescent structure, this fluorochrome, is very simple. I will assure you that by synthesizing some model compounds we have proven that this is a fluorescent structure that can result. Presumably, phospha-

tidyl ethanolamine is the main amine reacting but proteins
and nucleic acids will also react. I would like to indicate
that biochemical studies of these compounds can be made by
taking membranous organelles of the cell and exposing them
to oxygen. Many of you here in this room have done a large
number of studies along these lines. We have observed some
of the reactions, for example in mitochondria, using techniques
similar to those of Hunter's group. When mitochondria are
freshly isolated they have very little fluorescence. When
they are peroxidized they develop a large amount of the fluorescence similar to the fluorescence of the age pigment.

Here are some examples of the fluorescence of some of
the pigments we obtained from Dr. Siakotos and they are compared
with that of oxidized cephalin.

Let me perhaps explain the fluorescence by showing another
example. In this diagram the purple stands for the excitation
spectra. The green stands for the fluorescence spectra.
The fluorescence and excitation spectra of this type of pigment
are fairly simple; i.e., they do not have much definition.
One can differentiate these from other pigments very easily
because of their solubility properties and also because of
the maxima of the two spectra. The way we get the majority
of the pigment, as in the case of age pigment, is to do a
chloroform-methanol extract, much of this pigment is soluble,
presumably due to phospholipids, then we transfer that sample
to chloroform to remove the lipoproteins, then take a spectrum
of the chloroform layer directly. Because of the quantum
yield of this type of fluorescent group, one can get analyses
in parts per billion or even up to parts per trillion. It
is an extremely sensitive method. The fluorescence spectrum
is taken by sweeping the fluorescence monochrometer and when
you find the maximum you usually sweep the excitation mono-
chromator to find the excitation maximum. Quantitatively
then, one can express the results in terms of the fluorescence
of the total sample. Fluorescence must be measured with reference to a standard because fluorescence spectra are not like
infrared or ultraviolet spectra, i.e., they are relative to
the instrumental parameters. In terms of quantitation we have
recently been exposing mitochondria and microsomes to oxygen
and allowing them to peroxidize. Here are some spectra showing
the peroxidation expressed as fluorescence, although we measured
oxygen absorption and TBA reactants also. These mitochondria
came from vitamin E-deficient animals and these animals had
been fed a simulated human diet with the recommended level
of vitamin E (the bottom line) so they didn't peroxidize.
The middle group had the average U.S. level of vitamin E,
in other words, the average vitamin E in a U.S. diet was simulated for these animals. The fluorescence then develops as
a function of the peroxidation of the membranes. It doesn't
matter so much which membrane you are speaking about because

all of them that we have looked at undergo peroxidation and
finally formation of fluorescence. The amount of fluorescent
pigment formed is approximately one molecule out of 1,000
peroxidized. In other words it is formed in tracer amounts.
The only advantage to it is that it is so easily measured.
The amount of fluorescence formed does correlate with the
other parameters of peroxidation. One can get fairly good
correlations of fluorescence with the other measurements of
lipid peroxidation. Of course, the simplest system would
be to peroxidize phosphatidyl ethanolamine which also gives
this fluorescent pigment. I wonder if there are some questions
at this point?

Dr. Zeman: Yes, could you repeat again... Is the fluorescence the direct result of peroxidation or rather the formation
of the Schiff-base which crosslinks your substrate?

Dr. Tappel: Yes, it is the latter. You have to go through
the stages of peroxidation; break down of the chains presumably
yields carbonyl compounds. The carbonyl compounds react with
amines to form Schiff-base products.

Dr. Ingold: I gather that the fluorescence developed
in oxidizing pure unsaturated fatty acids don't have exactly
the same maxima fluorescent spectra as when the oxidation
is carried out in the presence of amines.

Dr. Tappel: Yes. We haven't looked at much of that
but peroxidizing polyunsaturated lipids alone, without the
presence of amino compounds, have very low-level fluorescence.

Dr. Malone: This is not specific. One would get this
type of reaction, as measured by the fluorescent compound,
from almost any combination of amines plus polyunsaturated
fatty acid derivatives.

Dr. Tappel: That is correct. There seems to be very
little in the way of specificity to the reaction.

Dr. Horvat: This is well known that when you get more
than two double bonds separated by a methylene group (1,4
diene) oxidation, at least auto-oxidation, goes quite rapidly.
The more double bonds, the faster it goes. I believe enzymatically they should go at about the same same rate. Is that
true with hydrolases?

Dr. Tappel: Yes.

Dr. Horvat: I don't know about lipid oxidations but
the products from the auto-oxidations are very specific and
very well defined. There is a great mass of information on
just where those allyl peroxidases break down and I'd show

43

you the scheme that is usually given, but Dr. Ingold, being
a physical organic chemist, can probably throw a little more
light on this. This has puzzled me for years. I have been
working on it for about 6 years. We have been trying to correlate
development of all flavors in types of stored foods. All
you need is linoleic acid and of the total lipids maybe half
a percent, after the material has been dehydrated. For those
of you who have forgotten, this is the structure of linoleic
acid and it can be either an ester or a glyceride. The glycerides
are a little more stable than the methyl esters. The first
assumption is that either ionizing radiation or peroxide extracts
a hydrogen atom and the double bonds conjugate and you get
the two isomers (free radicals), depending upon whether this
pair of electrons shifts in, or the other and that is the
origin of so-called 9 or 13-hydroperoxide. This radical then
picks up oxygen in the system to give us the peroxy radical
which later abstracts another hydrogen atom and continues
the free radical chain. Only very specific things are found
from these oxidations. The way they are usually illustrated
if you go to the literature is that you have this cleavage
occurring from this alcoside radical to give hexanal and,
true this is the major product from all of these oxidations,
but when you look for the other end of the radical, if the
cleavage was that simple, you should get a good slug of product
from the vinyl end of this particular reaction but there seems
to be no evidence here. The malonaldehyde is a thing I rather
doubt is produced, or if it is, is a minor product, because
I think the evidence is on paper--I don't want to mention
who did it--but a great deal of effort has gone into it.

    Dr. Malone: I was going to ask Dr. Tappel about the factors
controlling the rate of this process. It seems to be a chain
reaction--the distance between double bonds or the configuration
cis trans across the double bond affects the reaction rate.

    Dr. Horvat: I would like to hear from Dr. Ingold on
that.

    Dr. Ingold: As far as this scission goes, you are con-
siderably more likely on energetic grounds to finish up with
the conjugated aldehyde $CH_2C=CC=CC=O$. Of course, this is
an equally good precursor for the unit that gives the fluorescence in these bodies. There is no necessity to invoke malonaldehyde. Any conjugated aldehyde will do just as well to
give this fluorescence. Furthermore, with a conjugated aldehyde
you can still get polymerization of one protein to another
protein because you are going to finish up with something
that is still difunctional. There is still the other end
of the conjugated aldehyde that has very weak, very labile
hydrogens because they are adjacent to a conjugated system;
thus, they will come off very easily under free radical attack.
This other end of the conjugated system will form a peroxide

link which can then cleave in exactly the same way to put
another aldehyde unit on and hence pick up another protein
unit. I think that this would be quite consistent with what
has been observed. I'm not sure that it matters whether malonaldehyde itself is involved, one would have things that
structurally can behave the same way and cross link two protein
units. This is in addition, of course, to the normal crosslinking of polyunsaturated fatty acids which occurs by a
preliminary oxidation to give a conjugated system to which
peroxy radicals add to give polyperoxides.

Dr. Zeman: Dr. Tappel, perhaps you could summarize this
somewhat expanded view of Dr. Horvat, Dr. Ingold and yours.
What I have in mind is that we have something on paper which
I can also understand.

Dr. Tappel: The point that Dr. Ingold was making is
that the fluorescent product can come from any conjugated
dicarbonyl. It doesn't have to come from malonaldehyde.

Dr. Zeman: Let me ask you this, do you isolate other
aldehydes or dialdehydes?

Dr. Horvat: Actually you get dicarbonyls from linoleate
oxidations which would work beautifully in this type of thing--
they have been isolated by about 50 oxidation chemists from
all over the world.

Dr. Zeman: I might point out that this is for us simple-
minded morphologists a rather significant fact because, as
you know, morphologists require for their technology fixed
tissues. If indeed aldehyde or dialdehyde should be generated
in a chemical reaction within the cell then we would have
a very toxic and damaging molecular species which could fix
and thus denature biological molecules.

Dr. Malone: I think this is interesting and extremely
important. There is one long-chain polyhydroxyamine that
is a component of a large number of compounds, particularly
in brain. I am speaking of sphingosine hydroxyl groups of
carbon atoms one and three and a primary amine on the second
carbon. The unsaturated double bond is located between the
fourth and fifth carbon atoms. Would such a molecule be very
susceptible to this type of change that you are speaking
of?

Dr. Tappel: I would think as susceptible as a monoene
essentially.

Dr. Zeman: Dr. Malone is now drawing the structural
formula of sphingosine, an aminoalcohol.

45

Dr. Tappel: Dr. Ingold, would you say that a monoene would oxidize like that?

With the OH on the carbon adjacent to the double bond the hydrogen that is attached to that particular carbon will be extremely susceptible to free radical attack. One would then get an alpha hydroxy hydroperoxide adjacent to this C=C. This would give you a carbonyl function in that position. I perhaps didn't make something clear earlier. I didn't intend to say that malonaldehyde isn't the important species. It may very well be. The energetics of the cleavage of the peroxidized linoleic acid is such as to give you a conjugated carbonyl function. This will be favored by several kilocalories over the other form of cleavage.

Dr. Witting: In regard to Dr. Horvat's original question as to the effect of structure, my impression is that this has been in the literature for about 30 years under the heading of Bolland's rules. They worked that all out in terms of what effect various groups adjacent to double bonds have on rates of oxidation. Your comments on the products of oxidation refer to a relatively anhydrous system. We also have to be concerned with some of the products that Shoenstein has shown to occur in an aqueous system. Since presumably at the interface you would have the possibility of that type of product formation; whereas in the relatively anhydrous system you tend to accumulate most of the alpha, beta unsaturated aldehydes and the corresponding doubly unsaturated aldehydes. In the aqueous system, as I remember, you also find quite a bit of oxygenation of double bonds so that polyfunctional oxygenated aldehyde compounds accumulate. These would be presumably quite reactive then with the amino group of the protein. Let's distinguish then between aqueous and non-aqueous systems.

Dr. Ingold: One of the principal differences between an aqueous and non-aqueous system is that the cleavage of alkoxy radicals (produced from hydroperoxides) is much faster in the aqueous system than in the non-aqueous system.

Dr. Witting: I think one of the points Shoenstein made in reviewing that in Lipid Research a year or two ago was that where you have a lipid in an aqueous phase some products are out of contact, because of polarity with the main lipid phase and some products, therefore, accumulate that would not normally be found in quantity in a non-aqueous system. I am just talking in terms of the products that tend to accumulate rather than the course of the reactions.

Dr. Tappel: I think we can resume at this point. When we diverged from the story we were focused on the question of where does the formation of fluorescent products get us since these products have been observed by the pathologist

particularly for a long period of time. I think they get us
to the point of how we can incrimate polyunsaturated lipid
peroxidation in the process of their formation. As lipid
peroxidation forms the fluorescent products, then it must
also be damaging the tissues in its immediate proximity.
It has been shown in a number of laboratories and quite a
bit in our own that such molecular damage is something in
the order of that sustained from ionizing radiation, being
of a similar oxidative type and perhaps in a lower yield but
nevertheless being a very damaging reaction to sustain in
the living body.

Going back to the pigments that Dr. Siakotos has isolated,
we have looked at a number of them. They all have the fluorescence spectra of the type that correlated with this conjugated
Schiff-base and also the excitation spectra are of the same
type. Slight differences in fluorescence-excitation spectra
we are not ready to interpret as having any great significance.
There is a whole family of fluorescent compounds that can
derive. I think it is sufficient to say that we can measure
these at this time and we can relate these to lipid peroxidation.
Of the recent batch of fluorescent lipofuscin pigments, whether
you call them lipofuscin or ceroid--I don't think I would
differentiate them as a chemist at this point--that Dr. Siakotos
has isolated, here is the spectrum of a brain age pigment.
This pigment has the typical fluorescence in about the 430
nm region and excitation around 360 nm. These happen to be
very good regions of the spectrum to work in, incidently,
because you can get in very much light at 360 nm and most
photomultiplier tubes are most responsive at 430 nm. Thus,
it is an excellent fluorescence methodology.

Here is the spectrum of another pigment. This comes
from liver. It suffices to say that all of Dr. Siakotos'
pigments look alike to the spectrophotofluorometer, except
for small differences in amounts and sometimes we can pick
up vitamin A. Incidently, when there is vitamin A present,
this polyene is readily photo-oxidized in the chloroform solvent
upon exposure to ultraviolet light.

Dr. Zeman: What happens then?

Dr. Tappel: Then it is destroyed and it loses its fluorescence, so it is a very convenient assay method. In analyzing
Dr. Siakotos' pigment we get about 10^{-5} grams of pure fluorochrome
per gram of dry weight. You might say the fluorescent pigment
is only there in trace quantities but I think it is sufficient
to link it back to lipid peroxidation. In another example
quantitation of fluorochome was done on extracts of the testes
of aging mice, which I will bring out in a discussion of further
experiments, we found about 10.6 mcg/g of dry weight. The
pigments are quite enriched with fluorescence as compared

to whole tissue as you might expect.

I would like to provide evidence that this free radical process does go on in vivo and that it can be inhibited even in so-called nutritionally complete animals by adding vitamin E and other biological antioxidants. This is a design of an aging experiment in which we presume, following the same hypothesis as Dr. Harman, that polyunsaturated lipids cause damage through the free radical oxidants. This is a general damage which may express itself in aging deterioration. Particularly, we are going to measure it through the formation of fluorescent pigments that are formed. This is the design of the experiment.

The next slide will show the basal diet which was essentially a normal protein test diet. It was a fairly well balanced diet. We provided a vitamin E equivalent--I put it in human equivalents to make it easier to understand--of 24 mg/day. That works out for the mouse to about 30 mg/kg of diet. We used CD_1 strain of mice, starting with retired breeders just to get the experiment going.

The reason I bring out these antioxidant nutrient mixtures and the results of the experiments is that these are very similar to the antioxidant mixtures that are being used on the Batten's disease children. We classify the antioxidants in a practical way so that one mixture might be used now in man and another mixture might be open for future application. We used mixtures of antioxidants because the literature on vitamin E and related nutrients suggests that one could get synergism, for example with vitamin E and vitamin C, and the effect of the sulfur amino acids by putting in methionine, and that further use of a food antioxidant, butylated hydroxytoluene, you should get homosynergism with vitamin E, with higher amounts of antioxidants. There is considerable nutritional information on selenium acting somewhat analogous to vitamin E. These are all very long stories but in essence we are using very high levels of vitamin E, the equivalent of a gram or two per human, in this case, the diet which we called #3 has 0.2% BHT. This is, of course, a very high amount, bordering on the subtoxic level of BHT.

Dr. Rider: What is the toxic level?

Dr. Tappel: I would say that from the toxicity studies that have been done, Professor Harman has performed long-term feedings of animals, that 0.5% total diet and up would be toxic. The one toxic effect that I remember is that there is a general growth depression, I can't remember any others.

Dr. Harman: At the level of 0.5% by weight of BHT in the diet, with feeding started right after weaning, you find a depression in body weight of about 10% as compared to controls.

48

At that level you don't tend to see anything else. The livers
of mice receiving BHT tend to be a little larger than the
controls because of an increase in endoplasmic reticulum,
but no overt signs of toxicity.

Dr. Zeman: Is this 0.5% of the total diet or of the
free fatty acid?

Dr. Harman: Total diet.

Dr. Tappel: Very high levels.

Dr. Rider: Would someone interpret that in terms of
the amount in the diet of a human? How many milligrams or
grams?

Dr. Tappel: How many grams per day per human would that
be?

Dr. Harman: A half a per cent by weight for mice translated
to the human diet would be something like 25 or 30 grams of BHT
per day, a tremendous dose of BHT.

Dr. Tappel: So the amount we have suggested for the
human, though above the FDA suggestion for protecting foods,
is nevertheless very much in the safe range.

Dr. Zeman: Perhaps there has been a misunderstanding,
but we have been giving 200 mg/day to our patients. Some
of our patients have received that amount now for perhaps
2 years. Charles has been getting 400 mg daily, I think.
Of course, these are grown children and we would not expect
any toxic effect, because from what has been said here, we
are well below the toxic limits with this medication.

Dr. Tappel: That is correct.

Now just to mention the effects of antioxidants on the
aging parameters--here we have the diets; basal, that emphasizing
vitamin E and that emphasizing vitamin E and BHT. There is
no protection in terms of mortality and possibly we had even
a slighter increase in decline of the population. I'm not
sure how significant these are, we are still interpreting
the data. We did not in essence save any animals from the
normal death time by feeding them these antioxidants. In
terms of performance tests, there was a little better performance
in the vitamin E group. There was a considerable dispersion
of the population after they were two years old, however,
and had been on the diet for sometime over a year. In terms
of kidney function, which is not a highly selective test,
it looked as if this group had better concentratin of urine,
a test that you can apply to mice. These all have great limita-

tion I might say.

Dr. Zeman: How about the mating behavior?

Dr. Tappel: These were all males.

Our main objective was to look at the fluorescent molecular damage. It turned out that the organ of choice, because it has high polyunsaturated lipids and it deposits pigment, was the testes. These are three typical spectra of fluorescence of extracts of mouse testes at 3 ages-3 months, 10 months and 23 months. Plotting these data out, of course we studied a statistically significant number of animals, we get this type of correlation of increase of fluorescence as a function of age. It seems to be more exponential than linear. There have, however, been very few studies in this type of area.(see Figure 13, page 158)

We also measured the pigment formed in heart as a function of diet. The top curves are for the basal diet, the middle curves are for the vitamin E diet, in other words intermediate in antioxidants, and the dotted curves at the bottom were those containing BHT also. In other words, as a function of increased antioxidant, even superimposed on this normal nutritional diet that didn't have deficiences, we were able to depress in vivo the formation of this fluorescent pigment. Because of dispersion in the data, that in the heart was not statistically significant.

These are the spectra of the testes and here the top values statistically were significantly different from the bottom ones. There was again quite a dispersion of the data and this is a major problem in animal experiments. There is though on the average much more pigment developed in animals fed the basal diet and feeding antioxidants seems to depress the pigment formation considerably.

We did find in all tissues examined, in fact all tissues of human and animal origin that we examined, these pigments.

This shows the figures for an intermediate period when the animals were about one year old and had been on the diet for one-half year; already the decrease by the BHT had begun to show up.

This shows extracts from testes of the animals when we terminated the experiment. In this case the antioxidants had depressed the fluorescent molecular damage to about one-half. This was significantly lower than the basal.

I think these studies are interesting from the standpoint of application of antioxidants because by using this methodology of measuring fluorescent molecular damage, I think we have evidence that it is lipid peroxidation going on in vivo; the damage accumulates as a function of age, and it can be depressed even for animals on a normally complete nutritional diet by increasing the level of antioxidants.

Dr. Harman: I would like to make a couple of comments. In regard to the age of animals, you started with animals that were originally breeders. How old were they at that time?

Dr. Tappel: We tried to get a good start by taking 9-month-old breeders.

Dr. Harman: Just by chance at one time we carried out an experiment in which we started animals on antioxidants, not after weaning as we usually do, but at about 9 months of age, and the effect was considerably less. Secondly, we felt as you did that by combining antioxidants we might get a synergistic effect. We have combined BHT with vitamin E as you did and also 2-mercaptoethylamine (2-MEA) with vitamin E. I can't explain it, but the mortality rates were markedly decreased as compared to those with BHT or 2-MEA alone. In other words, a combination rather than being beneficial was deleterious. I don't know what this means.

Dr. Holman: Have you done the experiment which shows whether or not antioxidants in the diet can reduce the amount of pigment once it has been formed?

Dr. Tappel: No, we haven't done that. It would be very difficult to do in an aging experiment because the pigment develops fairly slowly and then there is the dispersion of the animals. Some animals have high pigment and some have relatively low pigment.

Dr. Harman: I would like to comment in regard to Dr. Holman's question. To my knowledge there has been only one or two studies reported in which age pigment was claimed to disappear or decrease in amount--in aged guinea pigs given a compound known as centrophenoxine.

Dr. Zeman: I can amplify further. We are still being left in suspense as to whether these experiments really did what they claimed to do. The principle investigator in this study, Dr. Nandy, worked with Bernie Strehler for a year and tried to duplicate the feat in Los Angeles. Dr. Tappel, do you know anything about the outcome of those studies? The results are forthcoming very slowly and, although these experiments were carried out two years ago, nobody--including Bernie Strehler--has been able to get any final data on this. We have treated patients with centrophenoxine to no avail.

51

What can be concluded from this is the following. (1) Maybe
we didn't have the right dose or we didn't give it long enough.
(2) It is possible that even if you do remove the pigment
this doesn't heal the damage produced when the pigment was
formed. That would go along with Dr. Tappel's hypothesis.
(3) The drug is not effective in removing the pigment from
the human brain. This is where we stand on the centrophenoxine
story and I just wonder whether the data which is extant in
the literature really warrants further efforts in this area,
perhaps with the exception of tissue cultures or something
of this sort.

Dr. Harman: I would like to add just one more bit of
information in regard to centrophenoxine. We have fed mice,
starting after weaning, a tenth and two-tenths per cent by
weight of centrophenoxine in the diet; the weight of the animals
was decreased somewhat at the higher dose levels and the life
span in both cases was depressed as compared to controls.

Dr. Witting: We have tried some work with centrophenoxine
too. On examination of the tissue by fluorescent microscopy
and electron microscopy, we couldn't find any effect attributable
to the drug.

Dr. Ingold: I think this is an appropriate time to make
my only contribution. I read over with great interest, and
I confess without much understanding, a large part of the
articles you sent me, Dr. Zeman, and it seemed that as a chemist
the only thing I could do, not realizing that Dr. Tappel had
given you all types of advice, was to think of possible treatment
or dosages and things to give to patients. I'll come on to
the antioxidants in a moment. One possibility that did occur
to me (now that we know from Dr. Tappel's work that one of
the polymerizing functions is an aldehyde) was to offer the
aldehyde with something more reactive than a simple amino
group. The only thing I could think of was hydroxylamine.
I looked this up in an Encyclopedia of Chemistry and Technology
and I found that it was somewhat toxic but it had been used
to control convulsions. Furthermore, it yields an inhibitor
of peroxidations. I can go into that for the chemists if
anyone is interested separately and not bother everyone else
with it. I did wonder whether perhaps the convulsions had
been in any way related to the Batten's disease convulsions
but I had no way of checking that in a limited time. To go
on to the antioxidants....

Dr. Zeman: Hydroxylamine?

Dr. Ingold: Hydroxylamine. I have photostated the relevant
pages out of the Encyclopedia of Chemistry and Technology.
I can give you the reprint.

Dr. Menkes: We have a much better known agent for aldehydes

52

aldehydes and that is isoniazide. We have used this for years and years.

Dr. Ingold: Does it work in the process? Does it stop....

Dr. Menkes: ....TB....

Dr. Witting: If the hydroxylamine would work, it would also have another effect. I don't know if you are aware that hydroxylamine has been used as an assay reagent for hydroperoxides. You get an evolution of nitrogen and formation of water with the reduction of the hydroperoxide group. If you were able to get it to a membrane interface, any peroxides that came to the interface would be destroyed by the hydroxylamine.

Dr. Ingold: Yes. There are all kinds of problems with it but it has been used medically. If you go after the aldehyde there is one big disadvantage. You are going after the second step of the peroxidation. Obviously, this is a very poor choice compared with going after the free radicals that carry the peroxidation chain along--one is much better off to attack them. The best possibility would be some synergistic mixture of additives that would inhibit the oxidation at every possible stage. BHT (butylated hydroxytoluene) is an excellent antioxidant. It has a methyl group on the aromatic ring. This methyl group can sometimes be replaced with advantage by other groups. Thus, one achieves a greater solubility in water if instead of a methyl group one uses a methyl amino group CH_2NH_2 (such a group might also trap the aldehyde). Dimethyl aminomethyl $(CH_2N(CH_2)_2)$ and various other amino groups have been used in place of methyl. These compounds have been administered to human patients and so there must be some data on them in the medical literature. They were being used by the Russians 8 to 12 years ago by a man called Emmanuel (who is actually a chemist) to try to control cancers. The prevailing theory at that time--I don't know whether it is still operating-- was that cancer was in a large part a free radical process and the Russians were trying to get very high dosages of hindered phenols into cancerous tissue. They used this trick of taking BHT and modifying it by putting amino groups on so they had methyl amino compounds which made them much more soluble. There were all kinds of games that were played with this-- again I could draw structures but I don't think there would be much advantage to it at this point.

There is another way one can change BHT to improve its efficiency. The methyl group can be replaced by a methoxy group to give the hindered paramethoxyphenol; i.e., 2,6-di-t-butyl 4-methoxyphenol. This compound is about four times as efficient an inhibitor as is BHT.

phenol and an unhindered phenol. The chemistry of such systems is quite well understood. In many systems one knows what are the most efficient inhibitor mixtures. In lipid-type systems, such as hydrocarbon oils, the most efficient synergism occurs when compounds such as 4-methoxyphenol or 2,4,6-trimethyl phenol are combined with BHT or presumably with the 4-methoxy butylated compound. I assume (on this basis) that this is the reason why vitamin E, which is structurally related to 4-methoxyphenol and to 2,6-dimethylphenol, normally synergises very well with BHT. It's very nice to see that Dr. Tappel and I obviously agree on the kind of mixtures that you should use when you want to prevent oxidation.

There are other synergistic mixtures--one could try using phenols that are known not to be harmful in the diet. Propyl gallate, I believe, is quite safe but this has a low fat solubility. However, if the length of the ester group is increased from propyl to ortyl or hexadienal one obtains fat soluble galates. These compounds would probably synergise well with BHT.

The other point I wanted to make was covered in diet #3 with the selenium. There are basically only two ways of stopping oxidation. One is to trap the free radicals that carry the chain. This is done with BHT or an unhindered phenol or better still by a combination of the two of them. The second method is to decompose the peroxides that initiate the chains. Selenium is known to be a fairly efficient peroxide decomposer. I don't think one necessarily knows in what form in the human body selenium exists but organic selenium compounds, many sulfide compounds, many phosphorus-containing compounds are all quite efficient peroxide decomposers. The compound that I was thinking of as a peroxide decomposer for this hypothetical treatment was thiodipropionic acid (or something similar) that allows you to get in a good hefty dose of sulfur.

Dr. Miquel: I would like to add a few words. Hochschild has shown that Drosophila live up to 30% longer when BHT is added to their food. Now we are testing this and other antioxidants on our flies. It seems to me that we could easily test some of the other compounds discussed here. Of course, investigations on Drosophila would not be so time-consuming as those performed on rats.

Dr. Zeman: I hope that we are all aware that this discussion is really concerned with two different, independent variables--one being the amount of fluorescent pigment deposited in specific tissues and the other one the mortality. I would like to ask Dr. Harman, do you have a correlation between the amount of pigments and mortalities as observed under these experimental dietary complements?

Dr. Harman: We haven't actually looked at pigment formation in connection with mortality but it is apparent from Dr. Tappel's work that we do not see a correlation between pigment accumulation and mortality rates. In this connection I would like to point out that Dr. Strehler has done work on the Japanese in connection with age pigment in that population as compared to our own. Mortality rates in these two countries are pretty much the same and yet the pigment accumulation in the brains of the Japanese is much higher than our own.

Dr. Barber: One observation with regard to the synergism, besides the dual chemical role here, the synergism with E and BHT might indeed get into a membrane solubility problem in that E does give you a nice long tail to hook it into different interfaces than BHT would. Thus, you might be getting a dual protection here with respect to the micro-environment itself.

Dr. Siakotos: Dr. Ingold, what would you consider the best chemical approach to breaking this amino protein crosslinking in trying to recover the original compound possibly?

Dr. Ingold: I can't think of any easy way of doing that.

Dr. Witting: Can you think of any way of doing it in the test tubes so that we can get at the structures of these things.

Dr. Ingold: No.

Dr. Witting: Dr. Tappel, I think you said, not here but somewhere else recently, that you'd managed to isolate some of this crosslinked lysine from tissue.

Dr. Tappel: Yes. The question that Lloyd Witting posed essentially is, "Has the crosslink been identified?" We did this with ribonuclease, an enzyme whose structure is well known. We found that the crosslink was apparently at the lysine epsilon amino group, the most reactive amino group that reacted to form this conjugated Schiff-base, and actually two ribonuclease molecules were crosslinked.

Dr. Witting: This is test tube then, you haven't actually isolated it in tissue.

Dr. Tappel: Right. So then it could be hydrolyzed and the lysine bonded by the Schiff-base reactant could be identified. This was pure material.

Dr. Witting: I thought you had done this in tissue. If you had I was going to ask if you had looked for desmosine, isodesmosine or paradesmosine.

55

Dr. Tappel: No, but it is interesting that the collagenous materials to which you are referring....

Dr. Witting: These occur naturally in collagen but presumably they might also occur in the system generating pigment.

Dr. Tappel: Yes, it's the conjugated crosslinking element of elastin. These crossbridges have similar structure and fluorescence. They occur primarily in elastin but also in aged collagen.

Dr. Zeman: What is the crosslinking agent?

Dr. Tappel: It is usually an oxidized lysine to form a carbonyl and then it undergoes Schiff-base condensation with another lysine. It is very analogous.

Dr. Witting: I was wondering if you have ever looked for these in a tissue that was forming pigment as opposed to a collagen.

Dr. Tappel: No, we haven't as yet. I might comment on the fluorescent pigment. We can find this fluorescent pigment in all tissues but we don't know what it relates to. Thus, we have to be very stringent with our models and make sure that we understand the processes that are going on to form the pigment.

I'd like to comment on the suggestions of Dr. Ingold because he has had quite a bit of experience and has brought forth many good suggestions which I am sure would take us a long time to evaluate. It is interesting that in such an evaluation, though, that one does live under the restraints of present knowledge, in part, and also of what is known of the nutrition or toxicology of the proposed compounds. We used all of this to come forth with these ideas. We chose selenium and sulfur, notice we had methionine in our mixture, to generate and to put into the body both the sulfides and also the sulfhydryl compounds. We were seeking ultimate inhibition in order to break the free-radical chain reaction, to decompose the peroxides, to get hymosynergism and to trap the free radicals. As you say, go in all directions.

Dr. Ingold: I realize that. It is interesting that your ideas and mine as to the best mixture of antioxidants are in very close agreement inspite of our completely different backgrounds.

Dr. Tappel: I guess there are no more questions.

Dr. Harman: I would like to make just one more comment in regard to lipid peroxidation, at least in regard to mortality

rate. The studies that we and others have carried out, there
was one reported in Experimentia several years ago by someone
from U.C.L.A., would suggest that with adequate amounts of
vitamin E in a normal diet (i.e., sufficient to prevent overt
vitamin E deficiency) that there is very little effect of
dietary lipids on mortality rate. In mice, going from a diet
containing 5% saturated fat, such as lard, to one containing
20% safflower oil as the sole source of lipid, one finds at
most about a 10% difference in mortality rate--the mortality
rate being higher with the polyunsaturated fat. Although lipid
peroxidation may influence formation of age pigment, etc.,
it has a relatively small effect on mortality rate in mice.

   Dr. Zeman: There is a disease in which it is assumed
that a high concentration of dietary polyunsaturated fatty
acids does indeed significantly reduce the life span and this
is the so-called yellow fat disease of cats. I wonder whether
anyone has had experience with this condition. What is at
the bottom of this? Incidently, Dr. Koppang has also studied
this condition in dogs. Animals that are exclusively fed
on fish rejects which contain a high concentration of polyunsaturated fatty acids develop lipid peroxide autofluorescent
pigments in practically all storage fat depots. When you
then look at such an animal at autopsy, the subcutaneous fat
rather than having a somewhat gelatinous whitish appearance
is a bright yellow. This is a change which the pathologist
is familiar with to some extent and which has erroneously
been called starvation fat that occurs in people who live
on relatively small quantities of saturated fatty acids in
prisons and nursing homes, become quite emaciated, and their
body fats become apparently peroxidized and polymerized.
To make the full circle, it has been observed in patients
with Batten's disease that their storage fat depots also transform into pigments, especially in body fats which are associated
with organs of high metabolic turnover such as the heart,
to a lesser extent in the lymph nodes and in certain parts
of the bone marrow. It appears to me that here we have an
observation that would tend to support the assumption that
low concentrations of saturated fatty acids may indeed prime
the process of polyenic fatty acid peroxidation. I wonder
whether Dr. Ingold could make some remarks with respect to
the energy requirement of these thermodynamic processes.

   Dr. Ingold: I feel fairly sure that a fully saturated
fat or fatty acid could not auto-oxidize at the temperature
of the human body. The rate at which it would be attacked
by a peroxy radical would be so low that the peroxy radical
would wander off and find something else to attack. You must
have at least one double bond in order to get any kind of
a reasonable rate of oxidation. Why a low level of saturated
fats should lead to a yellow coloration indicating oxidation,
I have no idea at all. The yellow color itself does sound

like something which I commented on earlier in Dr. Tappel's talk--that pure unsaturated fats give a yellow color when oxidized. I was asking in order to make sure that the fluorescent species he identified was not the same and to assure myself that it did have nitrogen in it.

Dr. Zeman: Perhaps I should rephrase my question. Do we have to look at the thermodynamics of polyunsaturated fatty acid peroxidation somewhat similar to the nuclear fission reaction which does require a critical mass? In other words, if we were to have a mixture of polyunsaturated fatty acids and saturated fatty acids, would the relationship between these two types of fatty acids in any way influence the rate of auto-oxidation? To put it differently, would a high relative concentration of saturated fatty acids protect the unsaturated fatty acids from peroxidation by perhaps dispersing the focal concentration of the polyunsaturated?

Dr. Ingold: I think that the answer is that you would get a linear correlation in the ratio. The more saturated fat relative to unsaturated fat that you had, the lower would be the rate of oxidation. The saturated fat would act as an inert dilutant and so the radical that was looking around for something that it could attack would be forced to stay around longer because there would be relatively fewer molecules that it could attack. It would therefore have more probability of meeting up with another radical. The overall rate of reaction would be reduced. I think you would find, if one could do the correct type of experiments, an almost linear correlation. The more saturated and the less unsaturated fat you had, then the lower would be the rate of oxidation.

Dr. Holman: I would like to confirm what Dr. Ingold has just been saying, that the rates of oxidation do depend upon the degree of unsaturation. There is literature on this, quite voluminous and quite old.

To answer a question that came up several minutes ago-- the relative rates of oxidation of oleic acid methyl ester versus linoleic acid methyl ester is 1:2. Each additional double bond roughly doubles the rate of oxidation. Therefore, the more polyunsaturated a thing is, the faster it can oxidize. I think Dr. Witting can confirm this, that he has a correlation of rate of oxidation to the iodine number of a mixture. Now if this be the case, when we load up an animal with polyun- saturated acids, we are predisposing him to oxidation. I am taking this opportunity to get rid of alot of old reprints. I brought some along which indicate that you can influence the polyunsaturation of the lipids of the brain in the rat. The more linoleic acid in the diet, the more long chain ω:6 acids in the brain. The more ω:3 acid is fed, the more poly- unsaturated ω:3 acids are found in the brain. The picture is not nearly as dramatic as it would be in other tissues. Heart and liver show these responses much more dramatically but the effect of dietary fatty acid upon brain composition fatty acids is shown in general.

Dr. Malone: I noted in this paper--I was about to ask-- this was on mature animals?

Dr. Holman: Yes.

Dr. Malone: Were you able to influence the composition in terms of saturated or unsaturated fatty acids when such feeding experiments were carried on with immature animals?

As one changes the composition with respect to polyun-saturated fatty acids, one changes the composition with respect to saturated fatty acids to some small degree. Under arachidonic acid in Table I there seems to be an erratic shift from around 19% up to 25%.

Dr. Ingold: I would like to make a short comment. The relative ease of oxidation of the unsaturated fatty acids that you mentioned is completely what one would predict, isn't it? A single double bond has much less activating ef-fect on the hydrogens on the adjacent carbon ($C=C=CH_2$) than when you have a methylene interrupted system of double bonds ($C=C-CH_2-C=C$). Once you have a methylene between two double bonds in the linoleic system then, if you go on to a linolenic system, all you are doing is just doubling the number of methylenes per molecule that are in an activated position. Linolenic acid is therefore about twice as readily oxidized as linoleic acid, but the latter is much more readily oxidized than oleic acid.

Dr. Menkes: What would you expect cholesterol to act as a....

Dr. Holman: Much of the excess polyunsaturated fatty acids (linoleic in a normal diet) will go into the adipose tissue. Tissue phospholipid fatty acid composition is normal with respect to polyunsaturated acids at an intake of 1-2% calories linoleic acid. Above this intake the surplus will pour over into the adipose tissue. The turnover time in the human being of neutral lipid linoleate is of the order of 26 months, so that for a very long time after a change in diet either towards a saturated fat or away from fats, anti-oxidant requirement will be determined by composition of the adipose tissue, not of the diet. It is the 26-month half turnover rate which can cause difficulties in interpretation. I think we should realize that we aren't necessarily what we are eating at the moment. We are what we ate in the past.

Dr. Zeman: This is exactly the point I was striving for. I didn't make that very clear but I felt that it was possible that if the polyunsaturated fatty acids might have a longer retention time in the storage fats than the saturated there might be some type of a relative shift. At any rate people kept on low fat diets for a long period of time do show this yellow fat whereas people who have a normal American high calorie, high saturated fat diet, do not show this phenomenon.

Dr. Witting: I'm going to confuse the situation a little more because one of the peculiarities of tocopherol and one of the things that makes it a good biological antioxidant is that it isn't stored as fat per se. It's stored generally speaking with phospholipid, your microsomes and mitochondria. The problem with many of your synthetic antioxidants is that they go with fat per se, particularly something like DPPD which is a beautiful antioxidant except that it has the nasty habit of getting rid of pregnant female rats which has made it very unpopular with some government agencies in terms of using it in nutritional experiments. The antioxidant that will be with your phospholipid, will turn over relatively rapidly, the surplus will start out in adipose tissue and turn over very slowly. You can create an imbalance by withdrawing both at the same time, the antioxidant will deplete before the source of unsaturated fatty acids.

Dr. Zeman: Dr. Barber, would you say something about your system?

Dr. Barber: I'd better take a few minutes to try and insert this story with some perspective. My general interest has been in lipid peroxidation, but it has been in lipid peroxidation as it is studied in membranes rather than in pure lipid systems. After several years of looking at peroxidation in subcellular membrane systems it became rather obvious that there are a number of observations that we can report as semi-truths. Once reported it gives us a certain model upon which we can build where many of the things that we have talked about in terms of lipid peroxidation apply primarily to pure lipids. However, we have to add some parameters when we put the lipids in with proteins and talk about membranes. I think Paul McCay will probably get to another part of this story when he presents his material. You don't normally find peroxides in living animals except at very low levels but if you take tissues out, grind them up and expose this membrane material to air in the presence of ascorbate, you can get considerable lipid peroxidation to occur.

What we have shifted our attention to and what I am going to talk about specifically now are two systems that we have been working with, primarily to demonstrate the effect of

60

the lipid protein interaction on the peroxidation process.
I think ultimately, if we are going to talk about lipid peroxidation in animals, we are going to have to worry about what
is happening to this interrelationship between the lipids
and the proteins. One of the things that is obvious very
early when you look at this system is that proteins are very
protective to the unsaturated lipids when they are associated
in membranous structures. I am going to say some things as
if they are absolutely true only because I want to go through
some of this material rapidly and I will come back to how
semi-true some of them are.

If you do things to destroy the integrity or to hasten
the destruction of the integrity of a lipid protein complex,
so that you get dissociation of the complex, you increase
the rate at which peroxidation occurs. You take a membrane
system out; you aerobically incubate it; then you add detergent-
like solubilizers. Chemical agents which break up hydrophobic
bonding alter peroxidation. The lipids are away from their
normal hydrophobic environment and this hastens peroxidation.
If you do the reverse experiment, that is you maintain the
integrity of the membrane chemically by crossreacting with
glutaraldehyde, for example, which crosslinks proteins, you
protect the hydrophobic environment of the lipid system and
you completely inhibit lipid peroxidation by this method.

We've done this in essentially two systems. One is of
historical significance and the second system, which we are
rather excited about now because we believe we are a little
closer to membranous structures, is more recent. The first
system consisted of structural protein from membrane and
phospholipid micelles which we prepared from the same membranes.
We isolate microsomes and prepare a protein fraction from
microsomes by solubilizing in detergent, stripping the lipids
off, and precipitating with 12% ammonium sulfate. We then
get a protein out of this which is very interactive with phospholipids in the micelle state. If you look at the peroxidation of the phospholipid micelle, you get a certain kind of
kinetics. If you now react the micelles with structural
protein you find there is a great difference in the kinetics
of the peroxidation. The kinetics of the peroxidation that
you note are very similar to those in the intact membrane.
In looking at the kinds of association that you have between
the structural proteins and the lipids, you find that these
are primarily hydrophobic interactions. They are not dissociated
by high salt concentrations. They have no pH sensitivity
for dispersion. The interactions are non-ionic; they are
essentially hydrophobic, with the primary interaction occurring
between the long fatty acid chains and the proteins. We did
considerable work on this particular system. We examined,
for example, the efficiency of vitamin E versus BHT as antioxidants. This is where we picked up one of the major differences

between these two antioxidants and we support Dr. Witting's point on the distribution of vitamin E. Certainly vitamin E is distributed biologically in these membranous structures presumably through the long hydrocarbon tail that is present because you do get the hydrophobic interaction in the normal membranes. I think you not only get good protection from free radical mechanisms here, but you also get hydrophobic stability from such a long chain inserted into the membrane. If you add BHT to these systems, it is not incorporated and it doesn't inhibit. It remains in the soluble phase. What we do here is to interact the antioxidant with the complex, spin out the complex, and then look at the peroxidation of the complex. If you put fat soluble side chains on the antioxidants, they inhibit the system; you put in the long tail inhibitors, they do indeed act as antioxidants in this system whereas the BHT and BHA do not.

Recently we have gone over to a new system whereby we solubilize membranes into lipoprotein particles, get rid of the detergent, then by use of divalent cations we reaggregate this system. What you do is simply get a nice soluble membrane system out, remove the detergent, put in the divalent cation. This gives you vesicular structures which look somewhat like intact microsomal vesicles. We have been playing with this system and we played with it primarily to look at this hydrophobic-hydrophilic kind of interaction. What you find is that if you look at the lipoprotein particle, the peroxidation kinetics are very rapidly approaching almost what you get in pure lipid states. If you now add magnesium and you bring these things down as vesicles, giving you again what we call the membrane reaggrated system, you again reestablish the peroxidation kinetics of the normal membrane. This implies that in normal membranes certain sites do not see oxygen. However, if you blow this apart into a soluble system, then you increase the rate simply because you have more sites available.

We have done such things as treating all three preparations with phospholipase C. Phospholipase C acts by removing the base and phosphate. It destroys lipid peroxidation. Wallace has already shown that if you treat membranes with phospholipase C you get a red shift. People interpret this red shift as an increased hydrophobicity. What it looks like is that phospholipase C cleaves the charge groups off. You then have a much tighter lipoprotein particle. We are interpreting this as the mechanism whereby we are inhibiting the peroxidation. What we have done is hydrophobically protected this system so that now during aerobic incubation you are not getting the peroxidation that you normally see in the non-phospholipase C treated materials.

We have also done the glutaraldehyde and DOC studies

on this system. Again it indicates that anything that you
do to reduce hydrophobicity you indeed increase peroxidation.
Anything you do to crosslink or protect this structure inhibits
lipid peroxidation.

Out of this we are generating a model of lipoprotein
units for membranes which is compatible with the Benson model
where you get the phospholipid tails deeply buried in the
globular protein structure of membranes. It's now well established that most microsomal protein is not in the beta
configuration but are globular in nature. Since you can isolate lipoprotein soluble units containing the same phospholipid to protein ratios that you have in the intact membrane,
the membranous elements are falling apart into small heterogeneous units which have altered characteristics with respect
to peroxidation. We interpret the changes in hydrophobicity
as responsible for the protection or acceleration. Bringing
this back and trying to add something in terms of the peroxidation story and tying it into Batten's disease is somewhat
difficult. One explanation is that peroxidation happens
during the time of lipid turnover. These are the times when
those fatty acids are not under the hydrophobic protection
of a membrane. It may be that during certain critical periods
of development you have high rates of turnover. Thereby,
if the lipids are not protected in other ways, they will be
undergoing peroxidation and you will be seeing products of
this peroxidation. As long as these materials are buried
in the membranes you do get a great deal of protection and
the additional vitamin E and BHT would be helpful. It would
seem to me that what these antioxidants are working on are
the fatty acids which happen to be at some point in transport
or turnover where they are not getting the protection of the
primary structure that they normally see in the membranes.
When you look at the kinds of things that can affect the localization of phospholipids there may be certain kinds of genetic
diseases which sufficiently alter primary protein structure
where you get marked changes in either the rates that the
phospholipid turns over or changes in the degree of protection
that these things have buried in membranes and so on. What
you don't look for is this peroxidation process occurring
deep in the normal membrane but look for it associated in
some way with the dynamic structure that is evolving in terms
of membrane morphology and membrane biochemistry because these
things are turning over at rather rapid rates. I think phospholipid half-time turnover is 100 hours and so your protein
turnover is somewhat less. Nevertheless, this means that these
components are turning over about every 4 days, so you are
going to have alot of mobility within the system. I think
it is during these periods of mobility that you will be getting
your peroxidative attack. If anything genetic happens to
alter the structure of the protein which allows for the deep
embedding of the long side chains of the phospholipid, then

then these are the kinds of things we have to look for to explain peroxidative mechanisms in membranes.

Without getting into a lot of data, which I can show if you want, why don't we just see how this model fits with your ideas of Batten's disease.

Dr. Menkes: I think what you are outlining is very interesting, that you have two essentially different means by which you can get these pigments in aggregated forms. One is by itself so to speak, that is through the weakening of the lipid-protein bonding by alteration of the protein structure or a mechanism that causes them to be subject to oxidation as the lipid-protein bond breaks.

Dr. Barber: Let me add one more point to this from the other side.   We have done considerable detergent work but people in San Diego have been working with chaotropic agents which destroy the proteins.   They get the same accelerating effect destroying protein structure that we see destroying hydrophobic bonding.   You get an acceleration of peroxidation.

Dr. Menkes: If this is one form, you would see the particle having included in it a considerable amount of protein; if they peroxidize with the whole globular material in it.... Another way would be by the presence of some easily peroxidizible lipid, a polyunsaturated aldehyde, some derivative of sphingosine, etc.   In itself, I don't necessarily see that it would have that much protein.   I could correlate with what Dr. Siakotos has, what is a heavy particle which has a lot of protein in it, than what is a lighter particle which is more lipid.

Dr. Barber: In other words, you would take his two pigments as being different in origin.

Dr. Menkes: Yes.

Dr. Barber: Dr. Siakotos and I got into this a little bit during the break because I do think we are going to have to come to this.   We are going to have to learn whether or not these pigments are coming from different places.   Certainly there is heterogeneity in the pigment.   As we know there is heterogeneity in even different membranes within the cell, certain membranes are high in iron, for example. One thing that we have done through this study is that we have done differential fractionation on microsomal membranes. These are heterogeneous structures.   What we have come up with is that if you just do a simple ammonium sulfate fractionation of your lipoprotein particle system, and you drop down to 10% ammonium sulfate, you get a large amount of material from the membrane solubilized material.   This is your most hydrophobic material, coming down with a very low ammonium sulfate. These particles won't peroxidize. They are the ones that aggregate in the very large particles in the presence of magnesium. As you get up to 25% to 45% ammonium sulfate, these particles peroxidize very well and they do not reaggregate as well. We are working with membranes with a whole series of particles that are very different. You can separate these particles on acrylamide gels and you have many, many different kinds of particles. Again, when we start talking about general lipid peroxidation, I think we are going to have to study it at this level if we want to talk about membranes. If you want to talk about pure lipids, etc.--yes, the literature is good and certainly the mechanisms are known. I think we work with the same mechanisms in biological systems but I think we have the added complexity of the way these things are interacting with proteins, especially hydrophobically. I would like to get some of your comments on this type of thing because I do think structural protection is probably a primary antioxidant in biological systems.

Dr. Malone: I would like to ask Dr. Menkes' comment at this point. In one group of genetic disturbances, the amino acidurias, the work of Moser and Prensky several years ago suggests that in this type of inherited defect, which results in abnormal amino acid pools in various tissues, the ultimate result is not the production of abnormal proteins but a cessation of protein synthesis. Would you care to comment, Dr. Menkes?

Dr. Menkes: Well, this is certainly the case. In many of these amino acidurias you don't have enough proteolipids formed. We were able to show this in PKU where one of the major proteolipid fractions is absent. Your talk is really very disturbing to a person like myself who looks at these things very naively. Here we are talking about the possibility that there is really something just wrong in the protein and that as a consequence protein-lipid binding is abnormally weak. Then where are you?

Dr. Barber: I agree with you but if that is the data, that's it.

Dr. Zeman: Just for the sake of the argument, could we carry that argument a little further and state that lipid-protein binding is not poor, rather that it is specifically deranged due to a faulty assemblage of the protein molecule which due to an abnormal configuration does not afford the protection against peroxidation which it does if normally formed? Then we can bring this down to a relatively simple polypeptide-gene relationship.

Dr. Barber: Yes, but that is what disturbs him. We

are talking about something that is far more complex and we're not stopping this with vitamin E....

Dr. Menkes: We don't know which protein we are talking about.

Dr. Barber: But the one characteristic of these proteins you isolate out is that they are very hydrophobic. If you look at the amino acid residues, they come up with very hydrophobic numbers--the lysines are very high and so forth. Tertiary structure on these proteins seems to indicate that the hydrophobic areas are concentrated internally on the chains so that they are perfect areas for interacting with the long side chains on phospholipids. When you look at nice curves in peroxidation in things like microsomes and mitochondria, what I think you are really measuring is the rate that this system is falling apart. I think as fast as it falls apart you're peroxidizing the lipid but I think you are measuring a rate here which measures what is falling apart because you put DOC in this system, it accelerates that; you put glutaraldehyde in the system, it stops it. These aren't antioxidants, these are just changes in structural configuration.

My remarks get to the in vitro peroxidation system which is non-enzymatic. I use the ascorbate-iron catalyzed system. Paul McCay works with an enzymatic system and it may be that he sees the enzymatic attack here at a different site. It may be that he can have different sites in this complex particle. The interactions with the long chains are such that the double bond is buried within hydrophobic carriers. It may be that in your system you can get these things peroxidized without falling apart. Again, this may be another dimension to it but at least in our system, the aerobic non-enzymatic peroxidation, it looks as if this is one of the primary reasons that you get the kinetics that you do.

Dr. McCay: I would just like to say that we have electron microscopic evidence that the microsomes do not fall apart in the system that we are working with. They stay intact.

Dr. Siakotos: I would like to go from membrane systems back to the pigment. I have two slides here. Part of our work with the liver was that we were getting these lipid globules off, as I mentioned earlier. If you will notice here, you see some black material on the edge of this lipid globule. If you blow an area of this up, you see this strange looking structure here. Now this brings us back to Dr. Sulkin who was here last time at this session. To me this looks like what we see is the beginning of a lipofuscin granule or some sort of a structure like that. Now these structures here have lysosomal enzymes--they have acid phosphatase and

some of the others--but they are in very low concentration.
I would like to throw this in--it's one thing to talk about
changes in membranes, it's another thing to talk about changes
in lipid globules or fat deposits, the lipid pool so to speak.
I was wondering if any of you would care to comment on this
type of phenomena?

Dr. Tappel: I would like to comment in a sense. I think
both peroxidations would be damaging but the one that most
people consider most damaging to the organism is peroxidation
in membranous organelles that are of great importance to that
cell. One would think of the microsomal or endoplasmic reticulum, the mitochondria, the lysosomal membrane, etc.

Dr. Barber: This essentially is a summary of the type
of thing that I envision going on with the lipoprotein particle
and aerobic incubation. We know, for example, that by treating with agents which will accelerate this type of process,
we do indeed hasten peroxidation. The kind of reaction going
on is one which involves the removal of lipids, some of the
crosslinking products interact with the element itself. I
look at the crosslinking agent simply as something which further stabilizes this given structure here to inhibit this
sort of opening up.

Dr. Zeman: I think that this discussion has arrived
at a point where we could stop in order to have a chance to
think further about it. Before we close, however, I would
like to amplify the apparent dichotomy which has now developed
between the oxidation of unstructured or non-structural lipid
contents in cells on the one hand, and the mechanism of lipid
peroxidation of lipoprotein membranes on the other hand.
We all know that there is a lot of free lipid around in normal
cells under conditions of health and disease. One of the
characteristics of the so-called aging pigment is the fact
that you always find, what has been emphasized by most electron
microscopists, little vacuoles in these polymerized fluorescent
pigments, which have been interpreted as containing soluble
lipids. The electronlucent appearence is due to the relative
solubility of those lipids. One of our more recent observations on these pigments concerned the possibility of demonstrating oxidases, peroxidases or catalases and to ask ourselves
the question whether these peroxidative enzymes exist in
the brain, perhaps bound to peroxisomes or microbodies as
suggested by Baudhuin and de Duve. For this reason we have
begun to use traditional enzyme histochemical procedures which
have been developed for the demonstration of such peroxidative
enzymes. The enzyme is usually revealed by the dimerization
of diaminobenzidine in the presence of an O_2 radical and the
dimerized diaminobenzidine becomes an insoluble compound
that has a high affinity for osmium tetroxide and therefore
can be almost selectively stained. Just using a system which

works well in the test tube and which Dr. Patel checked out very carefully, we incubated brain. The interesting feature is that we got only a reaction in the area of the lipid vacuole. Now we are by no means certain that we are dealing with peroxidase activity. Rather, it appears to me that we have revealed something which is much more mundane but perhaps more interesting in the context of our discussions here--namely that this little vacuole of relatively pure lipids is subject to peroxidation mechanism on its surface and this is generating sufficient quantities of peroxides to dimerize our indicator, namely the diaminobenzidine. Notice that there is no activity in the membrane or in the solid part of this pigment granule. Again let me point out this is an age pigment. It is only in the area of the otherwise unstained lipid vacuole.

Unfortunately we have not as yet had an opportunity to do the same reactions on a brain biopsy on a patient with Batten's disease because it is such a rare condition. Perhaps, Dr. Menkes, you do such biopsies, or Dr. Malone has a chance to do that, but I would very strongly urge that we find whether this is a suitable electron microscopic procedure to reveal peroxidation of lipids morphologically as we do biochemically with the TBA method, for example. This is what I would like to propose.

Dr. McCay: Not being a histologist or pathologist, I don't know too much about this area. I have a feeling about 5 or 6 years ago Carl Mason got involved in something along these lines, I don't remember the details of it. In terms of potential oxidation he went through a series of procedures where he found an increase of material of this type and it was related to potential rather than being there when he started.

Dr. Zeman: Does anyone know?

Dr. McCay: He was using a series of procedures where some potentially oxidizing reagents were involved, incremental pigment formation of some type there. As I remember these were lipids. As I say, I'm not a histologist and could very well be wrong.

Dr. Miquel: Do you have hydrogen peroxide in that system?

Dr. Zeman: Yes.

Dr. Miquel: Did you run controls without....

Dr. Zeman: Yes, but we did not do specific inactivation with amino triazole.

To summarize, we have arrived at a point where the real issue seems to center around the sites and location of lipid peroxidation with respect to the magnitude of damage and quantum yield if we may use this terminology. I would suggest that you keep this in the back of your mind and dream about it so that we can embark upon a discussion which would attempt to correlate possible genetic mechanisms as we understand them today with the disease producing increased rate of lipid peroxidation versus the apparent spontaneous age dependent accumulation of slightly different pigments. Inasmuch as Dr. Miquel with his flies has thrown down the gauntlet and Dr. Siakotos finds now that this is not age pigment but is ceroid and therefore carries implications of much greater biological danger and damage, we will have to resolve this apparent discrepancy or biological riddle that the aging process in flies can be more damaging than it is in human beings. With this end in mind, I thank you for your discussions and we'll meet here tomorrow at 9 a.m.

January 24, 1971:

Dr. Zeman: We will hear from Dr. Menkes who has done some elegant studies on brain cells cultured from patients with Batten's disease.

Dr. Menkes: What we did is proceed on the assumption that all this lipofuscin or ceroid is nothing but a fluorescent material and start looking at the metabolism of the brain cells in patients with Batten's disease. We felt the best approach might be, since this is a very slow disease, brain explants and watch these in terms of their metabolism, not over 30 minutes or 1 hour but over several days if possible.

We have a method by which we take explants from the brain, culture them in a serum supplemented medium. Then, after outgrowths are adequate, usually 8 to 10 days, transfer them to a chemically defined medium wherein we do the metabolic studies.

This is a picture of the usual outgrowth that we get from a rat brain. You can see that much of this is astrocytic material with their processes branching and rebranching. This type of a picture can be obtained, depending upon the age of the animal, within 2 to 8 days after its implantation.

Now, if we turn to humans for which this type of a study was designed, here is an outgrowth from a patient with Tay-Sachs disease, a 2-year-old child with Tay-Sachs disease. In contrast to the rat astrocytes, the cells are swollen. If you look very closely you can see that the lipid inclusions are present and these can be isolated and shown to contain the abnormal GM_2 ganglioside.

We can do this in a number of other diseases. To give

69

you an example, here is a patient with globoid cell leukodystrophy. You can see the multinucleated giant cells, characteristic for this condition, growing out very nicely in this
instance.

Here is a patient who has Batten's disease. You can
see the neurons on the bottom and also some on the top being
not the usual triangular shape but actually swollen. If you
look very closely you can see that it too has lipoid inclusions
in it. As yet we have not examined them for fluorescence.

In terms of metabolism the first question one asks, are
these cells really metabolizing adequately? The way we can
check this out is incubating these with C^{14} labeled mevalonic
acid. By the incorporation of mevalonic acid into cholesterol
you can see that these cells are metabolizing and taking up
mevalonic acid and converting them to stearols for at least
72 hours in a chemically defined medium. This is not in a
serum-containing medium because the moment you put serum into
this medium, they will take up serum cholesterol and will
stop utilizing mevalonic acid. This is one way of telling
that these cells are active.

The next question you ask, what do the explants do with
fatty acids? We have performed a series of experiments in
which we incubate explants with a variety of fatty acids,
mainly stearic and palmitic and try to show where the label
goes to and what the fatty acid is. Here for instance we
have a typical experiment with rats, adult and 17 days. You
can see the incorporation of $1-C^{14}$ stearic acid proceeds into
three major fractions--the first is the neutral lipid fraction,
the second is the glycolipid fraction and the third is the
phospholipid fraction. The lipids are fractionated on silica
columns.

Let me just give you the results very briefly because
we have to contrast these controls with studies we did on
Batten's disease. First of all let's use stearic acid. Stearic
acid will go to into the neutral lipids. Of the total labelled
stearate incorporated into cell lipids about 75% plus-minus
7% was in neutral lipids; in the glycolipids it was very little,
1.9% plus-minus 0.7%; and in the phospholipid fraction 23%
plus-minus 8%. There is a considerable variation here, as
any studies in tissue cultures would show. We have also
some studies showing that the incorporation into the neutral
lipid proceeds within the first few minutes after exposure
to the labelled fatty acid. Some of this is purely binding
of the free fatty acids to the membrane of the cells. In
the neutral lipid fraction the label is found in triglycerides
which contain about 41% plus-minus 10% of the label though
their concentration in brain is very low. You also have some
label in the diglycerides (8%) and a little bit in the fraction

which is monoglyceride plus cholesterol (3%). The remainder
is bound as free fatty acids to the membrane. As I said, this
binding of free fatty acids to the membrane is a very rapid
process and has been studied by a number of people and must
also occur in our experiment, even when we expose the cells
to the label and wash off the label as fast as we can which
is about 10 minutes or so, binding is complete by then.

Dr. Strehler: Is this Batten's disease?

Dr. Menkes: No, this is normals. This is a group of
rats. We don't have normal human brain. I should very briefly
elaborate on this and say that the incorporation of stearic
acid is a function of the age of rat brain. To our great
surprise, the maximum incorporation in rat brain is at 2 or
3 days of age. It reaches a minimum at about 15 days and
goes back up in adult rats. Fifteen days of age is the maximum
period of myelinization. The same picture is true for palmitic
acid. Whether this is a matter of oxidation or binding, I'm
not yet quite sure. Anyway, it's a function of age. The
palmitic acid will do essentially the same thing. If you use
lignoceric acid for these studies you will find that you will
get it more into the glycolipids.

The next problem is, what form are these fatty acids
in?

Dr. Siakotos: Dr. Menkes, what is the rate difference
between unsaturated and saturated fatty acids? Is there a
significant difference?

Dr. Menkes: I have this here. The relative counts....
If you express this in terms of counts per milligram of cell
protein you will find that linoleic acid, for instance, was
incorporated better than stearic but most of this is purely
bound to cells. You have to differentiate between a binding
and a true chemical conversion.

Dr. Siakotos: What you are saying is that the double
bond really makes no difference except the fact that you are
finding free fatty acids in lipid mixture.

Dr. Menkes: Right. It makes no difference except in
several ways. For instance, we don't see the age effect with
linoleic acid. There is no difference in the uptake by the
cell of linoleic acid with age.

As I said, there are two factors here. One is the binding,
and much of the linoleic acid is simply bound, and the second
is incorporation. We have for instance.... Well, in our linoleic
acid again the same thing occurs. It goes into triglycerides
to a similar extent except in the phospholipids there is a

71

considerable difference, more of it going into phosphatidal ethanolamine than stearic acid does. As yet we don't have the number of experiments for the linoleic as we have for the stearic and palmitic acids yet. We are playing around with the age factor which was very interesting in that there was no significant change with age of the tissue with the linoleic acid binding uptake.

Dr. Siakotos: What if you use a short chain fatty acid?

Dr. Menkes: I haven't done that.

Dr. Siakotos: Because the first step of the sole reaction is biokinase. They have a very nice optimum. Unsaturation makes a fair amount of difference.

Dr. Menkes: You would think that, say if we did a 10-minute binding study, your linoleic would be much faster but I haven't done 10-minute studies--which is the fastest we could do, expose the cells and wash off the medium because we have to be rather careful, otherwise we break down the cells. It takes about 10 minutes to get rid of the labelled medium. You would think you would get more incorporation. The trouble is that in 10 minutes the stearic acid that is going to be bound is bound already. We'd have to do much faster experiments than we can do on these things.

Dr. Siakotos: You are sure you can distinguish between the solubility phenomena and active incorporation.

Dr. Menkes: Yes. These all incorporated. As you will see some are not only incorporated but have been metabolized further. This table here shows the binding in stearic acid in 15-day-old brain, a very small amount goes to monounsaturated and di- and polyunsaturated fatty acids. This is far better now in 3-day-old brain as you will see in some of our other studies. The older, it seems to be the less active this conversion appears to be. Why this is, I don't know. Maybe we just don't have the right culture conditions for the 15-day-old brain. We would have thought that the chain elongation here would be the best because this is the time of myeliniza-tion. As it turns out, the younger they are, the better they metabolize the fatty acids.

Let's get back to the problem of what these patients show. First of all let's take something that we know the metabolic defect of. We have here a patient with Tay-Sachs disease. We know the metabolic defect so we can look at this. This is K.L. In her case when labeled stearic acid is used as precursor, 93% is in the neutral lipids of which the majority is bound, only 3% is in the triglycerides, and 0.7% in the diglycerides. In the glycolipids it's about the

same, 2.2%. Actually, interestingly enough, a considerable
amount is bound here in what looks like ceramide polyhexoside
fraction but that is another story. In the phospholipids
it is reduced by 0.4% of the radioactivity. As a whole the
total radioactivity uptake is quite poor. As you might expect
from diseased tissue, you are getting 6800 counts per milligram
protein which is about a quarter of what we usually run.
We usually run 20,000 to 30,000 counts per milligram protein.
Everything is depressed. Most of stearic acid is simply bound
to the membrane and very little is incorporated any further.
If you break down the lipids in which they are in, you find
that some of it is in phosphatidal ethanolamine, some of it
in phosphatidic acid and phosphatidyl choline. The uptake
of palmitic acid was a bit better. Again, much of this was
found in triglycerides which contained 26% of the total activity in the fraction, and in diglycerides which contained
5.3% so that this too is a bit depressed.

    Dr. Siakotos: You mean the first column in your table
is stearic acid?

    Dr. Menkes: Yes, this is stearic acid, this is palmitic
acid for K.L. with Tay-Sachs disease.

    Dr. Strehler: Do you have reason to believe that rat
brain cultures are good controls for normal human brain?

    Dr. Menkes: Of course not, but what are you going to
do?

    Dr. Malone: With respect to use of the cell cultures,
this is a model system and probably one of the best that we
have available, but one problem with working in this area
concerns changes in the quality of growing cultures. First,
as pointed out already, there is an increase in the overgrowth
of what looks like glial cells. Then with time an increased
primitiveness of the cell type appears. After a rather short
period of time one really cannot recognize specific mature
cell types. I feel uneasy about conclusions drawn in these
circumstances. How would you answer the objection that conclusions drawn from studies on cell culture really do not
reflect what is going on in the tissue?

    Dr. Menkes: I think the problem you mentioned is a real
one and this is what terminates our experiments usually.
I should have re-emphasized the incubating conditions. You
take the tissue from brain, you put it in a serum supplemented
medium for 2 to 8 days, depending upon the rate of outgrowth.
As soon as you get some astrocytic outgrowth, you remove the
original medium and do your studies on chemically defined
medium. Obviously the explant will deteriorate. Finally,

one obtains fibroblast overgrowth. We have just determined
that the best length for preincubation in the serum supplemented
medium is 8 to 10 days.

Dr. Malone: Are you using trypsin?

Dr. Menkes: No trypsinization. That ruins things unfortunately.

Dr. Strehler: Have you given radioactive glucose as
a precursor?

Dr. Menkes: We have used acetate. We are just starting
on the rats with acetate. Obviously the whole problem, going
back to Batten's disease, is the controls. I think your objection to the control, is it adequately controlled, the answer
unfortuantely is that it is not. I'm guessing what is an
age adequate control.

Dr. Rider: Dr. Menkes, if you have good rapport with
your neurosurgical department wouldn't it be possible to get
a small piece of brain, say from someone who has a brain tumor
or somebody who dies on the operating table?

Dr. Menkes: That is also not an adequate control. The
brain tissue of someone with a tumor is compressed, edematous.
I think this is a far worse control than a rat.

Dr. Strehler: Would the surrounding area be a suitable
control?

Dr. Menkes: All I can say is on our experiments on
microsomal and other subcellular fractions that we got enough
normal human data which were exactly like rat data so at least
with subcellular fraction we can get normal results from
humans that don't have anything very exciting; i.e., if you
take a severely retarded child and do this on it you can get
normal results which do correspond to the rats. This is the
only encouraging thing I have.

Dr. Zeman: Perhaps in order to proceed a little faster,
shouldn't we give Dr. Menkes time to finish the presentation
of his data and then we can have a more general discussion.

Dr. Menkes: Let me go on with a couple cases of Batten's
disease. Here we have patient A.P. who has been biopsied
and shown to have curvilinear body disease, whether we call
this Batten's disease or not is a matter of terminology.
Here we did two things. We did a stearic and a linoleic acid
incorporation. Using stearic acid, 94% of the label went
into the neutral lipids, 2.6% into glycolipids and 2.9% into
phospholipids. Now here was our very first surprise and probably

74

our first fluorescent herring. Instead of getting it into triglycerides, we only got 6.3% of label into triglycerides and, to our great surprise, 92% of the label went into the diglyceride fraction. We have not found any control that did this. This had an ultraviolet fluorescent band, this was the UV fluorescent area. This was very exciting at this point. Now let's look at the linoleic acid. Using linoleic acid, 51% of radioactivity went in the neutral lipids, 35% into the glycolipids (and I think this was an error), and 13% into phospholipids. If you looked at the incorporation within the neutral lipid fraction, 75% of the label was in triglycerides and very little was found as free fatty acids, only 3% as compared to what we usually get of about 30% to 50%. So this was very surprising. We went on to try and see in what form was the linoleic acid and what form was the stearic acid in. For this we had simultaneous controls. Here is stearic acid data, control, and patient A.P. Using stearic acid in the control, 84% of the label was in 18:0, 18:1 was 12%, 18:2 was 0.3%, 18:3 plus 20:0 was 0.5% and then a little bit more into other polyunsaturated and long chain fatty acids. Our patient K.L. had 64% in 18:0, 32% in 18:1, 1.9% in 18:2, and 0.5% in 18:3. This looks as if a little more unsaturated fatty acids were found than normal but it is not as striking as you will see with the linoleic acid.

In the linoleic acid, the control, 56% of the radioactivity was in 18:2, there was very little radioactivity in 18:0 and 18:1, 18:3 and 20:0, 9.0%; 20:4 and 20:6, 20.0% and 0.6%, respectively so you are getting a conversion of 18:2 to 20:4 which I think.... Dr. Holman, you were one of those who showed this in animal tissue.

Dr. Holman: I'm going to give most of that credit to James Mead.

Dr. Menkes: Now on A.P. here using labeled linoleic acid, again there is a small amount of 18:0 and 18:1, 64.2% of the label is still in linoleic acid; 20% in 18:3 here but only 2.5% in 20:4. There is about 1% in 22:4. This was a striking finding and goes along with what Svennerholm reported, that somehow or other, being converted to arachidonic acid (20:4). Unfortunately, we have not yet confirmed this.

This is about the point at which we are with this thing. We too may be chasing down a fluorescent herring, but I'm not sure.

Dr. Zeman: Dr. Menkes, we have some trypsinized brain cell cultures frozen away. Would you be able to do some of those studies on those cells?

Dr. Menkes: Let me say just one more thing. We also

have grown fibroblasts. These look as if they have some lipid inclusions. We are therefore doing the linoleic acid studies on them.

Dr. Siakotos: Dr. Menkes, one of the characteristics of Batten's disease is this mass destruction of neurons and what is left is really glial cells. I was wondering what attributes do you attach to these glial cells? Are they really what is responsible, loss of neurons in the presence of large population of glial cells? Is that really what is giving you the results or is it just these sick neurons that remain?

Dr. Menkes: I'll bet it's the glial cells that are active, metabolically, because we don't get neuronal proliferation at any time.

Dr. Siakotos: The other thing is that oxidized cholesterol linoleate has been identified by some authors as being the principal material that is found in atheromatous plaques in aorta. In vitro studies on oxide and cholesterol linoleate have shown identical spectra. This was published in Nature a couple of years ago.

The third thing is the presence of this high concentration of diglycerides. In my experience it is usually....

Dr. Menkes: Not high concentration. There is a difference between concentration and radioactivity. This is high uptake.

Dr. Siakotos: You can start out with triglyceride or phospholipid and end up very easily with diglycerides as an artifact. We had an animal that had 5% by weight diglyceride and when we checked our technique we could never substantiate this. It was actually always a trace except when our techniques were sloppy.

Dr. Menkes: This was from the triglyceride.

Dr. Siakotos: It usually derives from phospholipid and triglycerides.

Dr. Menkes: I should say one thing about your cholesterol esters. As some of you may have noticed, the original paper by--I think it was Gonatas (1963)--describing the juvenile lipidosis and the EM changes in Batten's disease, but he included chemical analyses and showed an increase in cholesterol esters. I always assumed that this was some myelin break down product. The child with Batten's disease on whom we performed an autopsy, also had a large amount of cholesterol esters. In this one we were certain there was no demyelina-

tion, certainly not to the extent indicated by the amount
of cholesterol esters. So in view of this we went ahead
and isolated the cholesterol esters and hydrolyzed them to
show that they were first of all cholesterol and weren't
some other peculiar sterol; and secondly showed that the
fatty acid composition was perfectly normal. Since then
I have done a patient with Kufs disease who passed away at
55. She too had cholesterol esters. So there is something
there about the cholesterol esters and the presence of lipofuscin material which I don't understand. Maybe you can
explain this to me.

     Dr. Zeman: Who, me? Well, I really cannot explain
it but it is well known that both cholesterol and cholesterol
esters do accumulate in the so-called membranous cytoplasmic
bodies of Tay-Sachs disease. Even so, there is no indication
that there is anything wrong with the cholesterol metabolism.
More importantly, however, is probably the fact that autofluorescent lipopigment bodies do indeed develop in the
liver and to a lesser extent in the brain in sphingomyelinase
deficiency and also in those forms of Niemann-Pick disease
in which sphingomyelinase is normal. Sphingomyelin nevertheless does accumulate together with cholesterol in the liver
of patients with the so-called Nova Scotia variant and also
of the Type II of Crocker and Farber. I am sure that Dr.
Malone is much more knowledgable about those diseases than
we are, but it is indeed fascinating to see that whenever
you do have autofluorescent lipopigments in large quantities
in parenchymatous systems, you do find increase in cholesterol
and cholesterol esters. Dr. Siakotos and Dr. Rouser have,
in addition to cholesterol demonstrated significant increases
in lysobisphosphatidic acid. It seems that there is a whole
spectrum of abnormal lipid profiles, even in those conditions
in which you can demonstrate a relatively simple and well-
defined lysosomal enzyme defect. The question which we really
have to address ourselves to in view of your findings, is
whether are these canonically conjugated changes in the lipid
profiles which are again "fluorescent herrings" which may
be UV absorbent or not, or are we dealing here with a simple
chance situation whereby the basic metabolic error produces
a diversity of epiphenomena. I think there is much to be
said for both. For example in subacute sclerosing panencephalitis,
a disease which now almost everybody believes is due to
a chronic, persistent measles virus infection, all sorts
of abnormalities in the profiles of sphingolipids have been
described. At the time when the virus was not foremost in
the minds of the people, these findings were accorded considerable significance with respect to the pathogenesis.
Very much the same is true with normal brain tissue of patients
with multiple sclerosis where also significant changes,
usually in the form of an increase in cholesterol and cholesterol esters, have been demonstrated. While I do believe

do believe that we are obligated to follow up those leads, it would appear a priori that the major question which has to be answered is really the relevance of these findings with respect to the etiology and pathogenesis.

Dr. Malone: I am in complete agreement with Dr. Zeman's comments. I would like to add a comment. We have been a bit too uncritical in thinking about these things. I know that at least I have the habit of thinking in terms of a primary disturbance which affects some moiety first. Then, this change sets in motion a disruptive breakdown of tissue or, more properly, membrane elements, followed by a series of secondary changes. It is very difficult to separate the wheat from the chaff, from the host of secondary changes-- you have mentioned the increase of lysophosphatides, the presence of esterified steroids (which are not normally present at all)--to pick out the basic derangement. For example, Amaducci has pointed out recently a marked increase in an enzyme system acyltransferase and suggested that this material in the periphery of MS plaques may have a role in the increase of esterified material. One tends to assume that these are all secondary changes and that they are part of the machinery for taking the tissue apart. Maybe we have been a little bit too comfortable with that assumption.

Dr. Menkes: We both agreed last night we should talk about these artifacts, the glycolipid...Bartsch's paper....

Dr. Malone: Oh, yes.

Dr. Menkes: Which certainly I can confirm, that there is an accumulation of glycolipids in Batten's disease.

Dr. Zeman: But it is relative.

Dr. Menkes: Yes, it is relative but it is certainly abnormal and again I've made the comfortable assumption, like you say, that this was a secondary change to some sort of neuronal disease, not anything primary.

Dr. Zeman: I should say that the case to which reference is being made by Bartsch has been originally diagnosed as a "myoclonic variant of cerebral lipidosis." The brain was kept for several years in a freezer under completely uncontrolled conditions. The brain was subjected to lipid fractionation studies. It was documented with techniques beyond reproach that there was an increase in practically all ganglioside fractions but particularly the two minor and one major mono-sialogangliosides and also the disialogangliosides and a relative loss of trisialogangliosides. Now this is something which I have also observed in Batten's disease and almost every case in which we did lipid analyses showed similar minor alterations. I have, however, not made the assumption that these are primary changes but they do correlate reasonably well with the observation that trisialogangliosides are predominating in the peripheral areas of nerve cells; i.e., dendrites and synaptosomes, whereas the disialogangliosides are enriched in the perikaryon. This has been clearly shown by McKhann. Indeed, one of the major features of Batten's disease is the enormous peripheral cytoplasmic loss of nerve cells. I think I have shown this before but I will show it again. It is a staggering thing when you look at the Purkinje cells of these patients and compare them with suitable controls. Here are Purkinje cells from the cerebellar cortex. This is a normal Purkinje cell. We use a relatively simple technique for demonstration of NADH diaphorase which is sort of a mitochondrial stain and does show the enormously rich dendritic ramification of a normal Purkinje cell. Down here is the cell body. Now here is a Purkinje cell in Batten's disease which is loaded up with lipopigment. This is the dendritic apparatus. If you do a spine count per unit per square area on these sections and use Abercrombie's formula for the three-dimensional reconstruction, this cell has a surface area which is about 1% of the normal cell. The larger portion of trisialogangliosides is in the dendritic spines which contain also considerable amounts of GABA and the GABA is severely reduced in brains from patients with Batten's disease.

Dr. Horvat: I would like to comment on the origins of fluorescence in the light of some experience which we have in the area of this type of material. I have been involved for the last year in using micro Raman spectroscopy; developing a technique where we can estimate quantitatively the number of cis and trans double bonds, first in fatty acids, secondly in terpenes and then other types of compounds. It turns out that the Raman bands due to the stretch of the carbon hydrogen on the trans and the cis carbon-carbon double bond in a molecule is about 50 wave numbers apart. Now these bands are not completely separated by the best spectrometers we have available today, so you have to use an estimate to obtain the peak areas either with a planimeter or you can go to an elaborate computer program. In attempting to get pure materials, one of our big problems in analyzing 200 microgram samples for a Raman spectrum is the presence of fluorescent materials. In this technique you have to use a powerful laser beam system to get the beam through this small tube that has grafted on one end a tiny, tiny lens. Any prior oxidation produces a tremendous fluorescence which obscures the absorption from these carbon hydrogen stretches. We then went to elaborate means to obtain linolenic acid in a form that did not fluoresce excessively. I would like to point out that I have a feeling that some of these things might be artifacts.

Dr. Menkes: I am sure they are.

79

Dr. Horvat: To prepare methyl linolenate from linseed oil we worked in high vacuum systems starting out with as fresh linseed oil as could be obtained. The oil was kept under nitrogen until work up but we still sometimes didn't succeed. I would just like to caution you on that. We found tremendous problems in this area.

Dr. Siakotos: Some time ago the average neurochemist took great delight in analyzing specimens that had been stored in formalin for 20 or 30 years.

Dr. Zeman: They still do today.

Dr. Siakotos: One of the strange things that we have found, we have 5 freezers at -76°C and 3 at -20°C, the conventional type of freezers that most chemists still use. I had a brain specimen that I brought from Baltimore which was always kept at -20° or in dry ice and when I ground this organ up some 3 or 4 years later, I found there was a major change in the physical properties of the lipids. I'm not saying that they all reverted to other compounds but the changes that one can obtain at -20° through enzyme action-- it appears that some of the hydrolases don't stop at -20° but they sure do at -76° and below. I would caution the interpretation of results unless you can show that no changes have occurred in specimens that have been stored for a long time at -20°, I would take these results with a grain of salt.

Dr. Malone: To simply confirm Dr. Siakotos' comments, we have begun storing white cells that we are interested in studying in liquid nitrogen. We found that storage, as you have mentioned at -20° or -30° C permits one to discover a whole series of marvelous enzyme deficits.

Dr. Zeman: We will now call on Dr. McCay who has developed yet another model system for the production of fluorescent lipopigments and he will now tell us about it.

Dr. McCay: I would like to make a few remarks before we start with the slides. After listening to the very interesting discussions that have been going on here, it's made me feel that the work that we are doing may have more of a bearing on the problems which have been discussed than I thought. If lipid peroxidation does have something to do with the formation of these fluorescent pigments in tissues, then it would seem that there are some very good mechanisms for the way in which these pigments can form in vivo without having to have very extreme conditions in order for it to occur. I would like to say something that struck me during the course of the discussion relating to the onset of the disease which does not start until the patient reaches the age of about 31 years. Obviously, if this is a genetic disorder, and the tissues of these individuals are normal up to that age, the biosynthetic mechanisms for the various enzymes must be pretty much intact, at least until that time is reached. It would appear that somehow the problem must involve, rather than the lack of enzyme or perhaps too much of an enzyme, some control mechanism goes awry. It is this point that I would like to stress in discussing the work that we have done.

There is a possibility that the peroxide production in tissues may be a consequence of normal enzyme activity occurring in various membranes. We got into this rather circuitously because we were interested in the process of oxidative phosphorylation. Beloff-Chain, et al had been studying an electron transport system in the microsome which oxidized TPNH in order to determine if the very large free energy change involved in the oxidation of this nucleotide by molecular oxygen might result in the production of ATP but it didn't turn out that way. What they did notice was that there was a stoichiometric excess in the amount of oxygen consumed during the oxidation of this nucleotide by microsomes. Hochstein & Ernster then observed what they believed to be malondialdehyde formation during this process and they presumed that there was a concurrent oxidation of the lipids in the microsomal membrane as a result of the oxidation of the nucleotide. We picked up this finding and in the course of the last 2-1/2 years we have elucidated some of the events that occur during the oxidation of TPNH by microsomes.

I would just like to briefly tell you what the incubation system is because it is a simple one. In the experimental system we have microsomes, 0.1 M Tris-HCl buffer pH 7.4, and TPNH (0.3 mM). The reaction requires iron as a cofactor but not unless the microsomes have been thoroughly washed. Ordinarily we add it just in case at a final concentration of 1×10^{-5}M to provide maximal activity. The cell sap of liver contains a higher level of iron than this. The control system is identical except for the omission of the 0.3 mM TPNH.

Dr. Strehler: Does this system also oxidize DPNH?

Dr. McCay: No, not this particular system. Microsomes will oxidize DPNH but this is not accompanied by the kind of lipid degradation which I am going to describe.

One can add a TPNH-generating system consisting of glucose-6-phosphate and glucose-6-phosphate dehydrogenase if you want to prevent depletion of TPNH and continue the reaction over a period of time. I have prepared a slide describing events that occur without spending too much time going into detail. We can visualize this part as representing an area of the endoplasmic reticulum, which consists of about 45% phospholipids and approximately 50% protein. Among the proteins is the DPNH

oxidase enzyme system for which there is very good evidence
indicating it is part of the drug hydroxylating system and
systems which perform a number of hydroxylation-demethylation
reactions. This system will function in the absence of any
substrate for hydroxylation. In other words all that is required
is TPNH, oxygen and iron. TPNH will be oxidized to TPN with
consumption of oxygen in excess of the amount required. During
this enzymic oxidation of TPNH, unsaturated phospholipids
represented here in the diagram undergo extensive alterations
consisting of peroxidating chain-cleavage of the beta position
fatty acids, primarily arachidonic. These are constituent
phospholipids of the endoplasmic reticulum which are peroxidized.
We have actually measured the formation of the peroxide intermediates. We do know that the peroxides formed are intermediate
in this process. These are unstable under conditions of incubation. They break down and form phospholipids with carbonyl
functions on the beta position of fatty acid which we presume
are formed by cleavage of the peroxide. At the end of the
reaction we extract the system by the Folch procedure which
gives you an aqueous layer, and a non-aqueous layer in which
one finds the phospholipids. In the aqueous layer we also
find carbonyl products which we assume are the split products
from the methyl end of the fatty acid chain. We also have
evidence that these same carbonyl-containing phospholipids
undergo a further peroxidative chain cleavage in which one
of the products of the cleavage is malondialdehyde. We have
what we believe is suitable evidence for the formation of
the malondialdehyde in this system. The products of the reaction
are phospholipids containing aldehyde groups on the beta position
fatty acid. There are no lysophospholipids formed because
the ester to phosphorus ratio remains unchanged. In the course
of this reaction (which is rather fast) we can lose in ten
minutes approximately 10-15% of the total fatty acids in a
microsomal membrane, most of which is arachidonic acid and
a small amount of docosahexaenoic acid which is also a constituent in the microsomal membrane. This reaction occurs
in liver, brain and muscle in humans and rat and in all other
species that we have looked at. As these products occur we
have evidence that they undergo polymerization--they can react
apparently with each other and also with amine groups in the
manner which Al Tappel described. At the end of the reaction,
when the lipids are extracted and examined by thin layer chromatography, we always observed material that doesn't move very
far from the origin or moved in a poor fashion which we now
recognize as high molecular weight lipids. These materials
also have a maximum absorption of around 365 nm and they have
a maximum fluorescence around 470 nm. They may have some
similarity to fluorescent pigments. The lipids in the control
system incubated without TPNH are usually normal-appearing
as in unincubated microsomes. We now know there are at least
3 different oxidoreductases present in mammalian tissues which
promote this kind of reaction. I might add that there is

evidence that all three of these oxidoreductases involve free
radicals in the mechanism of their reaction. I would like
to show you a thin layer plate (I must apologize for the quality
of this plate). This plate had to be charred in order to
show what I wanted to demonstrate. These are the phospholipids
from the control system which show the usual display of phospholipids from the microsomes. These are phospholipids from
the experimental system. What is to be pointed out here....
Actually the same amount of phosphorus has been put in those
spots. This represents 40 micrograms and this 80. The thing
to be seen here is this material which is always seen in the
experimental system, streaking out from the origin. This
does contain lipid phosphorus, in fact the only spots which
are present here except for these are phosphorus-containing
materials. We believe this is the polymerized material formed
from the reaction products. We have isolated the phospholipids
containing the carbonyl functions. We have obtained about
12 of them, which, interestingly enough, represents about
as many products as would be possible to obtain if there was
a cleavage of each double bond in arachidonic, docosahexaenoic
and linoleic acids because of the double bond position. The
other point I wanted to make is the.... This is the same
thin layer plate that you saw before but it has been sprayed
with ninhydrin reacting material. Again this represents the
control system lipid and this is the experimental system lipid,
40 micrograms of lipid phosphorus, 80 micrograms. From this
we can see on a qualitative basis that phosphatidal ethanolamine has decreased considerably in the experimental system.
We also have quantitative data for this that shows that the
amount of phosphatidyl ethanolamine remaining in the microsomal
membrane at the end of the reaction is about 50% of the control.
The control level is essentially the same as in unincubated
microsomes. At this point we observed that there was a structural change in the microsomal membrane which can be followed
during the reaction by observing the turbidity change in the
system as the reaction progresses. What I have done here is
to show the disappearance of arachidonic acid from the microsomal
membrane during the enzymic reaction, in which TPNH is being
oxidized. This curve is the turbidity of the reaction system
at 520 nm. This experiment was set up to show a relative
change in the optical density of the experimental system using
a control system as reference. The decrease in turbidity
observed (indicated by the change in optical density) was
about 50%, parallels the loss of arachidonic acid as the phospholipids undergo peroxidation. The turbidity change is indicative
of a change in the physical structure of the membrane. The
only thing I can actually say about this decrease is that
it is not due to any solubilization of the microsomes. They
do stay intact, at least according to electron microscopy.
The microsomes do appear somewhat different but the decreased
turbidity itself is not due to solubilization but rather to
some physical change in the membrane itself.

We observed that during the reaction tocopherol in the microsomal membrane is consumed. We immediately began to look for products by administering radioactive tocopherol to rats and waiting for it to be taken up into the microsomal membranes. The microsomes were then isolated and incubated in the same system that has been described. We then extracted the lipids and isolated tocopherol from the lipids. Two of the most common oxidation products (the dimer-trimer group and a tocopherol quinone) were observed. We also noted that the tocopherol in the experimental system was practically gone. Very little of it disappears from the control system as compared to unincubated microsomes. We did not recover the radioactivity in the dimer-trimer fraction nor in the alpha-tocopherol quinone fraction. All of these experiments were done using a large amount of carriers so that the materials were well protected from further oxidation from the moment of extraction on. We couldn't find the missing counts formerly associated with the tocopherol fraction until we eluted the alumina columns on which the fractionations were being done with acidic methanol. We then recovered radioactivity from the experimental system fractionation column which we then assume is the product of tocopherol conversion during this reaction. We do not know what this material is but it has some behavior that resembles tocopheronic acid or the seminal metabolite. The origin of this metabolite is not known but it is the only known metabolite of tocopherol that is excreted in the urine of human beings. So we have then during this enzymic reaction about 15-20% of total fatty acids of the phospholipids undergoing peroxidative chain cleavage and microsomal alpha-tocopherol is also largely consumed during this process.

On observing this we then wanted to know what effect the amount of tocopherol in animal diet would have on this peroxidative chain cleavage process. We placed animals on diets containing different levels of alpha-tocopherol and then measured the rate at which the peroxidative chain cleavage occurred. This is the per cent of total fatty acid consumed during the reaction (polyunsaturated fatty acids which undergo chain cleavage during this period of the reaction). This is the curve that one gets if the animals are on a diet containing 10 mg% tocopherol, this is 30 mg%, 60mg%, and 90 mg% of tocopherol in the diet. It appeared then that the rate of this reaction was governed to some extent by the level of dietary tocopherol. Furthermore, there was an initial lag period which was a function of the amount of tocopherol as well.

From this data then we assume that tocopherol was acting as a suppressor of this reaction presumably by reacting with free radicals produced by the enzyme in question, in this case TPNH oxidase. After the tocopherol in the membrane was exhausted, and we now know that the tocopherol in the membrane was exhausted in the first 23 minutes of the reaction, the attack on the membrane phospholipids accelerates.

One of the most difficult problems we had, was to really get firm evidence that free radicals were involved. We don't have conclusive evidence at the moment. We attempted to find an ESR signal during the reaction. We could not, but this is not surprising because no one has been able to find free radical signals during the functioning of the drug metabolizing system. If it is hydroxyl free radicals, presumably their half life is too short to accumulate to a concentration high enough to render a signal. The fact is that all of the reactions that I have talked about, the phospholipid cleavage, the conversion of tocopherol to a polar compound, are inhibited by a whole array of structurally unrelated free radical trapping agents. In addition, the TPNH oxidase system will promote the oxidation of sulfide which is another indication that free radicals are involved. To attempt to find out if we can show that such radicals would not only damage the microsomal membrane but possibly attack other membrane systems, we used washed erythrocytes from a donor animal. These were incubated in the TPNH oxidase system in an attempt to show a change in the fragility of the erythrocyte membrane. We got unexpected results in that the erythrocytes actually underwent hemolysis very quickly in experimental systems but not in the control. This hemolysis can be inhibited by any of these various compounds which are either free radical trapping agents or substances which readily undergo reaction with hydroxyl radicals. We assume then that the hemolysis must be caused by some kind of radical produced by the enzyme system which will not only attack the microsomal membrane but other membrane systems as well.

One other piece of information which I think may be worth mentioning, apparently I don't have that slide. If we isolate microsomes from an animal that has been fed on a high level of alpha-tocopherol such that the microsomal membrane is well protected during enzymic TPNH oxidation.... In other words, if you were measuring chain cleavage of polyunsaturated fatty acids, it doesn't occur at a significant rate until all the tocopherol has been destroyed. Then we get significant chain cleavage occurring at that point. If during this lag period erythrocytes are present, they undergo hemolysis. This would indicate to us that the enzyme system is producing free radicals during the time when no attack on the microsomal membrane phospholipids was occurring. Yet, they can still attack another membrane system which is not so well protected by tocopherol (or other antioxidants).

This experiment can be done in just the reverse way. Instead of using the microsomes which have been loaded with tocopherol, one can use oridinary microsomes in which the phospholipid cleavage begins almost immediately. Using erythrocytes from animals that have been fed high levels of alpha-tocopherol, one does not observe any hemolysis. In other words, tocopherol is an agent which protects membranes from the factor produced by the activity of the enzyme.

This is essentially the phenomenon that we are working on. In talking to histochemists I have learned that they have known, apparently for a long time, that histochemical examination of brain tissue has demonstrated that these fluorescent pigments occur in brain cells in specific loci where are found very active oxidase systems such as the NADH diaphorase system, succinic dehydrogenase system, etc.... In view of the pheonomena we have been studying and the fact that one does find this association between oxidoreductase enzymes and fluoescent pigments in vivo, I wonder if they may not have some relationship to each other?

Dr. Tappel: I would like to comment on Paul's very nice studies. We ourselves have experience in a very similar area because we use a system very much like Paul's but we use an initiator of iron and ascorbate. So it is primarily lipid peroxidation of the microsomal membrane. I am somewhat concerned about the fluorescent spectra that you indicate. You indicated a UV absorbance say of 360 nm, and that's the usual color of these pigments and the excitation spectra that I have indicated. This is one that we get from the microsomal system, having similar reactions as Paul with ascorbate and iron as the initiator. Then we usually get a fluorescence with a maximum around 430 nm, or if there is a vitamin A there it will tend to displace the spectrum. Vitamin A fluoresces at 475 nm, so judging from your fluorescent spectra you might have vitamin A in some of your products. That is a possibility. If this is there, it can be totally destroyed by UV exposure in chloroform solvent.

Another thing that sometimes shows up, depending upon the extraction, are the flavoproteins. These fluoresce at about 530nm but the fluorescent lipid peroxidation damage product usually is in the 430 nm region.

Another observation which we have which is very similar to yours is that as a function of oxidation measured by three parameters, oxygen absorption, beta-hydroxy butyric acid and fluorescence. The variations that it shows with the mitochondria are similar to the microsomes; i.e., from tocopherol-deficient animals as compared to say an animal getting the optimum amount of vitamin E, the relationship holds as you indicated.

Further, if you look at some enzymes like the TPNH cytochrome C reductase of the microsomal electron transport system, this decreases as a function of the peroxidation; i.e., the free radicals are damaging the enzymes as you might suspect.

I would like to congratulate you on your very nice studies.

Dr. Zeman: Dr. McCay, I would like to ask just one more question. If I understood your microsomal system correctly, your conclusions are that the lack of tocopherol is due to its consumption during peroxidation. If you introduce additional alpha-tocopherol into your system, can you then suppress the peroxidative cleavage and subsequent peroxidative polymerization?

Dr. McCay: Yes, Dr. Zeman. One of the slides was to demonstrate that. The slide that showed the effect of diet which protected the rate of cleavage in this way. The higher the level of alpha-tocopherol, the more the level of the alpha-tocopherol in the microsomes increases--it is a function of dietary level of alpha-tocopherol. The rate of cleavage is not only less, but also the lag period to the time when the cleavage actually begins is a function of the alpha-tocopherol content of the membrane.

Dr. Zeman: Of the concentration. In other words, you would then make a very, very strong point that one thing we have definitely to look for in Batten's disease is the alpha-tocopherol concentration in membranous subcellular particles such as mitochondria, ER, etc.

Dr. McCay: I would personally be very interested to know what the situation is. Further than that, I think another implication of this is the fact that there may be in Batten's disease a loss of control of some of these oxidase enzymes inasmuch as I believe there are changes in the ionic composition of these cells. Is that right? This may affect the control mechanisms regulating the activities of some of these oxido-reductase enzymes. Presumably a system like this ordinarily would not be functioning unless there was a requirement for some of the material to be hydroxylated or demethylated. It may be possible that it would function in the absence of an appropriate substrate with the result that it could attack it's own membrane system.

Dr. Zeman: Thank you.

Dr. Ingold: You've completely convinced me from every-thing that you have said that this is a free radical process. One simple test that could be used is electron spin resonance spectroscopy. I noticed you use diphenylamine as one of the inhibitors. I assume that you didn't look at the electron spin resonance spectrum while diphenylamine was there. When one has peroxy radicals formed in the presence of diphenylamine, then it is easy to pick up the spectrum of diphenyl nitroxide. It is a very nice, simple test for peroxy radicals.

Dr. McCay: Thank you. We will try that. We unfortunately don't have an ESR spectrometer. We use Bill Landgraf's instrument at Palo Alto and perhaps we will have an opportunity to use it again sometime.

Dr. Strehler: What do you visualize the next mechanism of oxygen attack to be in this case? Is a peroxide formed and then Fenton's reagent yielded an OH radical? In this case I don't see why you get two carbonyl groups at the point of cleavage.

Dr. McCay: We don't know whether or not two carbonyl groups are formed for each cleavage. We do get carbonyls in both the phospholipid product and in the water soluble products that form that we also isolate. In regard to the kind of radical, I would like to say that we considered the superoxide anion as a possibility in this system since it is known to be involved in several enzymatic reactions. Work of McCord and Fridovich and others have shown this and they have also shown that erythocuprein is a good inhibitor of superoxide anion dismutase and will inhibit reactions involving superoxide anion. At pH 7 sometimes it is written this way....

Dr. Ingold: The PK is about 4.

Dr. McCay: We obtained some purified erythrocuprein from Donald Hultquist at the University of Michigan to test in this system to see if it would inhibit it. It did not. So we presume then that if oxygen radicals are involved, and we believe they are, they must be the hydroxyl radicals. This appears to be reasonable knowing that this is a hydroxylating system that we are working with.

Dr. Ingold: The hydroxyl radical presumably is involved just in the initiating step, it being formed in the iron hydrogen peroxide reaction. Subsequently you get the standard autooxidation chain with alkylperoxy radicals as chain carriers.

Dr. McCay: Right. This would probably account for the strange stoichiometry of the system because for every mole of TPNH that is oxidized, we have an average of one polyunsaturated fatty acid disappearing and 4 moles of O_2 consumed. It's a little bit difficult to make clear but there is an average of 4 double bonds per mole of unsaturated fatty acid in this system. That is the way it works out. We presume that what this stoichiometry tells us is that for every mole of TPNH that is oxidized, one mole of polyunsaturated fatty acid is on an average attacked four times by O_2. Presumably this is a short term chain reaction that terminates itself.

Dr. Zeman: Would you need 1 or 2 moles of acceptor for your TPNH oxidation....

Dr. McCay: It depends on what the mechanism of the reaction is. We don't really know what the product of TPNH oxidation is in this reaction.

Dr. Zeman: I mean where do the hydrogens go? What are the substrates for those?

Dr. McCay: Presumably something like this.

Dr. Zeman: I see.

Dr. Menkes: Dr. McCay, you have touched on something which is only slightly related to Batten's disease and that is the mechanism of brain damage in Wilson's disease which is mainly localized in areas where you have a high oxidative-reductive enzyme content. You can see why the accumulation of cupric ion could interfere with this enzyme reaction.

Dr. McCay: Yes.

Dr. Harman: Isn't the level of this particular enzyme system quite low under normal circumstances? I understand that phenobarbital and a number of other agents will increase it.

Dr. McCay: Yes, that's right. The enzyme system is present normally. It is very active in liver. It's moderately active in muscle, and it's less active in brain. It can be induced to extremely active levels in liver by various drugs which can serve as substrates. It is always present in normal animals.

Dr. Harman: Do you know whether or not the activity of this enzyme system is increased or decreased in age? Also, are there any species differences in the level of activity and of the effect of age?

Dr. McCay: We haven't studied the activity of the system with respect to age.

Dr. Barber: Paul, we have looked at the TPNH cytochrome C reductase in aged rats. There are slight reductions in both liver and kidney. There is no change in the heart.

Dr. Harman: How about the rate of induction or ease of induction as opposed to age?

Dr. McCay: Part of this slide is not visible or easily visible to you but this does show the activity in various tissues in various animals. It is surprising that they are rather similar in rat, rabbit, chick, human, toad and the catfish.

Dr. Menkes: Did you look at the various parts of the brain?

Dr. McCay: No, only the total brain microsomal fraction.

Dr. Zeman: We conclude now the formal presentations relative to model systems and observations on peroxidative mechanisms. Unless someone else wants to add to the discussion. We will elaborate on some of the implications of this rather fascinating basic research as it might apply to further studies on Batten's disease. First of all I will call on Dr. Witting to present some of his observations.

Dr. Witting: This is probably a description of something that we are all working on one aspect or another of, the lipid peroxidation scheme. As you can see here (this slide is about 5 or 6 years old with the selenoamino acid still showing), formation of lipopigment is indicated. When we started working on this, we believed the people who said that the pigment was an intractable material and quite difficult to work on, and therefore initially concentrated on some of the rate limiting reactions and the dependence on polyunsaturated fatty acids. Of late we have switched over to some of the systems where the free radical generation is of importance.

I will run through a couple of old slides to show you what the basis was for these experiments. We were very simple-minded in some of our approaches and thought that the simplest comparison was between a beaker of fat and a rat to see how they compare.

This is one of the old experiments showing that as you increase in the unsaturation of the fat that you put into the rat, you have a pathological condition developing faster. This is the onset of creatinuria in the rat as a sign of nutri-tional muscular dystrophy. This is produced by both essential and non-essential polyunsaturated fatty acids.

I put in some of these slides on the slow models because I want to show you the differences between what happens in the test tube and what happens in the living animal over a period of time. Studying the muscle lipids you can put in all kinds of polyunsaturated fatty acids into the rat with dystrophy. Brain is peculiar in the situation we studied, that is encephalomalacia in the chick. There only the essential fatty acids are productive while the non-essential polyunsat-urated fatty acids are inhibitory. As the dietary level of linoleate was increased and as the amount of ω:6 polyenes in the brain mitochondria increased, the incidence of enceph-alomalacia increased. In reference to Dr. Zeman's previous slides, the Purkinje cells just about disappear in this con-dition.

90

If you do these experiments over a period of time and analyze tissue phospholipid fatty acids, there is not a generalized disappearance of polyunsaturated fatty acids. Basically, most of the polyunsaturated fatty acids disappear but characteristically there is an increase in arachidonic acid.

Dr. Menkes: As you increase the dietary linoleic acid?

Dr. Witting: No. This slide illustrates data obtained during the course of the development of nutritional muscular dystrophy in rats fed a single fat.

Dr. Menkes: This is with added dietary linoleic acid?

Dr. Witting: In this case both linoleic and linolenic acids were present. There are reasons for throwing in both. If you put in linolenic, you increase the level of the nonessential polyunsaturated fatty acids. If these are at a high enough level then you can follow their decrease, simultaneously one reduces the amount of arachidonic and it's easier to follow the increase.

Dr. Strehler: Is this with vitamin E and selenium deficiency or...?

Dr. Witting: Just an E deficiency.

Dr. Menkes: So this is also with E deficiency.

Dr. Witting: Well to get the nutritional muscular dystrophy in the rat you need an E deficiency.

Dr. Menkes: In addition to loading up with 18:3 and 18:2.

Dr. Witting: Yes. This changes the rate. As you increase the polys in the diet this occurs faster and faster.

Dr. Zeman: You made a more general point though. You made the point that a variety of diseases can be manipulated....

Dr. Witting: ....related to polyunsaturated fatty acids. The brain, at least in the chick, where you have the experimental model of encephalomalacia, is dependent only upon the essential polyunsaturated fatty acid.

I have here a few slides to show what you find in a chick with encephalomalacia. The major phospholipids don't change in concentration. You find a decrease, of course, in hexaenoic and an increase in arachidonic acid. The peculiar thing is that the decrease in docosahexaenoate is almost entirely limited to phosphatidal ethanolamine and the increase in arachidonic

91

increasing the level of tocopherol in the diet. Dr. Ingold might have some comments. If you work in a beaker and study the antioxidant activity of alpha-tocopherol, that is simply a beaker of ethyl linoleate with alpha-tocopherol in it, each alpha-tocopherol that is destroyed should be the termination of one free radical initiation. The upper curve will show you in how many cycles the chain reaction proceeded. In other words, for one termination from one free radical initiation, about 50 molecules of linoleate were oxidized. If this were arachidonic, it would be about 4 times that, say about 200 molecules per single free radical initiation for one tocopherol destroyed. For some peculiar reason, for which I haven't been able to get a reasonable explanation, the efficiency of tocopherol as an antioxidant increased with dilution. This results in a parabolic type curve relating peroxide formation to tocopherol destruction which has a minimum ratio of about 1,000:1. The thing that has fascinated me is, if you go through the literature and look at tissue tocopherol levels where the tocopherol levels are stated in terms of tocopherol per gram fat, not per tissue, most of your normal tissue tocopherol levels in adequately supplemented animals are in this range. Obviously, because of the coordinates here, powers of 10, you have some leeway but the body of its own accord seems to have arrived at something of an optimum situation. If we try to increase tocopherol rather than go to another antioxidant with synergistic activity, we are moving away from an optimum situation. Hopefully, our problem with something like Batten's disease may be in an area associated with problems of transport, storage or absorption and might be alleviated by simply flooding in more tocopherol and increasing tissue levels.

Dr. Zeman: Thank you. Dr. Ingold, would you have any comments?

Dr. Ingold: I don't think I have any important comments. Optimum concentrations of inhibitors are observed not infrequently and there could be various explanations in a system that is not too well defined. I suspect that one is dealing with varying extents of transfer with the phenoxy free radical that is formed from the tocopherol. The efficiency of the tocopherol also depends, of course, on the concentration of hydroperoxide that is present in the system. The reason for this is that the inhibition step in which tocopherol donates hydrogen to a peroxy radical is reversible. In other words, I'm not surprised at peculiar inhibition results when it comes to a rather ill-defined type of system.

Dr. Witting: Actually if you look at the curves which led to the one I showed on the slide, you destroy tocopherol initially, then you get to a point where the peroxide has accumulated to some fixed ratio to the residual tocopherol

level and at this point the reaction accelerates. If one
measures tocopherol destruction per lipid peroxidation, this
value drops to extremely low levels. The reaction proceeds
as if it were ignoring tocopherol.

Dr. Ingold: Tocopherol is a phenol and it wouldn't
matter if you put in any other unhindered phenol. You'd
find exactly the same results. All that is happening is that
at low hydroperoxide levels the peroxy radicals attack the
phenol to give a phenoxy radical and a hydroperoxide. The
phenoxy radical then will trap another peroxy radical. However,
as the reaction proceeds, or as the initial concentration
of hydroperoxide goes up, if you start with partially peroxidized
material, the inhibiting process becomes less efficient because
with an unhindered phenol it is in fact a reversible reaction.
So, although the phenoxy radical may be formed, it immediately
attacks a hydroperoxide molecule to reform the phenol and
to start the chain off again. Thus, it ceases to be an inhibitor. The efficiency of unhindered phenolic antioxidants
falls off with increasing concentration of hydroperoxide.

Dr. Zeman: Dr. Horvat will now make his remarks.

Dr. Horvat: First I would like to thank Dr. Rider and
Dr. Zeman for enabling me to be here. As I mentioned earlier,
I couldn't really see what I could contribute to this symposium.
I phoned several physicians and was able to get only a very
vague definition of Batten's disease. I knew it had something
to do with brain damage and I assumed it must involve lipids
or their deterioration or accumulation--but here I am, a simple-
minded organic chemist. I certainly would like to complement
the biochemists and physiologists who have presented so much
elaborate and basic work on what I consider to be an extremely
difficult problem.

I have only a couple of thoughts which I will throw
out for whatever they are worth. I have a feeling that this
ceroid pigment, although it may be a very high molecular weight
compound and extremely complex, actually may have a fairly
simple fluorochrome. I have a feeling that a good synthetic
organic chemist who has abilities in separating out compounds
could probably start with some type of peptide containing
lysine and work with some of the dicarbonyls found by Ed Day
at Oregon State from lipid oxidations. I think it (the dicarbonyl research) is about an 8-or 9-year-old paper. I feel
that a competent man who has a familiarity with the modern
isolation techniques might be able to get these fluorescent
compounds out as a homogeneous species, then measure the absorption and fluorescence. I think this might provide some
type of an insight into this, realizing that what Dr. Siakotos
is isolating is obviously much more complicated. Also, I
have a second feeling from the very elegant piece of work

that Dr. McCay presented that some of the products or gross
products from enzymatic lipid oxidations, the aldehydes, are
apparently the same as those produced from autoxidation of
lipids although they're attached to complex lipids. This
has been established by someone using soy bean peroxidase.
You get only one of the two possible hydroperoxides (I forget
whether it was the 9 or 13). This might account for an enzymatic
decomposition to produce these aldehydes. I think you people
are doing a tremendous job when you, the organic and mechanistic
chemists, really don't understand how linoleate hydroperoxide
breaks down. We have some gross observations. Further evidence
for the similarity of these two oxidations is: if you take
a soy bean, bring it up and within about 30 seconds take a
vapor sample and analyze it with a GLC flame ionization detector,
you will get about the same profile as you get from methyl
linoleate or the triglyceride of linoleate. The same type
of compounds are produced in both cases. I definitely feel
that you are on the right track there.

Dr. Zeman: Thank you.

Dr. Rider: I would like to ask a question. Do you
think that, for example, the ceroid itself which is obviously
very complex, could that be analyzed? If it were, would that
give you some clues as to what it came from, what it's precursors
were?

Dr. Horvat: That's usually the way it works. It may
turn out to be--this has been proposed, that these amino groups
are reacting with dicarbonyls. If you knew more about a simple
type compound and could get enough measurement on it so you
could really say this unit is in here, then you could, as
Dr. Siakotos hopes to do, have this analyzed by many experts
in different physical types of analyses. This information
would enable you to predict or make some rational assumptions
on its origin.

Dr. Rider: You mean how it got there?

Dr. Horvat: Yes. Whether or not you could control
it, I don't know.

Dr. Tappel: I would like to comment, Ralph, on the
structure of these fluorochrome derivatives. I have some
slides to try to illustrate part of the problem.

Firstly, there is a family of fluorescent products that
can derive. They derive mainly from alpha-keto carbonyls
and malonaldehyde. All of these products of lipid peroxidation
that come from the cleavage of the polyunsaturated chain.
The fluorescent entity is this structure RN=C-C=C-NR. In
other words, it is a Schiff-base in conjugation, whether the

conjugation involves another nitrogen, just a carbon or a carbonyl type group. This is the family of reactions that can take place. There are two approaches. One would be the analytic approach but since the R groups could be different on both ends, you have a high number of possibilities. The analytical approach of separation seems quite difficult. The synthetic approach is much easier and we are preparing a number of derivatives using different amines and different carbonyls....

Dr. Zeman: Just one second, Al. Are you saying that these five carbonyls you have here absorb and emit all at the same or pretty much the same wave lengths?

Dr. Tappel: That's correct.

Dr. Zeman: In other words, we cannot distinguish between them by fluorescent spectrophotometric measurements.

Dr. Tappel: No, because from a natural source you get mixtures of many of these. Then the spectra combine. Now we are very fortunate that there is no interference with the fluorescent spectra so that a simple extraction allows you to get at a measurement, even though you may have 10,000 times more other stuff. It's a very unique method in that respect. If one could interpret the fine structure of the fluorescent spectra, which usually doesn't show up very well in most measurements, then one might get at more specifics. Here, for example, is a reaction of a blocked lysine, so it's the reaction of the epsilon amino group of lysine with these various carbonyls, the ones that are likely to derive from peroxidation products. You see that most of the fluorescent maxima are in this region of 463 to 466 nm with excitation spectra 300 to 340 nm.

Dr. Zeman: Thank you.

Dr. Horvat: I think I should comment that Al Tappel is well on his way in synthesizing these type compounds.

Dr. McCay: I would like to ask Dr. Horvat, Dr. Tappel or anyone else who may have the answer, is there an agreed mechanism by which it is thought that malondialdehyde is produced from break down of polyunsaturated fatty acids? The last discussion that I heard about this by organic chemists ended in a complete disagreement.

Dr. Horvat: I think I will disqualify myself. I have rather strong feelings.

Dr. McCay: I would like to know what your feelings are, if you don't mind.

Dr. Horvat: I think the evidence for it is rather shaky.
There were two papers several years ago, I think one was in
Nature, where a 2,4-dinitrophenyl hydrazone derivative was
isolated and run on filter paper. It had roughly the same
retention time as the 2,4-dinitrophenyl hydrazone of malondialdehyde. I believe that is the sole evidence for the production or the actual isolation of malondialdehyde. Other
people may have more knowledge about this than I. I don't
know how specific that color test is, that is something that
has always bothered me.

Dr. McCay: May I show you some evidence which may change
your mind? We isolated the thiobarbituric acid pigment formed
in the enzyme reaction system. We also prepared the authentic
malondialdehyde thiobarbituric acid derivative and chromato-
graphed them on Sephadex columns at two different pH's. The
elution curves are identical. The elution curve at pH 7.2
is here and at pH 2.8 it is here. The pigment that we isolate
from the enzyme system is identical to that of the malondialdehyde derivative. This being a Sephadex column, we presume
that these have the same molecular weight, they are very close.
It would either have to be malondialdehyde or something very
close to the same molecular weight to have this kind of behavior.

Dr. Horvat: I guess I'm becoming a believer, enzymatically.

Dr. Ingold: Do you want to say anything on this, Al
or not? I was rather intrigued by this malondialdehyde and
went to the literature to see if I could find out how it was
formed and decided that the literature mechanisms were nonsense.
They just didn't make sense. If you want a suggested mechanism,
it is written down here.

Dr. Zeman: What we have here is an observation of Dr.
McCay's which seems to conclusively identify the carbonyl
in the fluorescent pigments produced by his system as malondialdehyde, a conclusion which was reached by Dr. Tappel on
different evidence. What we are missing here is a good organic
chemical explanation as to how the peroxidation of polyunsaturated fatty acids can indeed produce malondialdehyde.

Dr. Siakotos: Dr. McCay, what type of Sephadex do you
use, G-10?

Dr. McCay: Right.

Dr. Siakotos: Did the first peak come out with the elution
volume, in the front, with pH 7?

Dr. McCay: I'll have to study my material. We did
these studies some time ago and I'm not certain....

Dr. Siakotos: The reason I mention that is when you

change the pH, your material is retarded a bit and it is
known that Sephadex has a number of carboxyl groups on it.
I was wondering if this is really an ion-exchange phenomenon,
not necessarily molecular weight phenomenon.

Dr. McCay: I agree. Do you think that that would account
for a retardation of the pigment?

Dr. Siakotos: If you're using an ion-exchange site
at the other pH rather than just the pores, which is the
way it is supposed to work.

Dr. Zeman: Dr. Ingold is ready.

Dr. Ingold: The scheme is rather long, can I just go
through it?

We have a methylene interrupted diene here. One knows
that radical attack will occur on this position to give a
dienyl radical. The oxygen will add at the end of this system
to give a conjugated dienyl peroxy radical. The peroxy radical
will then attack another methylene unit and form a hydroperoxide.
We know that the hydroperoxides cleave either under the influence
of metals in their lower valency state or just for thermal
reasons and we get an alkoxy radical. Now I am not going
to say that this is the only mechanism by which the alkoxy
can react, and I think that while there is malondialdehyde
formed, it's a minor product but the mechanism for getting
to it is this one. You attack the chain at this position
and pull this hydrogen off in an intramolecular reaction to
give this species and a radical here which picks up oxygen,
becomes a hydroperoxide and itself comes back down now to
the alkoxy radical which can then cleave here at this position
and give you an aldehyde unit. Now it doesn't have to go in
this particular place. I've talked about it going this way.
Up at this end of the molecule, we have a conjugated diene
system which is a very efficient trap to which peroxy radicals
will add very rapidly. This is a fairly fast reaction at
least as fast as the attack on this initial methylene here.
A series of reactions then occur to give malonaldehyde. It
would be a minor product because there are many other reactions
that could have taken place at the various stages. One would
expect, I think, that one would be able to form other dialdehydes
as well as the malondialdehyde because one should also be
able to attack at the next position down.

Dr. Zeman: Have you figured out the yield of this reaction?

Dr. Ingold: There is no way of doing that.

Dr. Zeman: I mean theoretically.

Dr. Ingold: No.   There is no way of doing that either.
It is just going to be small.

Dr. Zeman: You say it would be a small yield. Why do
you say that?

Dr. Ingold: Because radicals can react in a variety
of ways and only a series of specific reactions can yield
malonaldehyde. For example, this particular alkoxy radical
is in fact just as likely to cleave in this position to give
you the aldehyde conjugated to this double bond system. It
will not cleave or will be very reluctant to cleave on this
side. So this is not a route that will give you malonaldehyde.
I think we went into this yesterday. You are not likely to
get cleavage on this side of the alkoxy group. Now any particular alkoxy that we form may cleave the wrong way or it may
abstract hydrogen not intramolecularly at this point but inter-
molecularly on another molecule in which case attack of peroxy
radical later on in this conjugated system would just give
you a saturated aldehyde, not a dialdehyde. So formation of
malonaldehyde depends on several reactions occurring in sequence.
As a consequence malonaldehyde is a minor product but there
is no way of saying how much of it should be formed and there
should be many other difunctional species formed. The mechanistic suggestions for its formation in the literature seem
to me quite incorrect because they rely on reactions that
just don't go in the right direction at all.

Dr. McCay: I was just going to say that we have calculated
that malondialdehyde rather consistently accounts for about
1/20 of the total oxygen consumed in the system. So whatever
happens must be fairly consistent in the process which would....

Dr. Ingold: The yield should be the same. What do you
have to say, Dr. Horvat, about that 1/20?

Dr. Horvat: I really can't comment. I haven't ever
seen it. Hexanal, pentanal, and heptanal are the major products
in auto-oxidation of linoleic esters. Also in most of these
oxidations you get quite a fair load of the decadienal coming
from the far end.

Dr. Tappel: Relative to the stoichiometry, using a system
somewhat different than Paul McCay's, in mitochondria and
microsomes we find the ratio of malondialdehyde produced on
a molar basis to be one out of a hundred peroxidations; the
fluorochrome derivative, again on a molar basis, one out of
about a thousand peroxidations. Of course, there are other
carbonyls and derivatives formed also.

Dr. Horvat: I think part of the problem on these things
is the unsaturated aldehydes and dienals, once they are formed,

don't stick around because they are subject to attack by cellular
enzymes and this is what makes it very difficult to unwind
the mechanism in this process.

Dr. Ingold: I think that this mechanism is correct
because it is consistent with the observation that one gets
malondialdehyde only from linolenic and so forth but you don't
get it with oleate or at least very little is formed from
oleate. That would be consistent with the necessity to develop
the diene structure first of all so that one could then cause
appropriate cleavage to get the dialdehyde.

Dr. Zeman: Thank you. Are there any more remarks,
discussions relative to the chemistry of peroxidation of
lipids? Then we would like to shift to a slightly different
aspect and concentrate somewhat more on Batten's disease.

What has transpired thus far, and I take the liberty
of summarizing this, is the following: there is reasonably
good evidence that the autofluorescent lipopigments have a
chemical pathogenesis which is closely related to the peroxidation of unsaturated fatty acids. This is apparently quite
a physiological mechanism as suggested by several of the presentations which have been made here. The difficulty in applying
this data to Batten's disease is the fact that in Batten's
disease we have very good evidence for a genetic factor.
What we require here now in our discussion is to develop hypotheses by which a mechanism, which can be considered to be
physiological for some biochemical reason, can be either enhanced or can attack systems which are otherwise pre-empted
from this lipid peroxidation and the ensuing damage. One
possible clue in this respect is the apparent dichotomy of
the pigments--one we call lipofuscin in which the product
of lipid peroxidation appears to indicate a genesis which
is qualitatively more related to storage fats and to fats
which may not be structural lipids in membrane systems. On
the other hand the pigments which have been isolated from
diseased tissues, particularly Batten's brains but also cirrhotic
livers, may very well turn out to be the product of lipid
peroxidation taking place in membrane systems and thus indicate
a much more severe interference with cellular function. This
assumption would explain the progressive loss of parenchymal
cells and the progressive loss of function. One obvious
situation which can be concluded from the studies of Dr.
McCay is the physiological protection of membrane systems
against auto-oxidation, and I must confess that we have perhaps
been remiss--not in our thinking but in our actions--because
no one has ever looked at tocopherol levels in isolated membrane
systems in normal individuals and in patients with Batten's
disease. This is something which is a must and should definitely
be done. I have gone so far as to spend $1200 in hiring the
services of an organic chemist to make these determinations.

The last I heard of him was that he had a jolly good time
in New Zealand on a Sabbatical. The other situation which
deserves more attention is the model system of Dr. Barber
and here we do find, at least from the point of hypothesizing,
that structural proteins may be formed in patients with Batten's
disease which do not offer the protection against peroxidation
of the hydrophobic chains that normal structural proteins
afford.

We have discussed the possibilities of collaboration.
This will be a future effort and we hope that we can definitely
implement the studies proposed.

A third area of possible one-to-one correlation between
a presumed polypeptide chain defect and the observed patho-
morphology and pathobiochemistry of Batten's disease, is the
realm of the GABA-degradating systems. We have observed a
significant decrease of GABA in all three brains affected
with Batten's disease that have been studied to this end and
with a methodology which inspires confidence in the data.
Dr. Strehler sometime ago made the promising suggestion as
to how this problem could be studied but again we have not
gotten to the point where we could do the necessary experiments.
It is, of course, axiomatic in medicine, and this may very
well be wrong, that the expression of genetic mutation is
reflected in protein transcription.

I will first call on Dr. Strehler and ask him to give
us some remarks and ideas as to how mechanism other than
transcription lead to genetic defects and what possibilities
would exist to explain the well documented phenomenon that
in the Batten syndrome a few rather repetitive patterns crystallize, namely clinically different forms--to some extent
also different as to the ultrastructure of the pigments.
We know a very rapidly progressive disease which usually begins
with generalized convulsions and leads to death or a complete
loss of cerebrocortical functions within a few years. A much
more protracted form begins with visual failure and has the
patient linger on in a state of slowly progressive dementia
and slowly increasing incapacitation in the motor-sensory
sphere. Finally we have come to recognize a condition which
begins in advanced adulthood, around age 25 to 40 years, different with respect to the dynamics, to the clinical evolution
and symptomatology from the former two. Yet, all these conditions are associated with the basic features of the Batten
syndrome, namely the consecutive accumulation of autofluorescent,
insoluble lipopigments and a progressive loss of parenchymatous
structures, in particular nerve cells, and their protoplasmatic
processes. In a nut shell then, we have 3 diseases which
can be distinguished clinically and to some extent morphologically. The first, the Jansky-Bielschowsky type usually but
not always begins in early infancy with generalized convulsions

and progressively and rapidly leads to severe incapacitation within a few years. These patients may die anywhere between ages 3 and 12 years. The Spielmeyer-Sjögren type is clinically distinctly different and affects children between 4 and 8 years with visual disturbances. Then it slowly but steadily leads to an intellectual decline and increasing motor-sensory difficulties, with a mean duration of the illness of 11 1/2 years. Finally, the very rare Kufs type affects adults and leads to death in perhaps 7 to 20 years. The last disease, though indistinguishable from the Spielmeyer-Sjögren type of the Batten syndrome morphologically, never leads to visual disturbances. Here are several parameters--distribution of the lesion, dynamics of the disease process, and perhaps age of onset--all of which are associated with parenchymatous loss and the accumulation of autofluorescent lipopigments.

Dr. Strehler: I brought along a listing of those things I thought were particularly exciting that have been developed in these meetings over the past two years. You have mentioned the three major items. Firstly, we really don't understand some of them, such as the GABA deficiency or the fact that there are several periods of onset of the disease. From the point of view of the programming of gene expression, I believe this is extremely suggestive. Thirdly, one should list Dr. Barber's extremely interesting demonstration that unprotected lipids (lipids that are not combined with the proper protein matrix) are much more susceptible to degradation than lipid in situ.

The thing which is exciting and may be significant about the GABA deficiency touched on during the last meeting, is the fact that GABA, in addition to being a natural depressor substance for certain types of synapses--an inhibitory substance (whose absence would be expected perhaps to lead to convulsions which are one of the symptoms of this disease)--is also an intermediate in the oxidation of between 30% and 80% of the alpha-ketoglutaric acid of brain tissue. As you know, this substance is a key substance in the Krebs cycle. The reaction that occurs in brain involves a transamination between GABA (gamma-aminobuteric acid) and the above-mentioned very close relative of it, alpha-ketoglutaric acid. The products of this transamination are glutamic acid and succinic semi-aldehyde (which is further metabolized by the mitochondria). Now, when decarboxylation of this glutamic acid occurs, one derives another GABA molecule. Thus, the GABA acts essentially as a catalytic intermediate in the oxidation of alpha-ketoglutaric acid; i.e., in respiration. It is likely that the decarboxylation of glutamic acid is caused by an enzyme. Therefore, one of the possibilities suggested by these facts and inferences is that individuals who develop Batten's disease suffer from a deficiency of the glutamic decarboxylase--possibly deficiences that express themselves at different stages of the life cycle.

I would like to suggest a possible mechanism for such a variable program of gene repression.

Preoccupation with the operon concept of control of gene expression during the first part of the 1960's tended to obscure the possibility that control of gene expression may be exercised by the translation apparatus a cell possesses. One idea is that if a message contains, for example, the word "AUU" at a particular position, such a message can only be translated if the enzyme necessary for the attachment of the appropriate amino acid to a tRNA which reads the "AUU" word is present. Such enzymes, called synthetases, are present in the "pH 5 fraction" and attach free tRNA's to appropriate amino acids using the energy supplied by ATP. Fundamentally, it can be seen that the kinds of products a cell produces at any given time (i.e., the message it can translate) will be limited to those message products for which the cell possesses a total complement of tRNA activating enzymes. Very recently a number of findings have clearly documented that a cell changes the kinds of genetic code words it is able to translate as it passes through its ontogenetic program. One of my students, Michael Bick, has shown that during the aging of soybean cotyledons (which age very quickly) there is an apparent loss of synthetase, an enzyme that attaches one of the tRNA's for leucine to this amino acid (between 5 and 21 days of age). This appears to be a programmed event. Even more exciting than this are some studies by the Ilans of Temple University. They showed that at the time an insect goes through its last molt, the cells in the epidermis have lost specific tRNA's and specific synthetases involved in the synthesis of chitin. The turning off of this ability to attach leucine to a particular tRNA results in the inability of these cells to make this material, a substance required for a further molt. Nevertheless, the message is still present in these cells. Thus, if one takes the synthetases and the tRNA's from either a "juvenile hormone" treated system or from an earlier chitin-producing stage, add these to a system which is unable to manufacture chitin proteins, the extract will cause the production of exoskeletal proteins.

These findings prove that the limiting factor in this system is indeed the formation of the proper set of translator molecules (charged tRNA's)!

Before I suggest a genetic basis for the various types of Batten's disease (in terms of onset) I would like to call your attention to the fact that a kind of thallassemia exists (an anemia which is found in various parts of the Middle East and elsewhere) whose victims produce perfectly normal hemoglobin, but in reduced amounts. Many kinds of hemoglobin abnormalities result from the substitution of one genetic base for another at one position in the DNA region that codes for hemoglobin;

104

i.e., either the last, middle or first letter of a word standing
for a given amino acid is changed. This frequently results
in a code word standing for a different amino acid; i.e.,
the one present in the mutant. However, in this particular
kind of thallassemia no change is observed in the sequence
of amino acids in hemoglobin; apparently a reduced rate of
production of hemoglobin results in anemia.

It was suggested some years ago by Itano that thallassemia
may results from a mutation that involves the substitution
of one word for another word standing for the same amino acid--
perhaps a mutation to a "poorly translatable" word in the
mutant cell type. It will be recalled that on the average
there are three code words for each of the 20 amino acids.
If "AUU" stands for an amino acid, "AUC" might still symbolize
the same amino acid but the ability to translate that word
might be greatly reduced because of limitation in the complement
of synthetases present.

I would like to suggest that certain forms of Batten's
disease are produced by mechanisms analogous to those Itano
has suggested for thallassemia but that the different onset-
time diseases differ from each other with respect to the time
at which a given word becomes untranslatable by the developing
system. A corollary of this hypothesis is as follows: some
words are probably used continuously throughout life; some
are turned on at a certain time and then subsequently turned
off; some may be brought into use and remain in use throughout
the rest of life; finally some are active at the beginning
of life and then are repressed later in life. One simple
mechanism for programming different patterns of activation
and repression of gene expression is therefore the sequential
and programmed production of the correlated synthetases.

Now let us consider the cases of normal individuals,
and a Class I (infantile), Class II (childhood), Class III
(adult onset) Batten's diseases. Suppose that the gene which
codes for glutamic decarboxylase (it could, of course, be
some other enzyme structure, but we will consider this possibility for simplicity) of a normal individual has a code
word which is perfectly translatable throughout life. Thus,
the normal individual will continue to make this enzyme.
Consequently, the respiratory activities of these mitochondria
which use this portion of the pathway will remain adequate
throughout life. For the infantile onset syndrome, we suggest
that a code word exists that is only translatable during prenatal
life and that the ability to read this mutant word is turned
off at about the time of birth. Such individuals (provided
they had a mutation in the message for glutamic decarboxylase
that was untranslatable after birth) would develop the symptoms
shortly thereafter. A mutation to a different code word,
one whose translation is repressed (i.e., at the time of the

cessation of the rapid growth stage of young children and never reinstated) would cause the development of the disease at this time. A third kind of mutation could result in a code word that is only turned off as adulthood is approached. In this case, the same syndrome would develop at that stage of life.

To summarize: in the normal individual we postulate the ability to translate key messages at all times. In case I the ability to translate the message is lost at birth. In case II the ability is still present at birth, but is repressed as mid-childhood is approached. In the final instance, the ability is lost as maturity is attained.

If there is repression of the ability to oxidize alpha-ketoglutaric acid through the Krebs cycle, one might well expect an inordinate accumulation of acetyl co-A, because in the absence of OAA (derived from alpha-KG oxidation) acetyl co-A cannot be incorporated into the cycle. Such accumulation should stimulate lipid synthesis. If lipid binding proteins are not synthesized at a rate sufficiently high to accommodate all of the lipid which is being synthesized as a result of this blockage of the oxidative pathway, one might well expect these lipids to exist in an "unprotected condition" (à la Barber) and be particularly subject to auto-oxidation. Loci of such initial damage would perhaps serve as nuclei for further degenerative reactions of the same kind--perhaps involving malondialdehyde or 1,2, diketones or whatever the important intermediates in lipid auto-oxidation are. The thing that binds these sets of observations together, a very fascinating feature of these diseases is that, although they have different times of onset, the symptoms are very similar. This similarity suggests that the same enzyme becomes deficient at different times, but for subtly different reasons. The model suggested above may account for this differential time of onset and perhaps for other genetic diseases which appear at particular times in the life cycle.

Dr. Rider: Did you say there was a build up of acetyl choline in these people?

Dr. Strehler: Acetyl co-A, acetyl co-enzyme A which can be utilized either in the Krebs cycle or in lipid synthesis.

Dr. Rider: Would that contribute to the build up of acetylcholine which might account for the convulsions which they have?

Dr. Strehler: I would suspect that the deficiency in GABA could account for the convulsions.

Dr. Zeman: Because it's a dendritic depressor agent

and it will prevent cellular hyperpolarization. That is probably a more logical explanation.

Dr. Rider: Wolf, as the cells degenerate do they give off acetylcholine?

Dr. Zeman: No. We have no evidence for that.

Dr. McCay: I think this is really a fascinating approach because of other implications too. If you can have an expression of a defect in this way, it might well also cause faulty building of structural protein in membranes which could lead to an inappropriate assembly. That is why I think the kind of studies being done by Dr. Barber are so important to be carried out.

Dr. Strehler: This would be a dominant mutation that results in defective structural protein that cannot effectively protect the lipid.

1   Dr. Barber: On a somewhat related issue, two people at U.C.L.A. working on the development of the retinal outer segments in frogs found an enormous lay down of the membranous discs in the outer segments 8 to 10 days after hatching. Associated with the membrane lay down is the initiation of the first electrical signals that you pick up out of the retina. One of the things that I have been thinking about is that in retrolental fibroplasia the oxygen toxicity could impair membrane development and be the cause of blindness. We are setting up experiments now to see if this does impair this very rapid membrane lay down that you see in the newborn. If you are getting oxygen toxicity via lipid peroxidation, oxygen is destroying the lipid profiles as these membranes are being laid down so rapidly. Therefore, you may be getting membrane destruction and this results in not getting the electrical signals out at the other end. The interesting observation of blindness versus sight in the age related diseases discussed here may be caused by the same kind of thing. You may be getting an impairment here at the very early stages when there is extensive membrane lay down; i.e., when the discs are formed in the outer segment. Once these discs are formed, as in older individuals, you may be getting a very much reduced turnover with respect to maintenance of lipid in this system, so you may indeed be bypassing the problem concerning the retina. The course of this blindness may be in another area where the turnover of the lipids is much higher.

Dr. Zeman: I think these are facts and observations which by looking at them with sufficient detail may turn out to be rather spurious but which would be extremely helpful in sorting out the probabilities of various hypotheses. In this respect even the most insignificant but yet repetitive phenomenon gains considerable significance with respect to

107

the development of testable and reasonable hypotheses. Unfortunately, however, we know practically next to nothing about the internal workings of lipoproteins and complex lipids as a function of time in any part of the body. We do know that during the spurt of development you have been speaking about something very dramatic does go on, but these are relatively restricted time periods as you pointed out during which chemical turnover is very high, but over the long range and especially when we come into the adult brain, we know very little. I wonder whether Dr. Malone could enlighten us further along these lines. Of course, you are working with rats and that might yet be different.

Dr. Malone: I am not certain whether I will be able to enlighten anyone, in fact I rather suspect that I will succeed in confusing things even further. Dr. Strehler's comments were extremely welcome and I must say in a certain sense rather worrisome. I presume that this would raise the possibility that instead of the simplistic view that most of us have been clutching to our bosoms of a simple static defect expressed in various ways, the possibility arises that what we may be dealing with is a far more complicated system of programmed enzyme systems which turn on and turn off at inappropriate times in a developmental sequence.

Dr. Strehler: I was actually implying that the program of turning on and off was perfectly intact and normal but that a particular message has a code word in it which cannot be translated after the inability to read that particular word is lost.

Dr. Zeman: Which would be the expression of the mutation.

Dr. Strehler: Yes. However, the mutation would be in the structural gene, not in the control gene.

Dr. Malone: We have been interested in the developmental aspects of brain chemistry. In capsular form, this is an organ or tissue with incredible morphological and biochemical complexity. It goes through a carefully programmed series of developmental stages in the fetal, neonate and early periods. A certain amount of this work has been done and reviewed by Seiler in Lajtha's Handbook of Neurochemistry. He has detailed some of the enzyme systems that come in during development. From the morphologic standpoint we proceed from a comparatively simple tissue by elaboration of cell processes; interlinking of processes and development of associational pathways. Biochemically, I mentioned the appearance, the differential rate at which various enzyme systems come in. I used the term at one point of a "critical" period in development and this, I think, again is being overly simplistic. We really should consider multiple "critical periods" at various times. At

any rate, development can be affected by a host of factors--
on the metabolic side for example, one may speak of changes
in this programmed series of events from a nutritional basis.
Benton, Carr and their co-workers described morphologic and
chemical parameters in animals that had been fed deficient
diets and showed that the normal sigmoid curve was depressed
and delayed. Their changes were related to the nutritional
status of the animal. We have been able to do the same thing,
to delay and depress the development curve by changing the
hormonal milieu, specifically the thyroid hormone. I would
also add at this point that the study of genetic metabolic
disorders, such as Batten's disease, have importance which
is out of proportion to the clinical incidence of the disease
entities. I like to think that the amount of information
that we are going to obtain from these cases will have enormous
fallout value. Ultimately we may hope to proceed from an understanding of pathogenesis to rational therapy. One example
of this progress is the work that Steinberg and others have
carried out in Refsum's disease. In this case a metabolic
error results in accumulation of an exogenous substrate.
More commonly, endogenous products accumulate. The examples
are numerous--the sulfatidosis, cerebrosidosis and the accumulation of the glycosphingolipids in Tay-Sachs disease. In
discussing pathogenesis in these disorders, a major problem
arises. This is the fact that it is really a major step from
our description of an enzyme deficit, with the accumulation
of substrate, to an explanation of the morphological changes.
How one may relate major tissue break-down to the simple
accumulation of a normal metabolic substance is an open problem.
I think possibly a great part of the discussion that has gone
on here of exposure of lipids to a catalytic chain reaction
so to speak may be very appropriate. I am very interested
in Dr. Barber's comments on this topic. In terms of the specific
metabolic disturbances, most of the ones which have been recognized are fairly well described, turn out to be on the catabolic
side of metabolism. One possible exception might be the
reports of the sulfotransferase deficit in globoid leukodystrophy. In discussing catabolic enzyme deficits, we face
an immediate problem. First of all, the best way to recognize
the deficit of an enzyme is to find the accumulation of the
substrates that the enzyme should be acting on. This is perhaps
a little bit old fashioned, but none the less it gives one
sort of a feeling of confidence. The problem we really deal
with is that so many of our demonstrations of these deficits,
we have taken frequently a leap in logic from the statement
that I do not find evidence of enzyme activity to the statement
that the enzyme isn't there. There is a tremendous gap here.
Further, our ability to deal with these enzyme deficits clinically is limited by solubility problems related to specific
substrates and frequently artifacts result. We have difficulty
presenting the substrate to our enzyme system in a physiological
fashion. We may use detergents to disperse lipid substrates

109

in one way or another, but we really can't get around the
fact that we are not displaying them to the active sites of
the enzyme in anything remotely resembling a physiological
way. One useful recent approach on this has been work that
Dawson and Sweeley described 2 years ago in the Journal of
Lipid Research. They suggested a sort of carrier for the substrate. These authors used filter paper discs, impregnated
with lecithin and then absorbed the specific substrate they
wished to expose to the enzyme upon this disc. The enzyme
and substrate-disc were incubated in a buffer. Then by various
methods (they happened to use gas chromatography of the TMS
derivatives of released hexoses) they assayed the activity
of the system. We have been working with this technique utilizing
white blood cells both cultered and fresh. We have found
that when the assay was used with white cells from globoid
leukodystrophy, we were able to show that in the cases we
studied, the activity was either considerably less, as seems
to be true with the heterozygote, or completely absent, as
seemed to be the case in two affected children, and present
in age-matched controls. We plan to continue with this approach
to examine the enzymatic hydrolase systems for sulfatides
and gangliosides. We are interested in setting up a series
of such assay systems that would, hopefully, have the advantage
of utilizing specific substrates and avoiding the problems
of research based on enzymatic deficits revealed by artificial
substrates. Then, in chronic cases, there is the problem
of an accumulation of substrates. The statement is frequently
made that because neurochemists have not shown that a given
class of substance is changed, one can exclude that particular
molecular species from pathological merit. This is true only
within limits. If we deal with a disease process which has
been fairly rapid and in which the deficit is fairly overwhelming, as seems to be the case for example in classical sulfatide
lipidosis, the relationship between enzyme deficit and substrate
accumulation is straightforward. In other circumstances,
particularly in disorders that evolve over years, I think
we may find ourselves faced with a whole series of nonspecific
changes. We have spoken of these at various times in this
meeting and I don't think it makes much point in reviewing
these in detail right now, but these changes do serve to obscure
and confuse the primary biochemical error. In other words,
secondary changes may obscure the pathogenic mechanism.

Dr. Zeman: Thank you very much, Dr. Malone. It is
indeed proper to point out that most of the better understood
genetically controlled disorders which involve the developing
nervous system are due to deficits in enzymes concerned with
catabolic activity. We mentioned the concept of lysosomal
diseases yesterday. There are indeed those who suggest that
in Batten's disease there also might be a similar accumulation

of a substrate which very rapidly, for reasons unknown, turns
into peroxidized lipopigment which then prevents us from really
demonstrating a major accumulation of a single compound.
One of the reasons why I have become somewhat discouraged
with this explanation is that we have never seen any evidence
for this. That is to say we have never seen evidence in very
early cases of this disease of a major lipid accumulating,
but it is only fair to state that with our analytical procedures,
we cannot demonstrate every single lipid. It has been correctly
pointed out that such compounds as inositol phosphatidic acid
and similar substances just cannot be demonstrated in fresh,
let alone preserved, tissue. This possibility still exists.
However, it is not very likely, and the argument I am now
presenting is somewhat circumstantial. There is one disease
in which we know the enzyme defect, in which we know the substrate that accumulates, that is GM_1 gangliosidosis. It is
in this condition that you invariably observe the simultaneous
presence of lysosomes that contain the non-catabolizable substrate plus some other compounds such as cholesterol and phospholipids, but in addition you can find evidence that some
of these lipid-containing lysosomes are transformed into peroxidized lipopigment. Something similar has been suggested
as a mechanism for lipopigment earlier in the case which Dr.
Menkes cited this morning, the case of Gonatas (1963). Again,
evidence has been presented that there is a transition from
lipid-containing lysosomes into residual bodies with peroxidized
lipids. This case, touted as an instance of juvenile amaurotic
idiocy or what we call here Batten's disease, however, is
an entirely different disorder clinically. Nevertheless,
the case could be considered to fall into the group of conditions
which we discussed here. On the other hand, we have had the
opportunity to study the ultrastructure of lipopigments at
various stages of the evolution of the disease and have essentially found no change and no evidence for a progressive
transformation of the contents of the tertiary lysosomes.
We could never muster sufficient evidence and therefore sufficient enthusiasm to follow up on this possibility. This
doesn't mean that it is ruled out. Yet, if you go to the
dog model (in English setters) where we have serial biopsies
and chemical studies beginning at the time of birth in ascertained homozygotes, we have no evidence that there is any
disturbance in lipids that are separable by present day thin
layer chromatographic procedures coupled with column fractionation.
Again, the criticism remains that we cannot really determine
all the lipids which occur in brain tissue. I suppose Dr.
Malone's point, not only being well taken, also should caution
us against arriving at a premature conclusion with respect
to the primary chemical pathogenesis of this disease. It
is for this reason that what we need is a reasonably applicable
and easily handled model system. This is why we will make
every effort to get the dogs into our hands so that we can
study them.

Dr. Barber: I would like to reinforce one point that
Dr. Malone made and that is in respect to the disappearance
of activity versus disappearance of the material itself.
When you start working with structually bound enzymes, membrane
associated enzymes, as opposed to soluble enzymes, these fall
into very distinct classes of stability and lability.   If
you isolate a microsomal fraction and look at glucose-6-phos-
phatase, for example, very minor modifications in the lipids
will cause very drastic changes in the enzyme activity, some
of which is easily restored with added phospholipid micelles.
You run the full spectrum where TPNH cytochrome C reductase
is somewhat intermediate and phosphatidic acid phosphatase
is extremely stable and withstands a great deal of mistreat-
ment.   I think that when you start looking at the structure
of a membrane, there must be differences in localizations
within substructures, some of which differ in lipid microenviron-
ments and are therefore probably considerably more sensitive to
lipid changes than things like PAPase which is probably more
deeply embedded in the structure and has less lipid involved.
When you look for a change in activity, therefore, you are
probably not measuring a change per se of the molecules available
but a change in the microenvironment.   This could alter the
solubility of a substrate or, because of the way that the
membrane lipoprotein structure is put together, it could be
changing the lipid, in a way that results in changing the
tertiary structure of the protein involved as the active
site.   When you get the structurally bound enzymes, you are
in a different environment than when you are working with
soluble enzymes.

Dr. Malone: If I may just add one note.   One thing
I think that in many of these disorders that has never been
ruled out in any fashion, is abnormal binding of the lysosomal
enzymes.   This goes back to some of the work of Dr. Harold
Koenig.   It relates to the manner in which these lysosomal
enzymes are tied, sequestered, or whatever term you wish in
the lysosomes proper.   I had always thought of them along
the classic terms, a sort of enzyme bag that migrated over
to the digestive vacuole, blended, released the digestive
ferments, and away the system went.   Dr. Koenig has postulated
that there is a sort of matrix and that the lysosomal enzymes
are embedded therein.   One might raise the question, coming
back again to the big jump between the statement "I cannot
demonstrate activity" to the statement "the enzyme is deficient,"
to the possibility that we could be dealing with a situation
in which the enzymes were there and were perfectly competent
but were so tied or bound or involved that they could not
act upon their proper substrates.   This is pure speculation,
of course.

Dr. Zeman: I would like to point out that even some
of the structurally bound enzymes seem to pass into the cytoplasm

and can be studied there, at least in very fresh preparations. When you look for instance at N-acetylhexosaminidase, which is supposedly bound, you get activity in plasma and you can even demonstrate isoenzyme deficiences related to the various forms of GM_2 gangliosidosis. You are saying that there are other possibilities and that our store of possible hypotheses is not exhausted by what has already been proven with a considerable degree of conclusiveness.

Dr. McCay: I think it might be pertinent to mention in regard to the inability to find any storage defect that it is not impossible that the feedback control mechanisms might be sensitive enough to prevent any real accumulation of any products for which the degradative enzyme is missing, but you might not see it or it might not be enough to observe.

Dr. Zeman: That's a point well taken.

Dr. Menkes: Or that the peroxidation is so rapid that you will never see it.

Dr. Rider: I have two comments, Wolf. One is if you are going to analyze for ceroid and see what it may contain and so forth, can you not analyze the whole part of the brain too in addition to this ceroid? Technically at this time what kind of studies can be done to analyze the brain or ceroids and see what kind of enzymes and what kind of substances or chemicals are present? It is like throwing out a dragnet in a sense but still I think you should look into all the things which we are capable of looking into and see if you can find some defects, such as Dr. Menkes has found with some of these uptake studies. I think that is very fascinating.

Secondly, Dr. Strehler mentioned the GABA. Is that feasible as a therapeutic agent? I have no knowledge whether this is given to people by mouth, if it is absorbed, if it can get into the brain, or if it could have some possible therapeutic benefits. If so, does anyone have any ideas as to how much a person could take or how to obtain it? I'd be willing to look into that aspect.

Dr. Strehler: You can give glutamic acid. If GABA comes from glutamic decarboxylation....

Dr. Rider: Glutamic acid has been used, I think in the past. I know we have used it and I am sure other....

Dr. Strehler: No effect, as I recall.

Dr. Rider: This was many years ago. Almost anyone that was retarded or had any difficulty in learning was given glutamic acid. There were some glowing reports. I think some Spanish doctors reported that it was of benefit. I think over the years that most people have pretty well decided that glutamic acid really has no benefit in any of these diseases.

Dr. Menkes: Let me add this on the subject of GABA. GABA has been used as an anticonvulsant by the Japanese. Its penetration into the brain is minimal in normal brain, but seems to be quite adequate once the blood-brain barrier is disturbed. I recall very distinctly a paper on this subject in a symposium on the chemical environment on the brain that was edited by Seymour Kety. There is a paper in there discussing the dosage of GABA used in seizures.

Dr. Rider: Could you send me a reference on that?

Dr. Menkes: It's in the book edited by Seymour Kety, published by Pergamon Press, "The Chemical Environment of the Brain." It was a symposium held about 7 or 8 years ago.

Dr. Rider: Do you think that would be a reasonable approach to this?

Dr. Menkes: No, I don't think so because we do know already what happens if you have glutamic acid decarboxylase deficiency. There is a disease, called pyridoxine dependence in which Dr. Scriver has some evidence that in the kidney GABA decarboxylase is defective. It requires far more pyridoxine than normal to be active. These children do have convulsions and are retarded but do not have the picture of Batten's disease.

Dr. Strehler: Various kinds of glycogen storage diseases are expressed in different tissues and it is very likely that different genes are involved in coding for the similar enzymes in different tissues of the same amount. The deficiency of say glutamic decarboxylase in kidney might not necessarily involve glutamic decarboxylase deficiency in the brain.

Dr. Menkes: Oh, they do have seizures. They do have severe seizures so you assume that it is also in the brain.

Dr. Rider: I happened to see an article in the paper that someone brought me about some woman that said her child had convulsions, that nothing seemed to help the child. The husband said that the body should heal itself and that they should go to natural products. They started to give their child large doses of vitamin B. The convulsions disappeared. They first stopped all of his medications. I wonder if that child may not have had this disease that you are talking about. Apparently they were giving him pyridoxine, that was one of the things that they mentioned, B complex including pyridoxine. The husband said just give him natural products and that will heal any disease in the body. This child improved.

114

Dr. Strehler: If there is no deficiency of glutamic decarboxylase in the "Batten's" dogs that you will hopefully be dealing with or in any biopsy material, then one still has to explain why there is such a low amount of GABA in the biopsies that you studied.

Dr. Rider: Wolf, you have two main problems. One is that you don't see a lot of these children and it is hard to get many good specimens--if they are biopsied, maybe you'll get a tiny piece. If you wait until autopsy, the specimen may not be fresh enough and so forth. The other thing is technically what can you do and what can you analyze for. Now if you get these dogs and they have a similar condition, of course, the amount of tissue available will be in a sense unlimited.

Dr. Zeman: The studies you can do are also unlimited. We do have to make some intelligent decisions as to what should receive which priority. What we will do in addition to what has been proposed, is to look at those lipids which might accumulate on the basis of a supposed degradative enzyme defect which have to be determined not only by TLC but perhaps by chemical procedures for various phosphatides. Furthermore, we will have to look very definitely into the metabolism, be it biosynthesis or catabolism of lysobisphosphatidic acid which seems to crop up all the time in various connections. We will definitely, and Dr. Siakotos has developed the procedures for this, isolate various subcellular particulate fractions of membranes such as microsomes, nerve endings, ER, mitochondria and so forth, and have Dr. Barber look at their potential for oxidation and have Dr. Fleischer look at their electro- phoretic pattern of structural protein. In the dog model, of course, this can be done very elegantly because we can use the same strain of dogs as the control animals in the form of heterozygotes. There is no problem whatsoever. Sticking to Batten's disease, there is very, very little we can do because, as you say, the material is exceedingly limited. We get perhaps a brain per year under variable conditions. We will have to go to the various mechanisms by which vitamin E reaches the intracellular milieu and is incorporated into membranes. We know very little, next to nothing about it. As I said before, we have not yet really measured alpha-toco- pherol concentration. I also believe that the studies of Dr. Menkes are very promising. He hasn't said anything as to whether he has observed any autofluorescent pigments in his cultural cells.

Dr. Menkes: I don't know. I have to get a fluorescent microscope.

Dr. Strehler: Is there any indication that there is a higher rate of conversion of glucose to lipids in these individuals?

Dr. Zeman: That has not been determined.

Dr. Menkes: I can do that very easily.

Dr. Strehler: In the explant. I was wondering if it might be done in vivo by perfusing radioactive glucose and looking at the level of CO_2 production. If there is a high level of lipid formation and if you label positions 1, 2, 5 and 6, you will get very little radioactive CO_2 out, whereas, if there is a high efficiency of the Krebs cycle, you will get a lot of radioactive CO_2 out.

Dr. Menkes: How do you label your glucose?

Dr. Strehler: I think 1,2,5, and 6 because the 3,4 position becomes the portion that is decarboxylated.

Dr. Menkes: ....measure the CO_2 production.

Dr. Strehler: Measure the relative CO_2 production maybe, using an intracarotid and intrajugular catheter.

Dr. Menkes: What are you trying to say here? I'm not sure what....

Dr. Strehler: Let's assume that there is a deficiency of the glutamic decarboxylase and that this metabolically backs up the mitochondria so that they accumulate excess acetyl co-A. This should drive lipid synthesis followed by auto-oxidation of non-membrane bound lipids. If that were the case, then the Krebs cycle release of CO_2 would be much reduced.

Dr. Menkes: Why can't we just measure glutamic decarb-oxylase in a renal biopsy?

Dr. Strehler: Well, this, as mentioned before, is based on the unwarranted assumption that one will observe the same enzyme deficiency in various differentiated tissues.

Dr. Menkes: I see. I'm not sure it would be.

Dr. Zeman: You are referring to the analogy of liver phosphorylase versus muscle phosphorylase deficiency and things like that.

Dr. Menkes: Yes.

Dr. Strehler: So one way to find out if there is an enhanced conversion of glucose to lipids, which I think is a little more direct actually than using oridinary lipid pre-cursors such as acetate or already preformed fatty acids because the brain operates mostly I believe on glucose. This fits....

116

Dr. Zeman: You could do those experiments in your tissue culture just by using the radioactive glucose and then do your lipid separation.

Has anyone else any suggestions with respect to how we can now attack the clinical problem of Batten's disease?

Dr. Harman: I would like to make one comment and ask one question. Assuming that this is a case of lipid peroxidation, some of the things that could be under genetic control are the factors which influence the rate. For example, serum copper varies from individual to individual; if this is measured in a given individual over a period of years it will be found to be essentially constant. Serum copper levels can be modified by increasing the dietary intake of copper. I suspect that serum vitamin E levels are also fairly constant in a given individual but, like copper, can be influenced by diet. Thus, some of the clinical manifestations of infantile, juvenile and adult type Batten's disease may be the resultant of both genetic and environmental factors.

I actually have two questions. First, is there a higher degree of hypertension in Batten's disease? Secondly, has anyone looked at the small vasculature in Batten's disease?

Dr. Zeman: The answer to both questions is yes. As a matter of fact there is always hypertension in the adult form of Batten's disease. This is significant to the extent that the non-affected members of the same subject do not show hypertensive disease.

Dr. Harman: This is interesting because a case can be made on theoretical grounds that lipid peroxidation contributes to atherogenesis (that was the reason I asked that question yesterday) as well as to hypertension. Lipid peroxidation products formed in the serum and the vessel wall could stimulate fibroblasts leading to the scarring down on the small vasculature, with subsequent development of hypertension. It is possible that the rate of oxidative polymerization is enhanced in serum in individuals with Batten's disease--due to an increased serum O_2concentration, etc. Your comment yesterday that yellow pigmented material is present throughout the adipose tissue in Batten's disease suggests that oxidative polymerization of lipid is widespread. It would seem that oxidation is not only taking place in the endoplasmic reticulum in the cell but also in adipose tissues all over the organism and in the serum. If this is true, then increasing the dietary intake of antioxidants such as vitamin E or butylated hydroxytoluene (BUT) may have a beneficial effect on individuals with Batten's disease.

Dr. Zeman: Thank you very much.

Dr. Miquel: I would like to ask one question. We are studying mammalian tissue cultures from nerve cells and astrocytes in collaboration with Dr. Tobias of the Donner Radiation Laboratory. We are investigating the effects of ionizing radiation on the glycogen of astrocytes. In our studies the glycogen content of glia is a very sensitive indicator of pathological conditions in the brain. Since we are set up for this technique, it would be very easy for us to study some of Dr. Menkes' tissue cultures to determine if there is an abnormal glycogen increase. We could also observe fluorescent pigment, as we are set up to do ultraviolet microscopy. If I could get a few tissue cultures, I would be happy to do these studies in collaboration with Dr. Menkes.

Dr. Rider: Wolf, I think one of the important things in this kind of a symposium is to try and get some cross-fertilization. If someone can do some special technique that another party isn't equipped to do, it makes sense to cooperate and utilize what each person can do best. There are so many approaches to this. I think that's a very excellent idea and cooperation is really better.

Dr. Zeman: Well, time is drawing to a close and I first wish to thank Dr. Rider and the Children's Brain Diseases Foundation for having made this conference possible and to Franklin Hospital for letting us use their facilities.

Our real thanks, however, are to you for having come to this lovely part of the country from the cold of the midwest and smog of the east.

What I certainly hope will issue from this meeting is that we will keep in touch and as soon as you develop new ideas or further data, that you will make those available to us. Eventually, we hope to establish a library or some sort of an information storage system where we can deposit much of the type of information presented here.

PARTICIPANTS
FOURTH ROUND TABLE CONFERENCE ON BATTEN'S DISEASE
SAN FRANCISCO, CALIFORNIA
January 15-16, 1972

Dr. R. J. Desnick
Department of Pediatrics
University of Minnesota Medical School
Minneapolis, Minnesota

Dr. E. H. Kolodny
Department of Neurology
Harvard University
Cambridge, Massachusetts

Dr. Jaime Miquel
Experimental Pathology Branch
NASA, Ames Research Center
Moffett Field, California

Dr. P. P. Nair
Biochemical Research Division
Sinai Hospital
Baltimore, Maryland

Dr. Michel Philippart
Department of Pediatrics, Neurology & Psychiatry
University of California
Los Angeles, California

Dr. J. Alfred Rider
President
Children's Brain Diseases Foundation
San Francisco, California

Dr. A. N. Siakotos
Department of Pathology
Indiana University Medical Center
Indianapolis, Indiana

Dr. Al Tappel
Division of Food Science & Technology
University of California
Davis, California

119

Dr. J. R. Wherrett
Department of Medicine (Neurology)
University of Toronto
Toronto, Canada

Dr. L. A. Witting
L. B. Mendel Research Laboratory
Elgin State Hospital
Elgin, Illinois

Dr. Wolfgang Zeman
Department of Pathology
Indiana University Medical Center
Indianapolis, Indiana

FOURTH ROUND TABLE CONFERENCE ON BATTEN'S DISEASE

Dr. Zeman: First let me express thanks to the Children's Brain Diseases Foundation, to Dr. Rider in particular, as well as to his staff for setting up this conference and for making it possible that we meet here. The past conferences were stimulating and beneficial to our thinking and to our efforts in shaping scientific approaches towards the study of Batten's disease, and I'm sure that this conference will be no less successful.

We have come together in order to discuss general aspects of Batten's disease, a group of disorders which have as a common denominator a twofold problem, namely, the accumulation of autofluorescent lipopigments and the cumulative damage to cells, in particular neurons.[1] These diseases, as you know, have been formerly lost among the familial amaurotic idiocies and have been frequently confused with conditions in which there is an accumulation of gangliosides.[2] This is not the case in Batten's disease, and so far we have not been able to develop evidence that these conditions (and there are definitely several different genotypes) have anything to do with a primary disturbance of the breakdown of complex lipids or lipoproteins. Instead, the primary problem in the pathogenesis is an uncontrolled peroxidation of unsaturated fatty acids which, by formation of carbonyls and lipid peroxides, produce in situ fixation of biological constituents that accumulate in the form of cross-linked polymers called lipopigments. Dr. Siakotos during the past several years has developed a procedure by which he is able to isolate these pigments in pure form, and he will now bring us up to date on his findings.

Dr. Siakotos: The pigment that is found in Batten's disease is arbitrarily called ceroid, and the pigment that is associated with tissue from aged individuals is termed lipofuscin. Lipofuscin is brown and ceroid is a bright yellow. Our first goal was to resolve these pigments and make a careful distinction on the basis of whatever parameters we could use. Fortunately, you could make these distinctions on the basis of specific gravity, in that ceroid from patients with Batten's disease has a very characteristic density and is quite a bit more dense than lipofuscin (that includes lipofuscin from brain, heart, and liver). In trying to work up new sources

121

of ceroid, since the tissues from patients with Batten's disease
are quite rare, we looked at the cirrhotic liver, in which
there is a pigment, again called ceroid, that has the same
density as the pigment found in brains of patients with Batten's
disease. This was our first goal, and once it was achieved,
we had enough pigment to characterize it chemically, to distinguish it from the other pigment, and to ascertain whether
there is anything unique to which we could attribute the pathological mechanism in this disease.   The neutral lipid components
are shown in Figure 1.

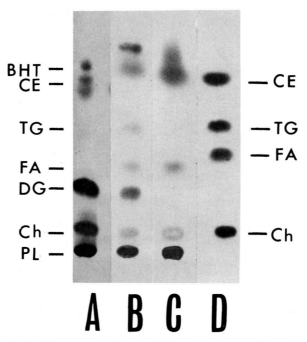

Figure 1. Neutral lipid compositions. Abbreviations: CE - cholesterol
          esters; TG - triglycerides; FA - free fatty acids; CH - chol-
          esterol; PL - Phospholipids; DG - diglycerides.
          A. Normal human brain lipofuscin.
          B. Normal human liver lipofuscin.
          C. Ceroid from cirrhotic human liver.
          D. Standards.

     We find some neutral lipid in lipofuscins. As you can
see, the characteristic lipid in these lipopigments is a lipid
polymer; there is a trace of cholesterol if you refer to the
standard. There is a fair amount of free fatty acid, but this
may be associated with these pigments as insoluble organic
salts. Other trace components are triglyceride and some minor

constituents. The principal neutral lipids in lipofuscins
are really free fatty acids, traces of triglyceride, and a
small amount of cholesterol.

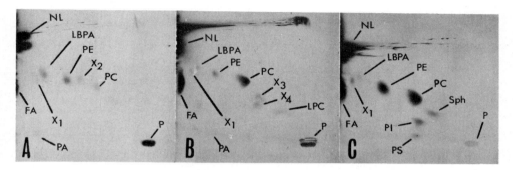

Figure 2. Polar lipids of different lipopigment preparations separated
by two-dimensional thin-layer chromatography on silica gel,
plain, with 10% MgSiO3 and the solvent systems (a) 65/25/5
chloroform/methanol/28% aqueous ammonia followed by (b) 3/4/
1/1/0.5 chloroform/acetone/methanol/acetic acid/water. Abbreviations: NL – neutral lipids; LBPA – lysobisphosphatidic
acid; PE – phosphatidyl ethanolamine; PC – phosphatidyl choline;
LPC – lysophosphatidyl choline; PA – phosphatidic acid; X_1,
X_2, X_3, X_4 – unknown compounds; P – polymeric lipid; PS –
phosphatidyl serine; PI – phosphatidyl inositol; Sph – sphingomyelin.
A. Polar lipids of brain lipofuscin.
B. Polar lipids of ceroid from cirrhotic liver.
C. Polar lipids of normal liver lipofuscin.

Figure 2B shows a separation of polar lipids from ceroid
of cirrhotic liver. As you can see, there are really very
few polar lipids or phospholipids. Phosphatidyl ethanolamine
and phosphatidyl choline appear as traces; the region for
sphingomyelin shows no material. What we noticed near the
origin were a number of high molecular weight lipidlike substances. At first we didn't think very much of this, but
then if we compare a corresponding separation of brain lipofuscin
(Fig 2A) we have very few minor phospholipids and again polymeric
material. We felt that this polymeric material was characteristic of these lipopigments. Figure 2C shows the separation
for normal liver lipofuscin. There are some trace components
of phospholipids, and P again denotes the region that is characteristic of polymeric lipids.

One of the things we noticed earlier was that these
pigments would bind very high concentrations of cations (Table
3); for example, ceroid binds more than three times as much
copper as lipofuscin; calcium and iron binding by ceroid are

123

much higher. On the other hand, zinc was much lower in the
ceroid pigment than in lipofuscin. This ceroid material has
a pH of the same order as strong cation-exchange resin the

Cation, ppm

	Cu	Mn	Ca	Fe	Zn
Lipofuscin	20	1.3	240	300	400
Ceroid	70	2	960	1500	110

Table 3.Cation composition of brain lipopigments.

equivalent of Dowex 50, which you know is a very strong sulfonic
acid resin. Based on what we know of the composition of these
pigments, it was unlikely that any of the materials that we
know would be binding with these cations in any significant
concentration.

When we partitioned the lipid extract on a Sephadex column
we found that lipofuscin, from whatever the source (heart,
liver, or brain), had in the order of 97% of the material
segregated in the F_1 fraction (F_1 being the regular phospholipid,
neutral lipids, and neutral lipid polymers) and about 3% in
this very strong acidic lipid fraction. In other words, this
was a lipidlike polymer, which has acidic properties. This
was not terribly surprising. The F_2 fraction is the one
in which the ganglioside appears, and there is no ganglioside
in the pigment. Much to our surprise, when we looked at the
distribution for ceroid, we found it to be quite different:
57% of the total lipid fraction came out on this very strong
acidic fraction F_2 , and only 43% was in the neutral lipid
or native lipid fraction F_1. This, as far as we are concerned
now, explains the very strong ion-binding properties found
in these pigments. In fact, in Batten's disease, our present
view is that this strongly acidic, lipidlike high molecular
weight polymer is the stored substance. This really accounts
for the material that is piled up in these brains rather than
a native lipid, such as in the sphingolipidoses, where sphingolipids accumulate. This is the state of our knowledge at
the present time. These pigments all have relatively high
concentrations of lysosomal enzymes; they also have relatively
high concentrations of an enzyme which is normally associated
with the membrane of myelin, i.e., cyclic 2,3-AMP phosphohydrolase. This has been considered a marker enzyme for myelin,
but it is also a marker enzyme for lipopigment. There is
no difference in the enzymes of these two pigments.

The main feature which distinguishes normal aging pigment from ceroid, the pigment accumulated in Batten's disease, is this very strongly acidic lipid polymer. This acts in some respects as an ion-exchanger by binding ions in the cell.

Dr. Philippart: Do you have any phosphorus or protein in that ceroid fraction?

Dr. Siakotos: We have started to characterize it. I haven't looked very closely. It has phosphorus in it, nearly 10% by weight.

Dr. Philippart: Do you find lysobisphosphatidic acid in this fraction?

Dr. Siakotos: No.

Dr. Kolodny: What is the carboyhdrate content of the 57% ceroid F_2 fraction?

Dr. Siakotos: We don't know yet.

Dr. Kolodny: Have you had any chance to evaluate the sialic acid content?

Dr. Siakotos: No, but there are no gangliosides there. The other interesting thing is that recently we have been working on melanosomes from melanoma and found the same type of polymeric material there, too. Melanosomes build up large quantities of zinc, and this has been known for a long time. These acidic polymers, apparently, are found in more than one type of pigment. The one we are concerned with here, of course, is the one in brain, i.e., ceroid. It does have the same type of polymeric lipid that is found in alcoholic cirrhotic liver as well.

One of the major problems that we have had, I might add, is that of having enough material to work with. (We only have 10 mg of total extract from a preparation of ceroid, and that has to be fractionated to do molecular weights and careful characterization of the polymeric material.)

Dr. Nair: Is there any distinction between the two, in terms of ultrastructure?

Dr. Siakotos: There is and there isn't. There are some forms of lipofuscin that look like ceroid, but there is really no distinction on an ultrastructural basis between ceroids. One may have one type, and another may have another type. But to pick up an electromicrograph and say that this is ceroid and this is lipofuscin is very risky.

Dr. Nair: Is there a distinction between pigments in different tissues, for instance, in brain or liver?

Dr. Siakotos: The pigment of brain, for example, has approximately four or five morphological species of lipofuscin; in heart there are only one or two, and in liver there are two at the most.

Dr. Tappel: Do you have something on the molecular weight of the polymer? Is it an oxypolymer? Does it derive from phospholipids?

Dr. Siakotos: It has approximately 10-20% phosphorus. But we have a very small amount of this material. We recently got a case, a complete autopsy, of a Batten's disease patient, and we have to be very careful what we are going to do with it lest we waste this material. We know that it has between 10 and 20% phosphorus, on a weight basis.

Dr. Tappel: Does it carry quite a bit of fluorescence in the total lipid extract?

Dr. Siakotos: We haven't investigated that yet.

Dr. Philippart: Was your material inspected for the presence of so-called curvilinear bodies?

Dr. Zeman: The answer is yes; the curvilinear bodies belong to the ceroid type pigments.

Dr. Philippart: Do you find the same appearance after isolating the pigment? After extracting it, do you still have the curvilinear bodies?

Dr. Siakotos: Yes.

Dr. Philippart: This would make it different from lipo-fuscin, which as far as I know is quite amorphous, although it may be associated with membrane material.

Dr. Zeman: Perhaps I can answer the question. The curvi-linear bodies (Figure 3) are distinct with respect to their identification as ceroid. It is superficially similar to the ceroid that we get from English setters[3] with neuronal ceroid-lipofuscinosis (Figure 4). However, Dr. Siakotos pointed out that not all patients with the clinical course of the Jansky-Bielschowsky type, who are therefore presumed to have curvilinear bodies, do show up with this type of lipopigment granules. Indeed, the first case from which ceroid was isolated,* did not show curvilinear bodies in the brain, only in kidney and

*This case has been reclassified as Haltia-Santavouri type.

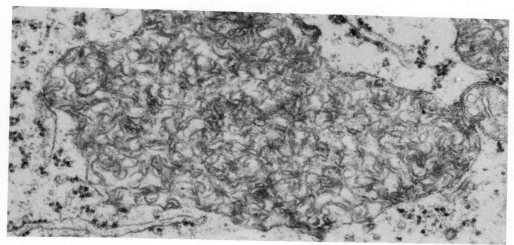

Figure 3. Neuronal perikaryon of 4-year-old girl with neuronal ceroid-
lipofuscinosis, Jansky-Bielschowsky type. Intraneuronal curvilinear body surrounded by a unit membrane. X 50,000.

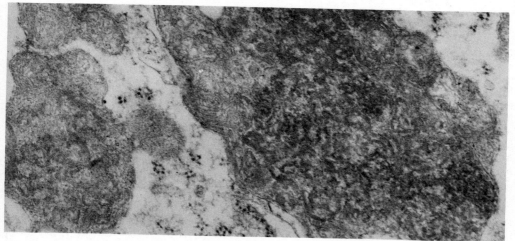

Figure 4. Neuronal perikaryon of 15-month-old dog with neuronal ceroid-
lipofuscinosis. The internal structure of the lipopigment body
shows a fingerprint pattern. X 50,000.

liver.[4]   The nerve cells contained a pigment with a granular
matrix (Figure 5) which in the isolated purified state as
well as in situ does not show curvilinear profile. It is
quite similar in appearance to lipofuscin pigment, although
the physiochemical features place it distinctly in the ceroid
group.

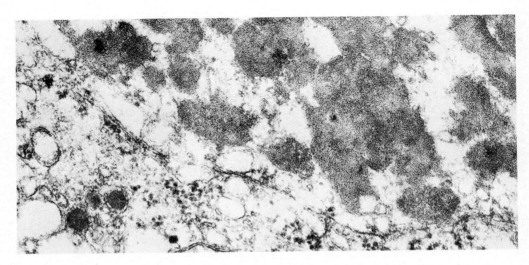

Figure 5. Neuronal perikaryon of 6-year-old boy with neuronal ceroid-lipofuscinosis, Haltia-Santavuori type. Several membrane-bound granular pigment bodies have displaced cytoplasmic organelles. X 50,000.

Dr. Siakotos: The ion-binding capacity of these pigments has always led to some confusion about morphology, because it tends to mask the fine structure. We first observed this ion-exchange feature of these pigments in brain pigment from English setters. All one could see was a hazy picture in the electron microscope. Then we thought it was cesium from the gradient material. When we treated it with Dowex 50, when the ions were removed, we saw a beautiful fingerprint pattern. This has been characteristic of all of the ceroids that we have found to date. In tissue, the ions will be bound, and so on careful study the fine structure presents a nonphotogenic appearance. That is perhaps one of the reasons the morphology has not been very useful.

Dr. Desnick: You indicated that lysosomal enzymes are associated with the pigment fraction. Specifically, which enzymes have you assayed? I'm curious to know why they are still there following extraction procedures.

Dr. Siakotos: We treat with Nagarse, which is a very strong proteolytic enzyme. However, this treatment does not destroy the enzymes; even in brain, there are 5000 units of acid phosphatase/mg of protein/hr (Table 4). This is the pigment that has been isolated. In ceroid there are 6400 units/mg/hr. These are very active preparations. In AMP phosphohydrolase, there are almost 4000 units. That is almost as active as pure myelin preparations. So these pigments

128

have the classical acid hydrolases that are found in lysosomes. Much to our surprise recently, other lipopigments have been found with the same type of enzyme.

These are the classical lysosomal hydrolases. They are all present, and this is the cyclic 2,3-AMP phosphohydrolase which is in all of these pigments. This is not true in the melanosome pigments.

| Enzyme | Brain | Lipofuscin, units/mg/hr | | Ceroid, units/ mg/hr |
		Liver	Heart	Brain
Acid phosphatase	5000	4500	420	6400
Cathepsin D	234	131	57	195
β-Galactosidase	230	170	120	253
β-Hexosaminidase	310	185	95	446
β-Glucosidase	420	24	4	n.d.
α-Glucosidase	13	9	1.5	9
α-Mannosidase	9	7	0.7	n.d.
α-Fucosidase	5	n.d.	n.d.	n.d.
AMP hydrolase	6200	525	350	3750

Table 4. Hydrolytic enzymes in lipopigments

Dr. Tappel: Just from the profile of the lysosomal enzymes, it appears that the hexosaminidase, which has normally 10 times the activity of β-galactosidase or the β-glucosidase, has rather low activity. I assume they are all specific activities, i.e., millimicromoles/unit of protein/unit of time. Can you make anything out of the profile?

Dr. Siakotos: In the melanosome, hexosamindase is low. We use basically the same approach to isolating the pigment, i.e., enzymatic digestion followed by the cesium chloride fractionation. Acid phosphatase is also there, but these other enzymes like β-galactosidase remain low in the melanosomes. I think this is a unique characteristic of these pigments and not a characteristic of the method of isolation.

Dr. Philippart: I wonder what type of substrate you are using for your enzyme assays. Since your pigment is fluorescent, I wonder if this interferes with umbelliferone fluorescence?

Dr. Siakotos: You mean will it absorb enzymes?

Dr. Philippart: No, will the pigment itself participate in the fluorescence of your assay?

129

Dr. Siakotos: No, we don't follow the fluorescence. We use the p-nitrophenol derivative, which absorbs in the 340 nm region, and that's not fluorescence.

Dr. Rider: By just looking at these values, there doesn't seem to be much difference between the lipofuscin and the ceroid, except the β-glucosidase and the α-mannosidase. Are these significant?

Dr. Siakotos: No, I don't think there is any significance to them. The β-glucosidase was not measured.

Dr. Rider: They appear to be very much the same.

Dr. Siakotos: The profiles are the same.

Dr. Wherrett: How do you solubilize the pigment to do the enzyme estimation?

Dr. Siakotos: That's done by Dr. Patel.

Dr. Tappel: He might use Triton X-100, which is known to be a very good detergent but which does not affect the enzymes.

Dr. Zeman: I believe we use Triton X-100 following ultra-sonification.

Dr. Kolodny: Did you measure the β-glucuronidase activity of the lipopigment? The reason I ask is that Ockerman has reported[5] elevations in the activity of this enzyme in the plasma of three patients and in post-mortem specimens of liver from two patients with Batten's disease.

Dr. Siakotos: I don't know whether Dr. Patel did measure that. Who reported that again?

Dr. Kolodny: Öckerman, in 1968.[5] He also reported increased activity of β-glucuronidase in autopsy specimens of brain cortex and spleen of one of the two cases he examined. In certain of the post-mortem tissues he also found elevations in the activity of acid phosphatase.

Dr. Zeman: Perhaps I should add that these patients all have increased serum levels of acid hydrolases as also reported by Öckerman.[5] I have seen a number of patients in Denmark, all of whom had an increased SGOT activity, and some of them (a statistically significant number) have an increased activity of phosphokinase. The point I want to make is that we have to be prepared to find a number of chemical abnormalities in these patients, for several reasons. For one, these patients are catabolically immensely active and in order to maintain their weight have to have enormous caloric intake, especially in the advanced stages of the disease. Secondly, there is significant breakdown of tissues which should both liberate as well as activate lysosomal hydrolases and other enzymes. Then, as in other lysosomal diseases, there is increased fragility of lysosomal membranes. I therefore do not consider this increase of β-glucuronidase as specific.

Dr. Desnick: I would like to comment further. The lysosomal accumulation of noncatabolized substrate may cause a morphologic response at the subcellular level. The cells may increase in the activity of membrane-bound enzymes per gram of tissue. This is consistent with the ultrastructural findings of an increased number and size of lysosomes in tissue from patients with documented lysosomal storage diseases.[6] Therefore, those tissues will have more lysosomes per unit weight and give you higher activity levels for various lysosomal enzymes. I think that might explain some of the results we have seen in the past in other diseases and in this case with respect to elevated lysosomal enzymatic activities.

Dr. Kolodny: However, not all lysosomal enzymes are elevated in lysosomal storage diseases. In Batten's disease, the increases in lysosomal enzyme activities are somewhat selective. We have looked at the lysosomal activity of two biopsy cores from the liver of a patient with clinically and pathologically proven Batten's disease, of so-called Spielmeyer-Sjögren variety. What we found by looking at several different lysosomal enzyme activities was that only three were elevated: β-glucuronidase, β-galactosidase, and β-N-acetylhexosaminidase. Our findings for these enzymes and for two of the enzymes with normal activity are shown in Table 5. They are in agreement with those of Ockerman. I would like to ask Dr. Tappel whether he can explain the selective increase of certain enzymes in lysosomal storage diseases.

| | % of control activity | | | | |
| | Post-mortem cases* | | Biopsy cases* | | Patient D.L. |
Enzyme	No.1	No.2	No.1	No.2	
β-Glucuronidase	222	275	222	161	169
β-Galactosidase	224	129	142	139	166
β-N-acetylglucosaminidase	117	131	105	96	149
Acid phosphatase	104	117	n.d.	n.d.	95
α-Fucosidase	124	46	n.d.	n.d.	95

Table 5. Liver enzyme activity in Spielmeyer–Sjögren Disease

*Data of Öckerman.

Dr. Tappel: That's a very good question, Dr. Kolodny. Thus far, there have not been enough studies in the literature to answer the important question that you raise. However, the profiles of lysosomal enzymes have been studied in some diseases associated with the accumulation, and it seems more like there is a general rise. So I think that Dr. Desnick points to the main problem, which is that when the biosynthetic route is stimulated to produce more hydrolases, it produces all, not specific ones, so the stimulation seems to be more general. The important point that we are developing here is that in catabolic activity and stimulation of lysosomes, which occur as far as I know in all catabolic activity, whether it's pathological or nutritional, you would expect a large number of lysosomal bodies with approximately the same complement of enzymes.

Dr. Zeman: Did you really answer Dr. Kolodny's question? He wonders whether these lysosomal hydrolases show either an increase which is specific for a given disease, or whether certain other hydrolases might be relatively depressed in relationship to others. Is there evidence that in a specific lysosomal disease, a repetitive enzymatic pattern with an increased or depressed activity of certain hydrolases occurs or not? Is the pattern specific for Batten's disease? Is there another specific pattern for β-galactosidase deficiency for GM_2 gangliosidosis, types A and O?

Dr. Tappel: To try to generalize a little, this question is very broad and also has been treated diversely in the re-search done heretofore. One can say that in various pathological catabolic responses, like muscular dystrophies, there are very large increases in lysosomal enzymes, and this may be on the order of a ten- to a hundred-fold increase in muscle. Herein the pattern seems to follow that of the phagocytes because they bring in the lysosomes, and they bring in all the lysosomal enzymes, catabolizing mainly protein. This occurs also in various types of starvation wherein the liver is being catabolized. Again, the increase seems to dominate the whole lysosomal hydrolase pattern. Recent work was done, for example, by O'Brien's group and by us in some of the diseases (Hurler's disease for example) wherein maybe ten or twenty lysosomal enzymes were measured.[7] It seemed that all lysosomal enzymes were increased approximately three-fold. There was no discernible change in profile. On the other hand, in the muscular dystrophies, in which some muscles do not have the aryl sulfatases, when these new populations of lysosomes come in, it appears all of a sudden; so you might say it goes up infinitely. I don't see any general answer except there most likely is an elevation of all the lysosomal enzymes. Until more precise profiles are made, I think one would view the situation with caution. There is great diversity of possi-bilities.

Dr. Zeman: Inasmuch as it is relatively simple to measure
many lysosomal hydrolases in one and the same specimen, we
certainly should address ourselves to the questions as to
whether it is sensible to study a large number of patients
and to study heterozygotes for enzyme profiles; and if so,
what tissues should we take? As I understand, Dr. Kolodny,
you measured the enzyme activity in the liver of your patient.
Unfortunately, liver is not an easily accessible tissue.
Admittedly, there are certain changes in the liver of our
patients, but there are also changes in the leukocytes[8] (Figure
6). Should we therefore undertake a screening study on leukocytes of as many patients with this disease as possible
and determine their enzyme profiles to see whether or not
there is a repetitive or perhaps even diagnostic pattern?
Do you think we should get involved in such a study which
is relatively simple?

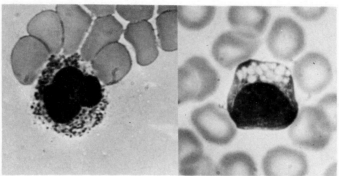

Figure 6. Leukocytes of 13-year-old boy with Spielmeyer-Sjögren type of
           neuronal ceroid-lipofuscinosis. The polymorphonuclear neutro-
           phil shows hypergranulation; the lymphocyte is vacuolated.
           Special Giemsa stain. X 920.

Dr. Tappel: I believe that there are certain indications
that this procedure might have success. The work of certain
investigators with vitamin A[9] showed that the breakdown of
lysosomes relating to hypervitaminosis A gave rise to a significant increase in β-glucuronidase in the blood, so blood
enzymes might be monitored. We've been pursuing a similar
pathway in terms of looking at damage to lungs when exposed
to air pollutant oxidants. The enzymes we have chosen to
look at include lysosomal enzymes from the alveolar macrophages;
that would include lysozyme as one of the enzymes that is
present in high concentration and also hexosaminidase, which
is one of the most easily measured lysosomal enzymes and the
one with the highest specific activity. In fact, I think
since it can be done easily and since you may very well find
increases in lysosomal enzymes, it seems like a good approach.
I suppose the other possibility is that in many pathologies
there is a phagocytic response, so there will be an increase

in lysosomal enzymes.

Dr. Philippart: I agree essentially with all that Dr. Tappel has said. In the major types of mucopolysaccharidoses which have been extensively studied, there is indeed an increase in most of the enzymes, but not all of them. For example, β-galactosidase has been frequently reported to be low in the liver at least. α-galactosidase is another example. Perhaps β-xylosidase and arabinosidase also tend to be on the low side. It would be interesting to find a way to induce lysosomal enzymes (either all of them or partly) because this might help treat the patients. So far we can't generalize because each disorder tends to have a specific pattern. For example, in GM_1 gangliosidosis Dr. Kolodny mentioned an increase in hexosaminidase. Here I think we have a reasonable explanation. There is accumulation of galactose and glucosamine in such tissues, and we have found with others that in the brain, fibroblasts, and the liver there is an accumulation of keratosulfate-like glycoprotein.[10] This might be a type of substrate which is able to induce a given enzyme. There is no indication that this results from an increase in the number of lysosomes, most of the enzymes may remain within normal limits.

Dr. Zeman: You mean most of the hydrolases?

Dr. Philippart: Yes.

Dr. Zeman: Hasn't Öckerman reported increase in lysosomal hydrolases in Batten's disease, too?

Dr. Philippart: I don't think he has studied brain. He analyzed mostly liver and skin fibroblasts, and I don't remember his results exactly.

Dr. Zeman: In other words, we should stick to one tissue if we were to do it at all.

Dr. Philippart: I would say each tissue has its own problems.

Dr. Kolodny: I would second your call for a systematic study of the white blood cell lysosomal enzymes. All of us recognize that this will probably not yield the primary defect in Batten's disease, but other benefits might result. For one thing, it might provide valuable clues for the recognition of heterozygous carriers of the disease. I would add that we have studied the white blood cells of our patient. I had no data of other workers with which to compare it, so that I chose to bring up the example of the liver, but again we found elevations in other enzymes--the three I mentioned plus α-mannosidase. It's very simple to do, and I think most of us have done it on perhaps 10 ml of venous blood.

Dr. Desnick: Yes, percutaneous liver biopsies have now become routine in most centers, and multiple enzyme analyses can be carried out on a small amount of tissue.[11] In addition to the leukocyte enzyme analyses, liver biopsies by competent individuals would be most helpful for the comparison of various enzymatic activities in different fresh tissues that are relatively easily obtained.

Dr. Zeman: Are you talking about needle biopsies?

Dr. Desnick: Percutaneous needle biopsies.

Dr. Kolodny: Our needle biopsy was carried out on a 16-year old boy who was quite far advanced in his disease, so that his degree of cooperation might have been less than ideal. Nevertheless, by carefully preparing and training him over a course of several days, he was able to cooperate fully. On the needle core that we obtained with a single pass into his liver, we were able to do a complete fatty acid analysis, lysosomal enzyme study, qualitative and quantitative neutral glycolipid determination, as well as light and electron microscopy. Therefore I support Dr. Desnick's thesis, and I feel, as he does, that white blood cells and liver biopsy specimens have value in studying Batten's disease.

Dr. Tappel: I would support both of these proposals in the sense that most of the lysosomal enzymes that are well characterized are from the liver. In 1968, when I last took a look at the number of profiles of lysosomal enzymes that were in the literature, there were actually only a few, but I believe that most of those that are available center around the liver, so that would seem to offer an advantage in that respect.

Dr. Zeman: As you know there is as yet no indication as to the basic biochemical defect--or let me say the causative pathogenesis--of Batten's disease. In other words, while we feel that the work of Dr. Tappel and others has established beyond doubt the intracellular pathogenesis of fatty acid peroxidation and pigment formation, we really do not know at the present time what triggers this particular reaction. By way of introduction, I will show you a very simple equation taken from Hartroft[12] which we have modified to some extent, that is, the rate of pigment formation dp/dt is related to the concentration of oxidants over antioxidants and to the concentration of polyunsaturated fatty acids (PUFA) over the concentration of saturated fatty acids (SFA):

$$dp/dt = ([oxid]/[antioxid])([PUFA]/[SFA])$$

Lipid oxidation goes on in most tissues at a very slow rate, but in these disorders the rate of peroxidation and therefore pigment formation is greatly increased. Whether this is a primary or secondary mechanism is, at the present time, completely unknown. It should be apparent from this equation (which is supported by experimental data) that a variety of variables or a combination thereof could be envisioned as a possible etiology of those conditions. Inasmuch as we have consistently found a very high concentration of bivalent cations and since bivalent cations are potent oxidizers, we have as a working hypothesis considered the possibility that at least some of the conditions which we call Batten's disease may be associated with a cellular siderosis. This assumption receives support from the fact that patients with Batten's disease, at least the few that we have been able to study, show low values of vitamin E in the serum and also a low activity of δ-aminolevulinic acid synthetase and dehydratase. Dr. Nair, who has been instrumental in establishing the role of vitamin E as a cofactor for this heme-synthesizing enzyme chain which ends with ferrochelatase, which, if deficient, could indeed lead to an accumulation of ferric ions in tissues, will now enlighten us on this problem.

Dr. Nair: Before I go into the subject matter of my presentation, I would like to briefly indicate the background to our work on vitamin E. Let us consider for a moment, lipids, in general, in tissues. There are a variety of lipids in tissues and in cells, such as triglycerides, phospholipids, and sterols, all of which occur in substantial concentrations. To a large extent, their functions in cells are known. In comparison to these "gross" lipids, there are lipids which occur in extremely small quantitities but which manifest themselves very significantly in terms of their physiological action. Trace lipids are defined as those lipids derived from our diet in small amounts which are essential for the normal maintenance of physiological processes. According to this definition, vitamin E is one such trace lipid.

Vitamin E deficiency is characterized by a variety of species- and tissue-specific syndromes (Table 6). This pleomorphism in the effects of vitamin E deficiency is further complicated by the fact that in addition to vitamin E, selenium, synthetic antioxidants, and sulfur amino acids prevent the onset of some of these syndromes. These observations have led several investigators to propose a number of mechanisms of vitamin E action.

Animal species	Syndrome
Rat Male	Sterility
Female	Fetal resorption
Both sexes	Liver necrosis (selenium)
Rabbit	Muscular dystrophy
	Myocardial degeneration
Dog and guinea pig	Myocardial degeneration
Chicken	Encephalomalacia
	Exudative diathesis
Primate	Macrocytic anemia
	Muscular dystrophy

Table 6. Syndromes resulting from vitamin E deficiency.

The purpose of today's presentation is to introduce a hypothesis, a novel and somewhat speculative one, which will seek to find a common ground for the different viewpoints on this subject. The idea that the deficiency of a single nutritional agent could give rise to several different, apparently unrelated, deficiency states in different animal species, led us to believe that this vitamin regulates a metabolic process or substance fundamental to all living cells. The demonstration of a nutritional anemia in deficient monkeys showed not only a nutritional requirement for vitamin E in a subhuman primate but also served to alert us to the possibility of heme or hemeproteins as an entity regulated by the vitamin E status of the organism.

Syndrome	Species & Characteristics	Reference
Macrocytic anemia	Rhesus monkey	Dinning & Day[13]
Macrocytic anemia	Rhesus monkey: Reduced synthesis of porphyrins and heme	Porter et al[14]
Macrocytic anemia	Man; protein-calorie malnutrition	Majaj et al[15]
Anemia	Immature brown trout	Poston[16]
Anemia	Pig	Nafstad[17]
Anemia	Rat; combined protein and vitamin E deficiency	Bencze et al[18]
Anemia	Premature infants hemolytic component	Oski & Barness[19]

Table 7. Historical review of anemias of vitamin E deficiency.

Table 7 shows the anemias observed as a result of vitamin E deficiency in several species. The evidence accrued over the last 13 years strongly suggests an aberration of heme biosynthesis.

137

Figure 7 is a schematic representation of the biosynthetic pathway to heme. The synthesis of heme is an attribute common to all aerobic cells, and it is initiated by the condensation of glycine and succinyl CoA, intramitochondrially. This step is catalyzed by the enzyme δ-aminolevulinic acid synthetase (ALA synthetase). The activity of this enzyme is negligible in nonhematopoietic cells. In other words, it is partially repressed when compared to that in hematopoietic cells, reflecting the relative demands for heme placed by each of these cell types. The second step in this pathway is mediated by the soluble cytosolic enzyme, ALA dehydratase, that condenses two molecules of ALA to give rise to porphobilinogen or PBG. The activities of these two enzymes either individually or in combination are rate-determining in this pathway. The terminal step in this pathway is performed intramitochondrially by the introduction of iron into protoporphyrin IX by the enzyme, heme synthetase, or ferrochelatase. The heme that is synthesized is now conjugated with numerous apohemeproteins that ultimately participate in a wide variety of cellular functions.

GLYCINE + SUCCINYL-CoA

⬇

(ALA SYNTHASE)

⬇

δ-AMINOLEVULINIC ACID

(ALA)

⬇

(ALA DEHYDRATASE)

⬇

PORPHOBILINOGEN

⬇   PORPHYRINS

PORPHYRINOGENS

⬇

PROTOPORPHYRIN IX

+ ⬇ Fe^{++}

HEME

Figure 7. Outline of heme biosynthesis.

138

Dr. Murty and recently Dr. Caasi from our laboratories have been investigating the biosynthesis of heme in the vitamin E-deficient rat. Rats (35-40 g) were maintained on a standard vitamin E-deficient diet[20] and sacrificed at various time intervals after they were placed on the diet. Our studies showed that in deficient animals, hepatic ALA dehydratase, catalase, tryptophan oxygenase, microsomal cytochromes b_5, P-450, and protoheme were significantly lower than those in control animals.[21][22] Since hepatic ALA synthetase remained unaffected, it was postulated that the primary metabolic aberration under these conditions may be at the enzymatic step involved in the synthesis of porphobilinogen (PBG) from ALA. The locus of the enzymatic defect was further studied by following the incorporation into microsomal protoheme of radioactivity from ALA-4-^{14}C and PBG-^{14}C, the two intermediates that serve as the substrate and product of ALA dehydratase. The ability to incorporate ALA-4-^{14}C into protoheme was significantly impaired in the deficient microsomes, an observation that was consistent with the concept of a defect in the step involving ALA dehydratase.

While these studies were in progress, we were also interested in the regulation of heme synthesis at the level of ALA synthetase, an enzyme which is normally in a state of partial repression in hepatic cells but can be induced by a variety of drugs (phenobarbital, allylisopropylacetamide) and steroid hormones.[23] Furthermore, the activities of this enzyme are significantly enhanced in hepatic porphyrias. Studies from our laboratories have shown that vitamin E prevents the induction of experimental porphyria[24] and causes a remission in human hepatic porphyrias,[25][26] presumably by counteracting the induction of hepatic ALA synthetase.[27][28]

The present state of our knowledge seems to indicate that vitamin E regulates the synthesis of heme and porphyrias. The primary site of action seems to be on the intranuclear elements of the cell, presumably on the synthesis of nuclear RNA. Our findings lend further support to the concept that trace lipids function as regulators of macromolecular synthesis.

Dr. Zeman: I believe at this point we might elaborate on Dr. Nair's observations, perhaps by way of speculation.

Dr. Siakotos: Dr. Nair, since lipids are primarily in the microsomal region of the cell, would you say then that what we see in Batten's disease may really be in fact a synthetic phenomenon rather than a degradative change? Would you like to speculate on that?

Dr. Nair: I think it could be a loss of control of regulation of synthesis, if you could look at it that way.

Dr. Zeman: Could you be a little bit more specific and perhaps try to give us the full picture of events of this hypothetical situation?

Dr. Nair: Perhaps there is an increase in synthesis of heme precursors; alternatively, perhaps the synthesis of heme is not fully consummated by the incorporation of iron into heme. These precursors could then possibly form aggregates. For instance, we know that cations, like iron, are increased in these lipofuscin-like particles. It is quite possible there is an increase in porphyrin polymers or defective incorporation of iron into protoporphyrin IX.

Dr. Zeman: Let's take one step at a time. It was my understanding that you did find a decreased activity of ALA synthetase in the plasma of the two patients we sent you, am I correct?

Dr. Nair: In the red cells, yes.

Dr. Zeman: In the red cells. How about in the plasma?

Dr. Nair: There are decreased vitamin E levels.

Dr. Zeman: Decreased vitamin E. Am I correct in assuming that you found the same situation in Dr. Kolodny's patient?

Dr. Nair: Yes. I'm not sure of the history of Dr. Kolodny's patient. Perhaps you could enlighten me on that.

Dr. Kolodny: It is a case that fits all the clinical and pathological criteria for the Spielmeyer-Sjögren type of Batten's disease.

Dr. Zeman: Just how much was the activity decreased?

Dr. Nair: Off hand I don't remember what those values are. Do you have those values?

Dr. Zeman: I think you reported about 30% or so.

Dr. Siakotos: Did you measure the enzyme? I think you measured the vitamin E.

Dr. Nair: The vitamin E and, I thought, the enzyme too; I'm not certain.

Dr. Zeman: Yes, you did determine the enzyme, too.

Dr. Nair: I remember that the vitamin E values were very low in three of them, as you have reported here. I didn't have the code to identify the samples.

Dr. Zeman: Yes, the vitamin E was about 40% of normal
in the two patients and 60% or thereabouts of normal controls
in heterozygotes.

Dr. Nair: I see.

Dr. Zeman: We sent you samples from two patients; one
control and one heterozygote.

Dr. Nair: Yes, that's one-tenth of the control; and
the lab control is 1.44 and 0.82; and the patient is 0.12.

Dr. Zeman: It appears that we have a significant decrease
in ALA synthetase. This may not be a genetically controlled
decrease, but it might be associated with the deficiency of
vitamin E. Can we nail that problem down?

Dr. Nair: It's possible that we can extend the previous
observation in the primate.

Dr. Zeman: Would it be a good control if we were to
send you the same erythrocytes and the same serum after treating
a patient with α-tocopherol for a certain period of time?

Dr. Nair: Yes. It should be a minimum of 28 to 30 days
before any change is noticeable, and, of course, we have to
follow the blood vitamins at the same time.

Dr. Zeman: Yes, I agree. But this is the first time
we really have observed an enzyme defect, with respect to ALA
synthetase; how about the dehydratase?

Dr. Nair: No, I don't have dehydratase values.

Dr. Zeman: But these two go together, don't they--dehy-
dratase and ALA synthetase?

Dr. Nair: Yes.

Dr. Zeman: That is the first time we have observed a
marked defect of an enzyme in any of these patients among
the many enzymes we have looked at, and it is on account of
Dr. Nair's very astute observations, namely, that the activity
of the synthetase and dehydratase is apparently governed by
the availability of vitamin E. Whether this is the direct
expression of some genetic mutation or whether the low vitamin
E values are due to an absorption deficiency remains open
to question. Perhaps you can address yourself now to this
question before we go further into the possible pathogenesis.
What would you propose we do in order to answer this question?
In other words, if we treat a patient for 4 weeks with high
doses of vitamin E, do we give it in the form of a water-

soluble or a fat-soluble preparation? How much do we give?
How should we set up the experiments?

Dr. Nair: Is there anything known about the absorption
of vitamin E in these patients?

Dr. Zeman: Nothing.

Dr. Witting: Well, may I ask a question here? I noticed
that a plasma tocopherol value you quoted for Dr. Kolodny's
patient is normal.

Dr. Nair: Our normal mean is from 1 to 1.3 mg/100 ml
in our lab.

Dr. Witting: Yes, but the published literature values
on samples from healthy subjects will usually cite 0.7 to
1.2 mg/100 ml as the normal range, and your value here is
approximately 0.8.

Dr. Nair: Well, we have been following it by GLC, and
our GLC values are somewhat lower.

Dr. Witting: Values obtained in these procedures always
tend to be lower than those obtained by conventional procedures
anyway.

Dr. Nair: Yes, they tend to be lower.

Dr. Witting: On the other hand, your population norms
are based on the Emmerie-Engel procedure,[29] and presumably
that would be the thing to which this 0.78 figure should be
compared.

Dr. Nair: I have a point here that normal levels of
circulating vitamins need not necessarily mean optimal physiological function; that's what we have seen. I don't think
the level of circulating vitamins could be taken as an indication
of sufficiency, as far as metabolism is concerned.

Dr. Witting: I was wondering about this value on Dr.
Kolodny's patient in that we had examined two of Dr. Zeman's
patients previously and had a low value on one and a relatively
normal value on the other. Do you remember what your determinations were on those patients?

Dr. Nair: We didn't have the codes; we just had one
to four samples we analyzed and sent. We didn't know which
of them were patients.

Dr. Zeman: These were the same patients; according to
Dr. Witting one had a normal value and the other a very low

one--about 0.4 mg %--and the mother had 0.8 mg%.

Dr. Witting: We had 0.4 mg-% on one of the children, but the values were around 1 mg-% for the mother and the other daughter.

Dr. Zeman: Yes, you had 1 mg-% on one of the affected daughters; this child died in the meantime. We seem to have an argument here; different laboratories have different standards of vitamin E. What procedure for determination did you use?

Dr. Witting: Ours was just a straightforward Emmerie-Engel determination.[29]

Dr. Zeman: And you, Dr. Nair, used the same technique?

Dr. Nair: No, we used our own GLC method,[28] [30] because we feel that gas chromatography is much more sensitive and specific.

Dr. Witting: This procedure, being more specific, will tend to give a lower value, which will create minor problems in comparing it to published figures of population norms.

Dr. Zeman: So we'll have to determine whether to use gas chromatography or follow the standard Emmerie-Engel technique.

Dr. Philippart: I have a question, perhaps for you, Dr. Zeman. Neuraxonal dystrophy has been compared with experimental vitamin E deficiency. Do you know if ALA synthetase has been determined in any of these patients?

Dr. Zeman: No.

Dr. Philippart: And the other part of the question, is the enzyme stable? Could you make reliable determinations on autopsy material, for example?

Dr. Nair: No, autopsy material cannot be used.

Dr. Kolodny: I believe that we should, in the systematic approach of this problem, try to answer Dr. Nair's question, which is: is there some deficiency in the intestinal absorption of fat-soluble vitamins, specifically vitamin E? I don't think we have, to date, any clinical evidence to point to any malabsorption difficulty in these patients. Do we, Dr. Zeman?

Dr. Zeman: No, we don't have any evidence as to that effect, nor do we know how biologically active is that substance which is being measured as plasma vitamin E. The other point is that we have never examined a large population, matched for sex and age, and considered circadian rhythm and dietary intake. We can do all of those studies on the English setters because we can maintain them on a very rigidly controlled regimen. Genetically, these dogs are closely related to each other because they are highly inbred. This is essentially what we propose to do. In fact we already have some preliminary agreement with Dr. Nair about doing these studies. The question to which we have to address ourselves is whether it is worthwhile to spend $5000 to do this type of experiment.

Dr. Rider: Well, it's a simple matter. I don't know how difficult it is to get your vitamin E levels, but it's easy to do a tolerance test, just as you would do a glucose tolerance, triglyceride tolerance, or any of these tests which are highly standardized. You know, you give them so much and you determine blood levels over the next 4, 5, 8, 12 hr. Depending upon how difficult it is to run your vitamin E levels, I think that would answer the question very quickly--whether there is any abnormality in the absorption.

Dr. Nair: If there is a defect in absorption of water-soluble vitamin E, then we could obtain a parenteral vitamin E from Roche; they have an IND on it, and we are going to try that very soon.

Dr. Zeman: Is that injectable vitamin E?

Dr. Nair: Yes, that's intramuscular. We have just gotten clearance to use that in human subjects.

Dr. Rider: Isn't U.S. Vitamin's Aquasol E water-soluble?

Dr. Nair: Aquasol E is water-soluble.

Dr. Rider: We have a bottle of vitamin E from Hoffman-LaRoche that is a powder.

Dr. Nair: That has a vehicle in it--some kind of vehicle.

Dr. Wherrett: May I ask: in human cases of vitamin E deficiency producing megaloblastic anemia, what are the blood levels?

Dr. Nair: Generally 0.1 mg-% or lower.

Dr. Wherrett: They're very significantly diminished?

Dr. Nair: Tenfold difference.

Dr. Wherrett: A group of astronauts was studied[31] who had, I think, a selective lack of vitamin E in their diet,

144

and they had mild anemia temporarily.

Dr. Nair: At least their blood levels dropped after the mission.

Dr. Witting: Generally speaking, you would not see vitamin E deficiency in the human. Gastric surgery or some types of malabsorption syndromes will, however, impair tocopherol absorption. In the Jordanian children[15] it was associated with the protein-calorie malnutrition, so I would say that was a grossly abnormal situation.

Dr. Rider: Of course, even if the vitamin E level is normal, it still doesn't tell you what it's doing to the tissue level. You could have just enough vitamin E floating around.

Dr. Witting: Well, of course, there again the liver biopsy would tell you.

Dr. Zeman: To return to the biochemical observations, it seems to me that there is indeed a discrepancy between the questionable decrease of vitamin E concentration in the serum, and the very definite decrease of ALA synthetase activity. The activity of the vitamin E-dependent enzyme is decreased significantly more than the concentration of vitamin E would suggest; one might be barking up the wrong tree by concentrating on vitamin E.

Dr. Nair: This brings us back to the same premise: Do we try to associate blood levels with corresponding decreases in enzymes all the time? Is there an uncoupling of blood levels and enzyme activity in certain cases? This is the question. Is there an individual variation? In order to elicit a certain response in enzymatic activity, in some patients we could expect a greater demand for vitamin E; is this a possibility? This is the question that I have. Can we just take blood levels as a definite indication of defect, or not?

Dr. Siakotos: I think it's been shown that it's really not the blood level or the diet level that counts, but rather the tissue level that counts--the membrane level.

Dr. Witting: But do you have any known situation where the tissue levels do not correspond to the blood levels? You're postulating something that has never been shown before. This is the question we're asking--is this a question of transport or of storage? Now there is one tissue that you could analyze for vitamin E that you could get painlessly and without any effort whatsoever, and that's adipose tissue. This is easier to sample than erythrocytes. You actually have adequate storage in the adipose tissue, you should have no problem in vitamin E transport in metabolism.

Dr. Rider: I might add that we've done a little of that ourselves, for the purpose of seeing whether a drug is localized in adipose tissue in neuritis. It's very easy to do. You can take an 18 to 16 gauge needle and just pick up the skin in the buttocks and put it in and put suction on it, and move it around to three or four places, and you can get fat out of that.

Dr. Witting: It's a little easier if you aspirate a little saline in and out.

Dr. Zeman: What is easier?

Dr. Witting: Hirsch's old procedure.[32] Put saline in the syringe, and you aspirate saline in and out and withdraw some fat cells with it. We used to do about 30 of these a morning every so often; it's very easy tissue to sample.

Dr. Nair: At least from our work we are assuming there are specific protein receptors, for instance, on chromatins. Is there a possibility that there could be genetic defects where the protein receptor is deleted? In that case we can give any amount of vitamin E but have no response at all.

Dr. Zeman: When you add extraneous vitamin E to these blood samples of low activity, do you raise the activity of the ALA synthetase?

Dr. Nair: Not in vitro, because this is not an in vitro mechanism. We have seen, or at least we have evidence, that vitamin E will have to get to the target tissue, to the cell; it has to be transferred into the chromatin, and thereafter a change is occurring before we can get a response to enzymatic activity. These are all tied in kinetically with the formation of RNA and with the synthesis of protein.

Dr. Zeman: Are there any further questions as to the methods or to the facts about vitamin E and ALA synthetase?

Dr. Tappel: I think Dr. Nair is to be congratulated on his very fine studies and, of course, we all encourage him to proceed. We should draw a distinction (I'm sure he wants to make it also) between what is experimental data and then what is hypothesis. This control at the DNA-RNA level is still a hypothesis; in fact, many of these results could be either running parallel with or resulting from lipid peroxidation. In vivo lipid peroxidation, I think, was provided with strong experimental evidence at the vitamin E symposium at which Dr. Nair was co-chairman.[33]

A couple of points I will cite. One is that the problem of catalase that Dr. Nair brought out is to some extent a

146

misinterpretation (I hope he'll correct that soon), because catalase does not really react very well with lipid peroxides. There is a glutathione peroxidase that does, but it's not a heme enzyme. Another problem, which I'm sure he'll want to face up to, is the fact that among the tissues that are easily peroxidized--and probably highly peroxidized--are the bone marrow cells, and this has been known for some time. So he is either dealing with a complicated problem, which has to be sorted out, of concurrent lipid peroxidation or a series of events of one following the other.

Dr. Nair: I agree with Dr. Tappel that this is a complicated question. We have a lot of data, but the interpretations are subject to changes as we go along. In fact, I'm sure we have enough work to do for the next several years before we can unravel this whole complex question. The only point I'd like to make at this moment is that there is definitely evidence to support a control mechanism exercised at the level of the synthesis of macromolecules, but this need not necessarily mean that vitamin E is not functioning as an antioxidant.

Dr. Tappel: For example, one point of evidence for control was brought out by Rao and Recknagel in a recent paper[34] referring to the complex situation at the level of microsomal RNA and protein synthesis; that is, when carbon tetrachloride is injected into animals, it can elicit an explosive lipid peroxidation in the microsomes, disorganize polysomes, and make drastic changes in protein synthesis. This is an example where peroxidative changes in the membrane can drastically affect the pathway of protein synthesis.

Dr. Zeman: It appears that we deal here with a specific situation. We have studied many lysosomal and microsomal enzymes and found them to have normal activity. For all I know, ALA synthetase is the first enzyme which has been shown to be significantly decreased in Batten's disease. I do agree that this finding may not represent a causative mechanism. I believe now is the time to have Dr. Siakotos' question answered: namely, what would be the mechanism to look for if ALA synthetase deficiency turns out to be a real and consistent finding? If we assume that this deficiency ranks relatively high in the chain of events, how would it facilitate lipid peroxidation and pigment formation especially in view of our related observations on high iron and calcium concentrations of the pigments?[35] Is that the question you asked?

Dr. Siakotos: The question really is: is the pigment a result of synthesis or is it a result of degradation of lipid components that were already there?

Dr. Nair: This is a question that we'll have to resolve jointly by isolating the material and looking at it carefully;

147

I think there is no other way of solving this question.

Dr. Kolodny: One point disturbs me.   ALA synthetase
is necessary for the synthesis of porphyrins and for the heme
moiety of hemoglobin.   If there is truly a deficiency in the
activity of this enzyme in Batten's disease, then affected
patients would be expected to manifest an anemia, yet this
is not one of the characteristics of the disease.

Dr. Nair: Yes, we would normally expect marked anemia
in these cases.

Dr. Rider: You mentioned your dogs; another simple approach would be to get a vitamin E level on the dogs.   Give
them some vitamin E and see whether they have a normal absorption.   You get a control and see if they absorb the vitamin E
normally or, even if they absorb it normally, how long the
blood level stays up.   It's possible that they might degrade
the vitamin E much faster.

Dr. Zeman: We have treated some of these dogs for as
much as two years with vitamin E, butylated hydroxytoluene,
and methionine and have not seen any change in the natural
evolution of the disease.   This is in contrast to the human
patients whom we have treated similarly, for we have the impression that we have at least slowed down and possibly even
arrested the progression of the disease for about two years.
Of course, these observations do not help to overcome the
current impasse.   The real question that remains--and I don't
think anyone of us has the answer--is, should we make an
all-out effort to clear up the vitamin E story; and if we
do so, what probability do we have that we make significant
observations in this area?   Again we come back to the initial
finding of decreased ALA synthetase activity in the erythrocytes of patients in comparison to controls; if this is so,
we should perhaps propose some sort of hypothesis as to how
such a decreased enzyme activity is compatible with a lack
of anemia and yet still does produce the disease.

Dr. Nair: We have to, first of all, look at heme synthesis
starting with the bone marrow--the stem cells of the bone
marrow.   It's quite possible that in the bone marrow and in
the stem cells there is adequate synthesis of heme, and there
is an adequate amount of ALA synthetase.   But with maturation
and release into the peripheral circulation, the half-life
of the enzyme might be affected, but by the time we get the
peripheral blood the level of ALA synthetase might be so low
as not to be detected.   The point is, what is the half-life
of ALA synthetase in the bone marrow and peripheral cells
of these patients?   It's quite likely that this is a totally
different type of ALA synthetase with a different half-life,
so it's quite possible that we would not find any anemia be-

148

cause of the significant decrease of half-life of the enzyme.

Dr. Kolodny: Would the findings with which we are all familiar regarding lead poisoning be of any help to us here? Dr. Siakotos has referred to the levels of certain metal cations that he found in pigment fractions from the tissues of patients with Batten's disease. In patients with lead poisoning there is an elevation in urinary excretion of δ-aminolevulinic acid. It is possible that the metal cations which accumulate in the pigment in this disease in some analogous way inhibit the activity of the ALA synthetase.

Dr. Nair: I would imagine that it would be much more pronounced as far as ALA dehydratase is concerned, as that is the enzyme which is directly inhibited by lead in plumbism. There are very few data on the effects of these cautions on ALA synthetase, so this is something that will have to be studied.

Dr. Philippart: Dr. Nair, could you tell us what's known about possible inhibitors of ALA synthetase?

Dr. Nair: It depends on which tissue we are talking about. For instance, ALA synthetase, from what we know at the moment, is a conglomeration of proteins with different catalytic properties and also different responses to various inhibitors. For instance, there is a clear demarcation between the ALA synthetase in hematopoietic cells and ALA synthetase in nonhematopoietic cells in the adult animal.

Dr. Witting: One point you didn't bring out when you were talking about the control exerted by heme compounds on lipid peroxidation in terms of destruction of peroxide--Paul McCay's data[36] come from the other angle; he considers the role of heme compounds in the degeneration of lipid peroxides. One might almost say that the decrease in heme synthesis in vitamin E animals could be related defensively to a necessity to reduce the activity of the mixed function oxidase system, which we would say generates most of the vitamin E requirement by leaking free radicals.

Dr. Nair: Microsomal drug-metabolizing enzymes are heme-dependent, and cytochrome P-450 is the functional component of microsomal mixed-function oxidases. There is direct evidence to show that in vitamin E deficiency there is not only a decreased level of cytochrome P-450, but there is also a decreased synthesis of its heme component.

Dr. Witting: McCay[37] suggested in one of his papers that perhaps one of the main functions of vitamin E in vivo was to act as a trap for the free radicals leaked from the mixed-function oxidase system, and that this--the leakage from this system--was a major source of lipid peroxidation. The cytochrome P-450 is an essential component of the mixed function oxidase system. Now if the animals become vitamin E-deficient then, they would be less able to cope with the leakage from this mixed-function oxidase system. Would it not therefore be reasonable to decrease the synthesis and lower the activity of the mixed-function oxidase system?

Dr. Nair: Yes, I assume it would be possible to lower leakage, but that's not what we find in our experimental situation.

Dr. Witting: Well, if you have less P-450 you'd have less mixed-function oxidase activity and presumably less leakage.

Dr. Nair: Apparently the protein is still there. It's not conjugated with heme. Do we know what the protein is doing?

Dr. Witting: Well, obviously we don't.

Dr. Zeman: Very well, the possibilities are many. Before we ever develop any testable hypothesis, we have to gain a firmer understanding as to how ALA synthetase and related enzymes behave in a variety of tissues, including erythrocytes, bone marrow, perhaps brain and liver. We will make such tissues available to Dr. Nair, according to his specifications, both from human and animal sources. The other question I have is what do we know about ALA synthetase in the Drosophila?

Dr. Nair: I don't know anything about that.

Dr. Zeman: Well, we have a Drosophila specialist here, Dr. Miquel, who, contrary to our observation, has been able to document that vitamin E does increase longevity in Drosophila. The most fascinating aspect of these observations is that the age pigment in Drosophila is not lipofuscin but rather ceroid, according to Dr. Siakotos' standards. I should also point out that Dr. Miquel tests the aging process not by the development of gray hair, which Drosophilae do not develop, but by monitoring the mating ability of these little creatures, for which he has devised a very ingenious test. I understand you cannot apply the test, Dr. Miquel; it has to be done by your female technician, is that correct?

Dr. Miquel: Right, right. We have one day of sex activities per week and we believe that mating is a very interesting parameter in gerontological studies. In previous investigations, life span has been the only endpoint, and the physiological condition of the animals has been ignored. However, it is well known that a reduction in metabolic rate or reduced

food intake may prolong life at the expense of decreased physiological performance. In our own investigations we rule out
undesirable physiological reactions by monitoring the negative
geotaxis and the mating and fertility of male flies.

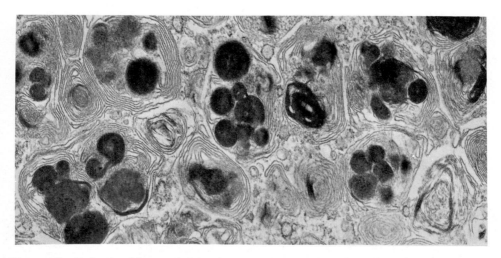

Figure 8. Splenic littoral histiocytes containing lamellated cytoplasmic
inclusions of ceroid X 21,000. From Miquel et al.[38]

For the benefit of those who were not here last year,
I will say that the connection between Batten's disease and
our Drosophila work is that we have been fortunate enough
to find in old flies tremendous amounts of a pigment which,
according to Dr. Tappel and Dr. Siakotos, is related to mammalian lipofuscins and ceroids. To document this point, I
will show an electron micrograph (Fig. 8) of spleen of a
patient suffering from "ceroid accumulation disease". As
you can see, the abundant dense bodies are somewhat similar
in structure to the "ceroid" pigment in the intestinal cells
of old Drosophila (Fig. 9).

Since our strain of Drosophila lives only about 4 months,
we can easily obtain old specimens for investigation of the
genesis and biochemistry of the "age pigments" present in
the various tissues. In view of the fact that fluorescent
molecular damage is particularly intense in the mammalian
testes, we are paying special attention to the reproductive
organs of Drosophila. Figure 10A shows a cross section of

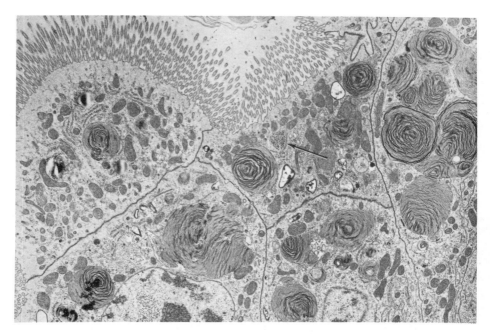

Figure 9. Mid-gut cell of an 84-day-old <u>Drosophila</u> showing numerous dense bodies somewhat similar to those of Figure 8. X 6,400.

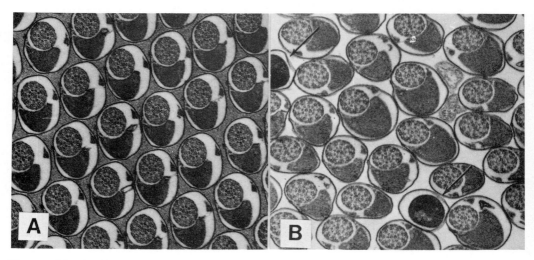

Figure 10. A. Spermatozoa in the vas deferens of a 7-day-old fly. This electron micrograph shows a cross section of the flagellum and of the mitochondrial rod. X 36,500. From Miquel et al.[38]

B. Cross section of spermatozoa in the vas deferens of an 84-day-old fly. The interstitial fluid is much less electron opaque than in the young flies. Also, some spermatozoa lack their axial filament complex (arrows) X 37,000. From Miquel et al.[38]

the sperm cells in the vas deferens of a young fly. The structures are very regular, and all the sperm tail cross-sections
are oval and about the same size. On the other hand, in old
Drosophila the arrangement of the cells is disturbed, and
occasionally the spermatozoa are lacking their axial filament
complex. In addition, the protein-rich fluid produced by
the accessory gland is absent in the old individuals (Fig.
10B). So far we have not looked at the sperm of vitamin E
treated flies. We believe that this vitamin may exert a protective action, in view of the observation that the treated
males are fertile until a more advanced age than the controls.

Dr. Zeman: For those of us who are not electron microscopists, let alone biologists, would you be good enough to
detail those structures in more specific terms?

Dr. Miquel: Okay, we have here, as I said before, a
cross section through the tail of the sperm cell. Note that
the spermatozoa have a very narrow head, unlike human spermatozoa,
which have a rather big head. It is amazing that the Drosophila
body measures only about 2 to 3 mm in length, and the spermatozoa are up to 1 mm long.

Dr. Zeman: And the tail is surrounded by a membrane?

Dr. Miquel: Yes, by a membrane--a cytoplasmic membrane,
of course. And inside we see this mitochondrion--just one--
the so-called "mitochondrial rod", and the flagellae.

Dr. Rider: Are there always two sperm cells?

Dr. Miquel: No. This is abnormal. Figure 11 shows
a pathological reaction induced by exposure of the fly to
γ-radiation. We have also investigated the effects of exposure
of the flies to high oxygen tensions and the protection afforded
by various antioxidants. Exposure during 48 hr did not change
the life span of the flies. On the other hand, longer exposure
times resulted in decreased longevity. Addition of 0.25%
of vitamin E to the medium resulted in some protection against
the oxygen toxicity. This correlates well with Dr. Tappel's
observations on the effects of vitamin E on rats exposed to
high levels of ozone.

In order to determine the physiological age of the flies
we have been using two parameters of vitality. One is "negative geotaxis", a rather involved name for a simple thing.
It is just the ability of the flies to move upwards when we
put them in a glass cylinder--a volumetric cylinder. As
you can expect, young flies tend to run or fly up very fast,
whereas old flies are rather sluggish. Our preliminary observations suggest that the decline in "negative geotaxis" appears at a more advanced age in vitamin E-treated flies.

153

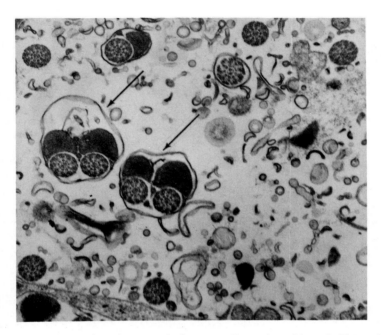

Figure 11. Spermatozoa in the vas deferens of an irradiated fly. Many
of the cell membranes are missing. Occasionally, a single
outer cell membrane is found surrounding two spermatozoa
(arrows) X 35,000. From Miquel et al.[38]

Another sensitive parameter of aging in Drosophila
is mating speed. When we house one male and three females
in a vial, the time until copulation starts is influenced
by the age of the male. When the male flies get old, even
if they keep the ability to mate, it takes them much longer
to start copulation. Male flies treated with vitamin E stay
in a better shape longer, as far as mating is concerned, and
keep producing offspring until a more advanced age.

Figure 12 shows the effects of vitamin E on Drosophila
longevity. This is part of a systematic study of the effects
of antioxidants on the aging process. So far we have checked
vitamin C, vitamin E, cysteine, methionine, glutathione, BHT,
and sodium bisulfite. We have observed extension of life
span only with vitamin E and sodium bisulfite. We could not
see any beneficial effect with vitamin C. On the other hand,
there were no toxic effects, even at doses as high as 1% of
the total food and water intake. Vitamin E, at the concentrations of 0.25% and 0.50% resulted in 12-13% increase in
both mean longevity and maximal longevity.[39] These results
are in disagreement with Harman's observations[40] on the effects

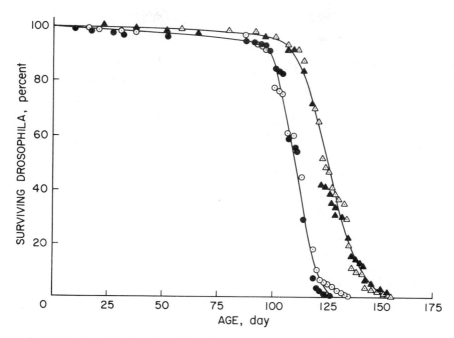

Figure 12. Effects of vitamins C and E on the longevity of adult
Drosophila melanogaster: From Miquel.[39] (o) controls;
(o) vitamin C, 0.25%; (Δ) vitamin E, 0.25%; (Δ) vitamin E,
0.50%.

of vitamin E and BHT on the longevity of the rat. In his
experiments, the antioxidants produced an increase in mean
longevity without change in maximal longevity.

Going back to our own experiments, it is interesting
to note that the extension of life span is not so marked when
vitamin E is given to the flies at the concentrations of
0.06% to 0.12%. The optimum effects are seen when the medium
contains 0.25% vitamin E, which would be equivalent to the
staggering dose of 5-10 grams for daily human consumption.
Since apparently vitamin E is not toxic, I think it would
be worthwhile to investigate the effects of very high doses
on humans, perhaps on Batten's disease patients. Obviously,
since our findings in Drosophila cannot be extrapolated to
human aging, further work on the effects of high doses of
vitamin E on experimental mammals is in order. Next month
we are going to start an experiment in which about 300 mice
are going to be treated with doses of vitamin E comparable
to those used in our Drosophila work. The cause of death
will be looked into, and we plan to perform some tests of
reproductive performance.

155

Dr. Zeman: Let me ask you one question. The per cent refers to what--the caloric intake, weight, or volume?

Dr. Miquel: The per cent refers to total food and water intake, i.e., per cent of the medium on which the flies live. In order to figure out the daily vitamin E dose for mice we disregard the body weight and food consumption. We have figured out the oxygen consumption of Drosophila, and by using this value for comparison with the oxygen consumption of a mouse, we arrived at a certain "comparable" dose of vitamin E which theoretically may afford the mouse as much protection against oxygen toxicity as the flies were getting in our experiment.

Dr. Rider: I think Dr. Zeman wanted to know whether when you said vitamin E 0.50% did you mean of the daily food weight?

Dr. Miquel: That was the percent of the food and water intake.

Dr. Rider: So it is one-half per cent of their intake.

Dr. Miquel: Of their intake, right. But by figuring out how much vitamin E the flies are taking per milliliter of oxygen we came to that tentative dose for possible human consumption.

Dr. Zeman: Thank you very much, Dr. Miquel.

Dr. Siakotos: Dr. Miquel, in Drosophila the pigment is really accumulated for the most part in the flight muscle, and the oxygen uptake of a flight muscle is very, very high, do you think it is fair to make this comparison to a human?

Dr. Miquel: Our more recent work shows pigment in every tissue of the fly.

Dr. Zeman: Have you started to collect those aged flies for us so that we can isolate the pigment?

Dr. Miquel: Well, we've been sending a few grams of old flies to Dr. Siakotos. We are saving some more.

Dr. Zeman: You mean vitamin E-treated flies?

Dr. Miquel: No, not yet. I think it would be very interesting.

Dr. Zeman: Are you collecting those?

Dr. Miquel: Not so far. You see, we have done repeated

156

experiments on the vitamin E effects on longevity to be sure that we were obtaining constant results. Now we are ready to start saving flies for the chemical studies.

Dr. Witting: When you were comparing your experiments with those of Harman[40] and Tappel[41] one of the problems that came up in those experiments was always the desire to get through the experiments a little faster and start with retired breeders or older animals. Have you, in your experiments with the flies, started at any time other than approximately birth to see if starting the treatment later had an effect?

Dr. Miquel: We are going to do that. So far we have been starting with adult flies, that's one day old, right after completion of the metamorphosis. But now we are going to take flies which are about 50 days old and see if we can still get life extension by treating them with vitamin E.

Dr. Witting: If you are going to try the mouse experiment, presumably you want inbred mice.

Dr. Miquel: We are going to use 10 to 12-month-old retired breeders and also 4-week-old male mice, probably C 57 BL/6J black mice, from the Jackson Laboratory.

Dr. Tappel: I might comment on the mouse parallel again, because it shows that chloroform-methanol-extractable fluorescent pigment increases with age. This fluorescent pigment forms primarily from membranes; it can be extracted from mouse testes, which as Dr. Miquel indicated for Drosophila and for mammals, forms the largest part of the fluorescent pigment as a function of age. The ages of the mice studied were 0.25, 0.83, and 1.9 years. The fluorescent pigment had a maximum around 430 nm. Now this is the same type of pigment that we can find in Drosophila, also in Siakotos' pigments, and in animals treated variously. The excitation spectrum is maximum around 370 nm. This allows fairly good identification of the pigment.[42] A few other criteria have been applied; for example, this type of fluorescent pigment, for which I can give you a partial structure, is not labile to ultraviolet light, whereas vitamin A is.[43] Another feature of it is that the fluorescence can be decreased by adding alkali and restored by adding acid, so we can get a partial identification by spectra and a few chemical tests; this is about as far as we've gone.

As with Dr. Miquel's experience, when we started our experiments with mice--and these were retired breeders--they already had been receiving sufficient dietary vitamin E, about 60 mg per kilogram of diet, and we had to add to their subsequent diets fairly large amounts of vitamin E, and other antioxidants, including butylated hydroxytoluene, which is synergistic with vitamin E, and sulfur amino acids, and even selenium. We aimed these studies at the question of whether or not these levels of antioxidants might be applied to the adults, and so we classified these as levels that possibly could be used. The first level (Table 8) is, for example, 1 g of vitamin E, a similar amount of C, smaller amounts of BHT, and 1 g of methionine, put on an adult human basis. For the mouse diet it's about that addition per kilogram of diet. These are higher levels up to 2 g of vitamin E and, like the level used in Harman's experiment,[40] fairly high in BHT; Harman went up to 0.5%.

| | Amt./adult/day | |
Antioxidant	Can be used now	Future application
Vitamin E	0.2-1 g	1-2 g
Vitamin C	0.2-0.7-1 g	0.2-0.7-1 g
Butylated hydroxytoluene	0.02% of fat (FDA approved)	Up to 0.2% of diet
Methionine	1 g	2 g or more
Selenium	0	0.05 ppm

Table 8. Antioxidants which may slow aging processes.

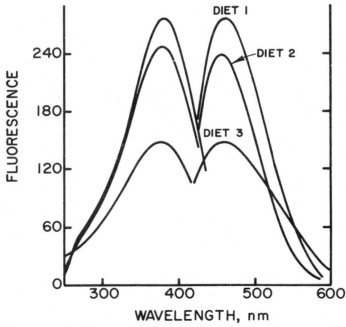

Figure 13. Fluorescent pigment extracted from mouse testes under dietary conditions given in Table 8.

Figure 13 indicates average results for the amount of
fluorescence extracted from mouse testes. We used a statistical
number of animals that had been on this diet for a year after
they were obtained as retired breeders. The highest amount
of fluorescence was found with the normal control diet. Diet
2 contained about 1 g of vitamin E/kg of diet; it produced
a small decrease in fluorescence, but it wasn't significant
because of the scatter of the data. Diet 3 produced a very
significant decrease in fluorescence; of course, this required
a huge amount of antioxidants. I guess the interpretation--
one held by, I think, Dr. Witting and myself--is that there
is probably so much slippage of peroxidation, because it is
a free-radical reaction, that peroxidation can take place
without termination by vitamin E, and so one would always
expect some peroxidation. Then, there is a very open question
I think as to what is the maximum amount of antioxidant that
one should apply to get optimum inhibition.[42]

Dr. Zeman: Dr. Tappel, thank you very much. Does the
intensity of fluorescence, which you mentioned here, follow
Beer's Law? Can we assume that this correlates with the
number of Schiff base bonds?

Dr. Tappel: Yes, exactly, right. Furthermore, there
is another interesting point, and that is the fluorescence
relates as a tracer directly to the amount of peroxidation,
so the amount of fluorescence that accumulates (and this
particularly works well for laboratory models) is directly
proportional to the amount of free-radical damage that has
taken place.

Dr. Witting: We've been running quite a few of these
fluorescent spectra lately. Your figures seem to indicate
a shift with age from an emission wavelength of 430 to 475
nm; as the amount of pigment decreases, the shift seems to
be toward 430 nm, and the higher values appear to be associated
with higher emission wavelengths. Do you have any particular
explanation of this? In other papers you've also shown doublets
with both absorption peaks present, with some absorption at
430 and some at 475 nm.

Dr. Tappel: Most of the characteristic spectra are like
this, and we haven't gone into any so-called fine interpretation, in part because of the limitation that we know it
is a mixture of pigments, probably deriving from malonaldehyde
condensing with phosphatidyl enthanolamine, but other fluorescent
pigments can be involved with the family of fluorescent chromophore groups. Also, there may be other parameters, like instrumental parameters, that could shift these peaks slightly.
Unfortunately in fluorescent spectra, although you can get
quite a bit of information out of this, the peaks are very
broad, and so we have somewhat lagged in the interpretation

of the fine changes.

Dr. Witting: You've done some synthetic work, of course, and determined the fluorescent spectra of the malonaldehyde condensation product. Have you determined the comparable spectra with the phospholipid basis?

Dr. Tappel: Yes, I have another slide in which I could show you the equivalent of that.

Dr. Witting: I was just wondering if that made a difference in the wavelength.

Dr. Tappel: Well, essentially, it doesn't. In other words, a phosphatidyl ethanolamine reactive with malonalde-hyde, such as would form in the peroxidation of phospholipids, will have fluorescence spectra essentially like those for the malonaldehyde-amino acid Schiff base.

Dr. Zeman: Now, we turn our attention to another aspect, which is in keeping with what was mentioned earlier; namely, that we must be prepared that a variety of different metabolic defects may trigger the peroxidation of unsaturated fatty acids, and Dr. Philippart is going to address himself to this problem. Before we ask him to present his observations, I would like a very brief discussion on the following problem. As you know, Recknagel[44] and Smith and Packer[45] described an enzyme called malonaldehyde oxidase. Dr. Arnason, of the University of Tennessee, has been working with this enzyme, and he feels that the enzyme is really much more active than Recknagel has found. He has come to realize that the limited activities which Recknagel described are apparently due to a poisoning of the enzyme system by its product, malonic acid. Besides the in vitro assay he finds that after a relatively slow period of 20-30 min the reaction comes to a standstill with more than 60% of the substrate not being oxidized. This raises the question as to whether malonaldehyde oxidase would be an enzyme to look at from the point of view that its de-ficiency could conceivably sustain lipid peroxidation at a rate that would be damaging to the cell because it exceeds its rate of repair. Perhaps Dr. Tappel can make a few remarks as to that fact.

Dr. Tappel: Yes, I'd like to, and perhaps I can illustrate the stoichiometry of the situation. What Dr. Zeman was bring-ing up related to the fact that malonaldehyde is formed as one of the products of the free-radical peroxidation of polyun-saturated lipids. One mechanism for malonaldehyde is in peroxidation itself, and in last year's symposium, for example, Ingold showed[46] how that was a likely possibility; the other source would be the decomposition of peroxides. It turns out that malonaldehyde is biochemically downstream from the damaging

160

reaction; so although it itself is a damaging species, I'm
sure it's not the most critical one. Then, also, the stoichiometry indicates that you can have, for membranes with the
usual composition of polyunsaturated fatty acids, something
like ten peroxidations with the formation of one equivalent
of malonaldehyde. This goes further in reactions like this,
if it's not used up by the oxidase system, and forms fluorescent
products which again are tracers downstream.

Figure 14 shows what this might be like in membrane
damage: peroxidation can be sweeping through the polyunsaturated
lipids in a membrane structure.[47] The peroxidation reaction
translates through the membrane, leaving peroxide (or hydroxide if it undergoes cleavage), and does a great deal of damage
without much production of malonaldehyde, though the key to
the question you raised is largely one of stoichiometry.
Malonaldehyde is only what might be considered one of the
semi-major products, and it's a good indicator of lipid peroxidation, but the damage has already taken place before it's
formed.

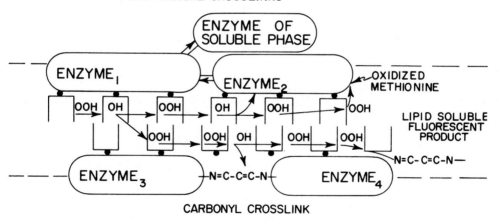

Figure 14. Schematic representation of peroxidation damage to membrane.

Dr. Zeman: Thank you. This is a very convincing argument.
Let me ask you this. If I'm not mistaken, the Schiff base
crosslinking reaction is, for all we know, an irreversible
reaction. Can we say the same about the peroxidation reaction
on proteins?

Dr. Tappel: Yes, that's right.

Dr. Zeman: In other words, if an enzyme molecule is
hit by a peroxide or hydroperoxy radical, it is inactivated
once and forever.

161

Dr. Tappel: Yes. For example, this illustrates a case that has been studied. A peroxidation translating through a membrane hits an enzyme, causes a free-radical abstraction of hydrogen, and that causes a free-radical chain reaction, polymerizing enzymes, so that the enzymes would be, in effect, covalently linked and inactivated (at least partially) for-ever. Then they would be abnormal. Another reaction has been studied: if the free radical hits some labile amino acid in an enzyme, it would oxidize into a new product--like oxidation of methionine--and that would be irreversible and presumably would not be repaired; the whole enzyme would have to be turned over.

Dr. Zeman: One further question. You reported membrane aggregation, for example, of mitochondrial and lysosomal membranes and of endoplasmic reticulum by malonaldehyde, and you found that this reaction would inactivate two moles of membranes equivalents per mole malonaldehyde.

Dr. Tappel: It could, right.

Dr. Zeman: Now what is the yield for hydroxyl radicals and other products of peroxidation?

Dr. Tappel: This, in part, hasn't been put on a very strong stoichiometric basis. Well, if you look at a hundred peroxidations, and Dr. Witting might check me on this, I imagine most of them would take place within the lipid and so damage the lipid, and only very few would in fact hit an enzyme. Now, when this is done in model systems, the highest yield would normally be two moles of enzyme inactivated per hundred peroxidations. So you damage a lot of the internal membrane lipids but not so many of the enzymes.

Dr. Zeman: It would take three hundred peroxidation events to produce one molecule of malonaldehyde?

Dr. Tappel: Well, one fluorescent crosslink. We also get malonaldehyde by reacting just with one amino group, but that doesn't produce fluorescence.

Dr. Zeman: Yes, it has to be the Schiff base, the imino-amino propene linkage.

Dr. Tappel: Right.

Dr. Philippart: What is the main source of malonaldehyde in normal circumstances?

Dr. Tappel: Well, unless it's formed metabolically, it's mostly scission products from peroxidation.

162

Dr. Witting: In December, at the New York Academy of Science Symposium on vitamin E, Barber[48] said that he had measured the activity of some of these dimeric and trimeric enzyme products and found that they still had a fair amount of residual enzyme activity.

Dr. Tappel: You still can have residual activity--that's right. What Dr. Witting is saying is entirely correct. In this model, although three enzymes might be crosslinked, they are not necessarily inactivated, so they can have some residual activity; one might have 20%, one 50%, and one 90%.

Dr. Zeman: How about enzymes having three and four crosslinks by a Schiff base?

Dr. Tappel: Again, they might have some residual activity. But they are all abnormal, so I imagine the cell would try to turn them over fast, also the damage is inside the membrane.

Dr. Witting: We looked at this type of reaction in a solution of a pure protein and a lipid hydroperoxide and found that usually there were specific lysine residues that were most susceptible to attack. Presumably, then, it would depend on the active site within the enzyme, whether it was near or distant from these lysines that were most susceptible to attack by the lipid hydroperoxide.

Dr. Tappel: Right, these nitrogens are presumably ε-amino groups of lysine; they're the most susceptible.

Dr. Wherrett: How much of the malonaldehyde generated can be volatilized, or is it a volatile product?

Dr. Tappel: You mean, like in a model system?

Dr. Wherrett: Yes.

Dr. Tappel: Yes, there are some papers, for example, one by Tarladgis,[49] which report malonaldehyde determination by distillation, so from biochemical products it can be volatilized.

Dr. Wherrett: Isn't malonaldehyde something that's picked up in the breath?

Dr. Tappel: I think there is sufficient evidence that one might pursue: I don't remember any specific papers. I believe that the plant biochemists have picked up products of lipid peroxidation, just as volatile, by GLC, so I think it would be good to pursue because of the high sensitivity of GLC.

163

Dr. Zeman: I take it from what you say that it may not be profitable to invest effort or time in malonaldehyde oxidase.

Dr. Tappel: That would be my feeling. Malonaldehyde certainly is useful as a measure of lipid peroxidation, so that might be pursued, and you do have to take account of the malonaldehyde oxidase system. In terms of stopping the damage, however, you really want to operate at the point of breaking the free-radical chain reaction. You may remember at last year's Batten's Disease Symposium, Ingold[46] was also very strong on that point.

Dr. Zeman: Thank you very much. Another possible mechanism which could trigger lipid peroxidation is suggested by the observation of Hagberg, Sourander, and Svennerholm[50] on one patient with ceroid-lipofuscinosis or Batten's disease. They found an unusually low concentration of long-chain ω : 3-fatty acids. They proposed that something was wrong with the chain-lengthening mechanism of ω:3-fatty acids which would produce high concentrations of linoleic acid, which in turn should trigger lipid peroxidation. This was the argument and, on the strength of these observations, some people have been looking at the fatty acid moieties of structural glycolipids in these disorders. Berra[51] from Milan has found that 50% of the fatty acid moiety of gangliosides in a case of neuronal ceroid lipofuscinosis consisted of linoleic acid.

Dr. Philippart: He found that in Kufs' disease only.

Dr. Zeman: In Kufs' disease, yes. Has he looked at other cases?

Dr. Philippart: Yes.

Dr. Zeman: Well, perhaps this is a good opportunity for Dr. Philippart to make some comments. I should mention that Dr. Philippart was the one who developed the procedures for culturing brain cells from patients with Batten's disease. He used his ingenuity to obtain viable preparations amenable to chemical studies.

Dr. Philippart: Thank you, Dr. Zeman. Just to close briefly on what I just said about Kufs' disease, we have studied one biopsy obtained from Dr. Martin at the Institute BUNGE. On the strength of the communication last summer of Dr. Bruno Berra, we have checked the ganglioside pattern. We had done that repeatedly in the past without finding anything abnormal, but that was the first case of Kufs' disease on which we had a frozen biopsy; the material previously studied was formalinized and thus practically useless. But in the case we are now studying the ganglioside distribution is markedly abnormal. In gray and white matter there is a large

164

increase in G_{D1b}. We have not found linoleic acid in these gangliosides as reported by Berra.[51] This is the first time I have seen such an unusual ganglioside distribution; I don't know if this is the primary disorder. Linoleic acid is a minor species which accounts for less than 1% of the total fatty acids in the brain and has never been reported in gangliosides. Linoleic acid would be highly susceptible to peroxidation.

The study I am going to present was devised to overcome the limitations of lipid analysis on either autopsy or biopsy material, in which lipid and ganglioside distribution has been repeatedly proven to be normal. We have developed a method to study lipid turnover in brain explants.

The experimental outline is shown in Figure 15. We use

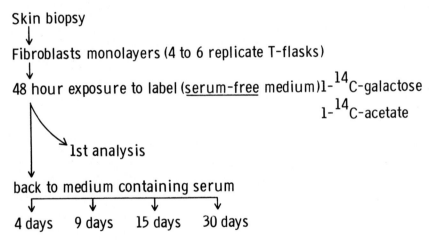

Figure 15. Experimental outline for the study of lipid turnover in brain explants.

the same scheme for skin fibroblasts and for brain. The main difference, of course, is that in the brain explant most of the cells do not divide. For the brain, we use a medium which inhibits fibroblast growth. We try to get T-flasks with a good monolayer of either fibroblasts or brain cells, and each flask contains a little less than two million cells, on average. We have confirmed the work done at the Wistar Institute[52] which showed that lipid in the growth medium will markedly depress lipid synthesis in the cells. This was shown in fibroblasts by Bailey,[52] and we were able to confirm that in brain explant.[53] Up to 95% of lipid synthesis in brain explant may be depressed by using serum as a medium. To overcome that problem we have developed conditions in which there is no serum. Another hurdle, however, is that cells from pathological samples

are more delicate than normal controls. They are more likely
to die or not to grow very well or survive for a lesser period
than normal brain explants. We have limited the exposure
to a labeled precursor to 48 hrs, and in this condition we
get good survival. These cells are incubated in a serum-
free medium which contains a high amount of glucose, which
is necessary for the brain. This precludes the use of
^{14}C-glucose, which is the best precursor of lipids in most
tissues, including brain. Under these circumstances, there
would be such a dilution of labeled glucose that it would
not be practical to use it in that type of experiment. For
that reason we have used mostly ^{14}C-acetate, which has the
advantage of being incorporated not only into lipids, but
also into mucopolysaccharides, and so on. We have also used
leucine, because protein metabolism has never been explored
in patients with all the variants of Batten's disease. We
used ^{32}P for exploring phospholipid metabolism. We have also
tried labeled triglyceride and a few other precursors. ^{14}C-
Galactose is an excellent precursor of glycolipids which in
the brain are cerebroside, sulfatide, and, to a lesser extent,
gangliosides. After 48 hrs in the serum-free medium, we analyze
the first batch of cells, and all the other flasks are returned
into a medium containing serum for different times, up to
6 weeks, or even longer. All brain experiments have been
done in duplicate.

The cells are first washed with isotonic saline to remove the labeled precursor which has not been incorporated.
No chemical is used for the extraction. Most enzymes used
to detach cells from the T-flasks contain carbohydrates which
interfere with further analysis so we add no chemicals or
enzymes. We just scrape the cells and then extract them with
distilled water by repeated freezing and thawing. On that
extract we can measure lysosomal hydrolases as well as the
radioactivity. Next, the cells are extracted with chloroform:
methanol (2:1) and we get the total lipids. Some of the lipids
were already extracted by the distilled water, but since we
fractionate the water extract with TCA we recover these lipids
and pool them with the total lipids. Finally, the insoluble
residue is dissolved in 1N sodium hydroxide, so that we have
an overall picture of the distribution of the radioactivity
in the whole explant.

We studied a brain explant from a Negro patient with
what we have to call, on a morphological basis, lipofuscinosis.
The patient had a sister similarly affected. Clinically,
they were typical for Spielmeyer-Vogt. The electron microscopy--
I don't have a picture of it here--was done by Dr. Cancilla
at UCLA, and all neurons and astrocytes were loaded with something that looked like pure lipofuscin in all sections. We
did not find much lipofuscin elsewhere. We studied skin
fibroblasts on these patients, but there was no accumulation

166

of lipofuscin there.

Dr. Siakotos: Are those lipid bodies, or are they crystal-line in structure?

Dr. Philippart: No, they're amorphous; they look like drops of oil.

Dr. Siakotos: Like drops of oil; but lipofuscins or ceroids don't look like drops of oil.

Dr. Philippart: Well, I'm not an EM specialist, so take my description for what it is worth. I was told it was typical lipofuscin by Dr. Cancilla. There were no lamellae, no finger-print, no curvilinear bodies.

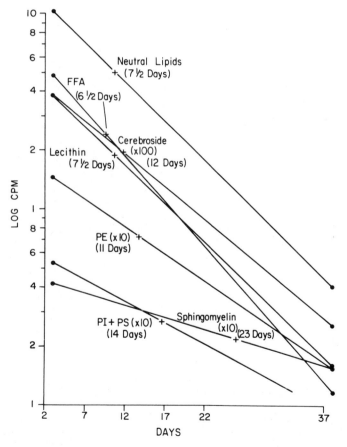

Figure 16. Half-lives of lipids in normal brain explants.

167

Figure 16 shows the lipid half-lives in a normal brain explant. This was obtained from a patient who was lobectomized for schizophrenia; he was 25 years old. All lipids were separated by thin-layer chromatography into 17 different species, including neutral lipids, glycolipids, gangliosides, and phospholipids. The lipid half-life under these conditions, with the use of ^{14}C-acetate, is 1-2 weeks. Sphingomyelin has a slower turnover of about 3 weeks.

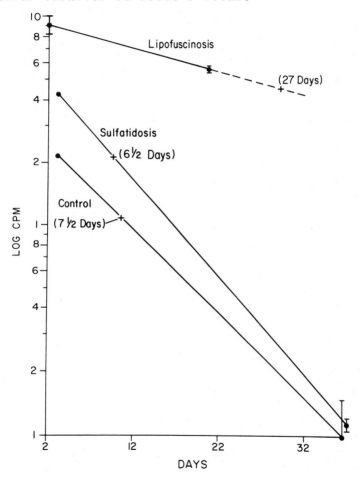

Figure 17. Half-lives of total lipid incorporated into brain explants from two lysosomal diseases.

Figure 17 shows the half-life of the total lipid fraction. In the control, the total half-life of the labeled lipids was 7 1/2 days. In a case of metachromatic leukodystrophy (sulfatidosis) it was quite comparable to the normal control,

168

and in the case of lipofuscin storage it was markedly increased (27 days).

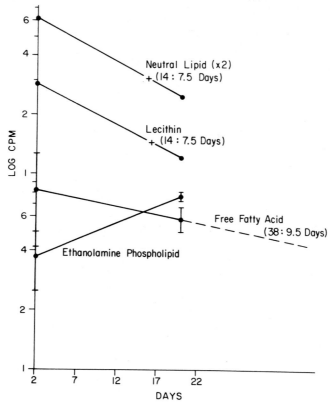

Figure 18. Half-lives of lipids in brain explants. Lipofuscinosis vs. control.

Now after fractionating the different lipids, we found (Fig 18) that most species, neutral lipids, phospholipids, and free fatty acid, have a markedly delayed turnover; ethanolamine phospholipid has an activity which goes up for 3 weeks, after which time the cells died.

We tried to check these findings in fibroblasts, but we did not find anything very striking. Figure 19 shows the distribution among the three main lipid classes: phospholipids, neutral lipids, and glycolipids. In a normal control, you have about 80% of the ^{14}C-acetate in phospholipids. This proportion was slightly decreased in the lipofuscinosis case, but this is probably not significant. However, the neutral lipids, which accounted for 15-20% of the total label in the lipids, were slightly increased in the lipofuscinosis case.

169

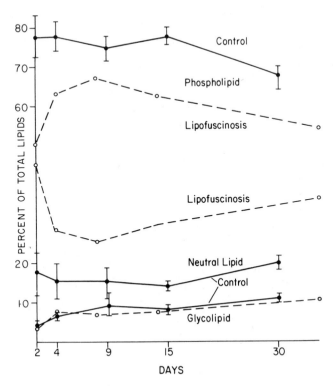

Figure 19. Incorporation of ^{14}C-acetate into lipid fractions from fibroblasts.

This correlated well with the electron microscopic appearance
of the cells, which showed an accumulation of triglyceride
in the fibroblasts. This, in fact, may be considered an
artificial situation. Most fibroblasts, if they are not
healthy or become old in culture, will tend to accumulate
triglyceride; this has been shown repeatedly by several workers
in the past decade, but nobody has offered a good explanation
for this phenomenon. What is unusual here is that we are
dealing with a young culture. We have obtained similar results
with fibroblasts of other types of lipid storage disorders,
such as Fabry's, Gaucher's or Niemann-Pick. All these lines
contain a larger amount of triglyceride and neutral lipids
than normal ones. This is probably an incidental finding
in these lipid disorders, but this may be significant in the
lipofuscin storage. However, there was no lipofuscin in these
fibroblasts, just oily droplets which were pure triglyceride.
It is possible to separate these oily droplets by ultracentrifugation and show that 90% of the lipids there are triglycerides.
If you incubate these cells with labeled triglyceride there
is little incorporation of the label into other lipids. The

glycolipid fraction in fibroblasts is a minor one; it accounts
for less than 10% of the total lipid. The distribution of
the different lipid classes remains quite constant over a
period of one month or even longer.

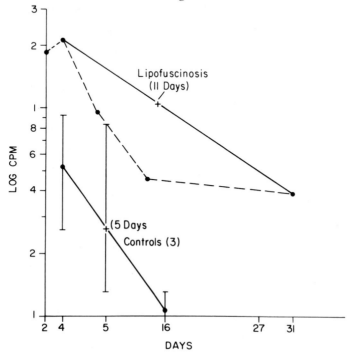

Figure 20. Half-life of acetate-1-^{14}C-free fatty acids.

Figure 20 shows the half-life of free fatty acid in the
fibroblasts from the patient with lipofuscinosis. Again we
found a slight delay, since it was 5 days in controls and
11 days in lipofuscinosis. Despite widespread variations
in the normal controls, this is comparable to our findings
in the brain, and on this basis, it may be significant.

In the brain, there was an increase of ethanolamine
phospholipids over a 3-week period. In fibroblasts (Fig.21)
there is a markedly decreased turnover, 21 days in the lipofuscinosis case against 6 days in the controls, but again
the controls have quite a large range of variation. This
recalls what we observed in the brain.

^{32}P incorporation was studied to check further the metabolism of the phospholipids. In controls, the lecithin activity
expressed as per cent of the total lipid count decreased regularly

171

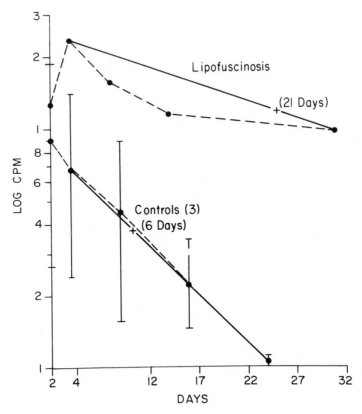

Figure 21. Half-lifes of acetate-1-^{14}C in ethanolamine phospholipid.

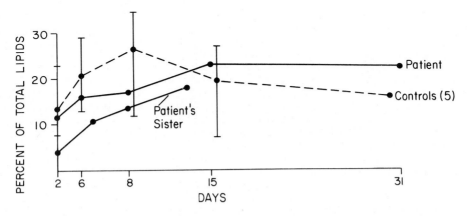

Figure 22. ^{32}P incorporation into ethanolamine phospholipid of fibroblasts.

over time, while during the first weeks sphingomyelin and
ethanolamine phospholipids increased slightly and then reached
a plateau for several weeks. In two patients with lipofuscinosis, there was no significant difference compared to the
controls. There was a slight delay in incorporation into
ethanolamine phospholipids, the maximum being reached only
after two weeks instead of one (Fig. 22).

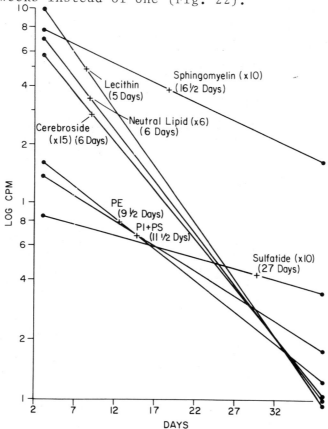

Figure 23. Half-lives of various lipids in brain explants from sulfatidosis.

In another type of lipid storage disease, metachromatic
leukodystrophy, which results from an impairment in the metabolism of sulfatide, all lipid half-lives are within normal
limits (Fig. 23), and only the sulfatide has a markedly
increased turnover, which is 27 days instead of the normal
8 to 9 days. Thus, here the block in the degradation of one
lipid species has no obvious effect on the metabolism of all
the other lipids. Of course, the sulfatide metabolism in
older patients or normal people after 2 years of age is quite

slow. Such patients may live for several decades with this
relatively minor impairment.

These findings explain why, in spite of the fact that
pathologists repeatedly showed there was lipidlike material
in the neurons of patients with Batten's disease, there is
no given accumulation of any specific lipid. Although lipids
are not normally turned over, the overall lipid pattern remains
unchanged. Such slowed turnover might explain why some of
the lipids which are not digested accumulate inside the lysosomes. These lipids could be more susceptible to oxidation
than they are within the original membrane. The fact that
we could not find striking abnormalities in the fibroblasts
emphasizes the fact that if we want to understand what is
going on we have to study the brain, at least for the time
being. This is a subtle disturbance, difficult to pinpoint.
Therefore I am trying to obtain more brain explants from other
patients. We had one patient with a typical curvilinear
variety, and we didn't find anything similar to this. At
least we now have some clues as to what might be going on
in these disorders.

Dr. Zeman: Thank you, Dr. Philippart.

Dr. Rider: Just a quick question on how difficult it
is to do these brain cultures. Does the culture maintain
its integrity long enough for you to do something, or does
it very quickly revert to a fibroblastic stage, where you
might say it's really not the same cell you have in the disease?

Dr. Philippart: No, the medium we use is specifically
designed to inhibit fibroblast growth, and generally we can
maintain explants with a healthy appearance for at least
two months. In that specific case I showed you we had obtained
from 100 mg of brain biopsy 36 T-flasks on which we could
experiment with a variety of labeled precursors. It is possible
to make very detailed lipid analyses and some enzyme studies.
Of course, when you can pinpoint some problem in lipids, you
can decide what enzyme you are going to study. We are studying
some phospholipid transferase, and so on. We have isolated
all the different lipid species, and we will make detailed
fatty acid analysis if needed. Of course, this is time-consuming
work.

Dr. Rider: I think this is a really tremendous approach
to the problem, because if this is true then you have almost
an unlimited source once you get the culture growing. I
don't know if you're familiar with the work of Menkes.[54]
I have a manuscript here which I don't think has been published.
I'm not an expert in this particular field; and, whether you
are familiar with it or not, you might take a quick look at

174

the discussion and summary and see how it fits into your work.

Dr. Philippart: Menkes' work has been focused on fatty acid uptake by brain explant. Mead's group[55] has shown that if you administer labeled free fatty acid, a fraction of a per cent will be taken up by the brain. We don't know exactly where it goes; most of it might very well remain in the vessel walls. Nobody has proven that it reaches the brain cells.

Dr. Rider: You might take a look at this discussion here--it's just a very short piece. I don't think that it has been published yet; he just sent it to me.

Dr. Philippart: This work on linoleic acid has been presented at the New York Symposium on Sphingolipid Storage Disorders.[54] It's not very convincing, since there was no significant difference between the controls and the brain of some of these patients.

Dr. Rider: Is it true then, from what you've shown here, that you feel that the cells do not handle some of these lipids.

Dr. Philippart: Yes, this suggests a phenomenon entirely different from the classical lysosomal disorders. By definition a lysosomal disorder is secondary to a specific enzyme deficiency. This causes an accumulation of one or several closely related components.[56] In lipofuscinosis, all lipids are involved, and no single hydrolase deficiency could account for that. However, this may result from either a single abnormality in the lysosomal membrane or in a switching mechanism. The one-gene one-enzyme hypothesis would thus be respected.

Dr. Rider: You still would have one basic enzyme that then affects the whole chain of things.

Dr. Philippart: Yes, the whole chain of things. It's difficult to understand why only lipid metabolism is involved here.

Dr. Zeman: Dr. Philippart, would your observation and data be in agreement with the assumption that some of these lipids, for which you have shown a considerably increased half-life, could be fixed in situ by crosslinkage and poly-merization on account of a peroxidation type of reaction?

Dr. Philippart: I don't think my data indicate that, but these lipids might be exposed to peroxidation. Of course, I am studying pure lipid species which have been fractionated. If they are bound together, it's in a loose fashion because we can separate them very easily. We did not find any evidence of denaturation or peroxidation.

175

Dr. Zeman: Oh, yes, I understand that.

Dr. Tappel: I think you probably are familiar with the various programs on cell type WI-38 which is used in cellular aging studies. It's been reviewed by Cristofalo[57] particularly, and one of the generalities that develops here is that there is a large increase in lipids as you go through cell passages-- in other words, related to cell aging. I believe that most of this work has been done by Kritchevsky.[58]

Dr. Philippart: In this case it's mostly triglycerides and, of course, in the brain you have very little triglyceride, all of which might derive from the vessels.

Dr. Tappel: Another characteristic of this so-called cellular aging, which is really increase in passage level, is a large increase in lysosomes, and this seems to be one of the dominant features relating to the decline of this cell population.

Dr. Wherrett: This postulate of decreased turnover of multiple lipids is out of keeping with your observation yesterday, Dr. Zeman, of increased metabolic rate in these patients in later stages.

Dr. Philippart: Well, not necessarily. The lipid metabolism is only a small part of the overall metabolism. It would be interesting to investigate how these patients use their energy.

Dr. Rider: I thought that one of the reasons for the increased metabolism is that it takes much more effort for them to do things. I think you can burn up a lot of energy just holding the muscles rigid. If you hold them rigid all day, when you move it's harder for you to move.

Dr. Zeman: Yes, I think we should not jump to conclusions because after all, as Dr. Philippart pointed out, the lipid metabolism is a relatively small part of the entire energy turnover in the body which, with respect to the brain, has a power rating of 20 watts, or something like this, in comparison to some 150 watts for the entire body at rest.

Dr. Desnick: Dr. Philippart might like to obtain brain tissue from classic cases in order to utilize his technique, to provide further understanding of the lipid metabolism in the brain cells of these patients. We should attempt to make appropriate tissue available to him. I would like to know if you've measured some of the various hydrolytic enzymes, and if enzymatic activities change with time in tissue culture.

Dr. Philippart: We determined about ten different lysosomal hydrolases--not only in brain, but also in fibroblasts, urine, and plasma. We didn't find any convincing abnormalities. It's not strictly normal; some enzymes are increased, and some are decreased. One of the main problems with lysosomal hydrolases, in human studies at least, is the wide range of normal activity which varies from 30% to 250% of the mean. It's very difficult to accumulate enough data for each patient to show a statistically significant difference. Another problem is to get reproducible protein determination in fibroblasts. If part of the fibroblasts stick to the wall, you might get falsely high specific activities. We are trying to standardize these techniques, but we are not yet too successful.

Dr. Zeman: I would like to focus the discussion on the determinants for the half-lives of lipids. Do we know anything about it? I mean, we accept the fact that we can measure half-lives of certain molecular species or subcellular organelles, but what is really the determining factor for the half-life. Do we know that?

Dr. Philippart: This is a complex question. My speculation is that most membranes are randomly engulfed into lysosomes which digest them entirely. Although this has never been emphasized by de Duve, who developed the lysosome theory, I think the normal turnover, to a large extent, results from the entrapment of all organelles and all parts of the cell cytoplasm in lysosomes where they are digested. If this holds true, it is a very neat mechanism to account for the fact that a wide variety of cell lipids and proteins are properly turned over, despite an enormous range of concentration. If a precise control of the degradation were to take place in situ, it is hard to imagine how the precise ratio of the hydrolytic enzymes could be maintained and constantly adjusted to the local needs. The problem of degradation is clearly different from the problem of synthesis. Most synthesis takes place in the microsomes, where controls such as feedback inhibition are known to occur. Membrane synthesis is probably directed by the availability of specific sites on specific membrane protein. If the membrane to be degraded is taken up as a whole by lysosomes (and we have some evidence to show that this might be the case[59]), we do not need to have precise adjustment of different hydrolases. The lysosomes possess an extensive battery of hydrolytic enzymes which share common properties such as acid optimum pH and resistance to cell proteases. In Niemann-Pick disease Type A, for example, sphingomyelin accumulates as a result of a profound sphingomyelinase deficiency, but other substances such as glycolipids that the tissue can degrade in vitro are also stored.[10] When a given lysosomal enzyme is deficient, we frequently observe that besides the corresponding substrate, other substances

also accumulate despite the presence of normal amounts of
enzymes capable to degrade them. Inhibitors may play a role
there. For example, it has recently been shown[60] that myoinositol
is a powerful inhibitor of α-galactosidase; there may be other
similar examples. I have the feeling that the decreased activity
of a few lysosomal hydrolases in the mucopolysaccharide storage
diseases may reflect such a type of inhibition.[61] In tissue
culture if you incubate your cells with mucopolysaccharides,
you will depress hyaluronidase activity; you can do that in
a test tube, too.[62] That type of situation is not likely
to be found in normal circumstances, where you have relatively
small amounts of material which are easily digested. Once
a storage process has been initiated, however, secondary phenomena may occur, such as peroxidation or physical interaction
of lipids on each other.[63] Under these circumstances a substrate
will not be easily available to the corresponding enzyme,
or the enzyme substrate interaction may become less than optimal.
Abnormal granules will be formed, and substances which could
be digested by the lysosome if they were accessible will pile
up. All electron microscopic evidence points to the reality
of such phenomena.

Dr. Tappel: I would like to reinforce what Dr. Philippart
just said. The lysosomes contain the apparatus for turnover
of membranes. In model systems we have studied the turnover
of myelin, the endoplasmic reticulum, and mitochondrial membrane, and by monitoring the total hydrolysis of protein and
lipids we found that they were in concert, both being digested
in these model studies. Another point which you mentioned,
which I think is very important, is relative to profiling
lysosomal enzymes. It is that of the diversity of the methodology and the diversity of the material, really something
that should be standardized, and it would be good if some
group did this. We came across this problem in our automated
methodology. When you standardize very well and run a profile
a multiple number of times, you can get a very high degree
of accuracy; but when you're working with random biological
samples it's much more difficult.

Dr. Siakotos: I would like to compliment you, Dr. Philippart, because in our search for other sources of ceroid, we
have had to work on the cirrhotic liver. There in the floating lipid fraction--that is, the so-called lipid droplets--
we thought we could detect quite significant changes in morphology in a cirrhotic liver as compared to a normal liver.
So your idea of changes in the metabolism of this lipid globule--
this so-called storage globule--in your system, I think, is
an excellent one. Perhaps those of us that always look at
enzymes as soluble proteins forget that really we're talking
about compartmentation and particles and membranes. I think
this is a point well put that you made.

Dr. Wherrett: I was interested in the increase in the phosphatidyl ethanolamine that you noticed.

Dr. Philippart: Yes, I'm very intrigued by that.   It's known that the main phospholipids, that is, ethanolamine and serine choline phospholipids, are closely interrelated.   We are trying to measure some of the transferases which transform them into each other.

Dr. Wherrett: I wondered if your chromatographic system separates lysobisphosphatidic acid from phosphatidyl ethanolamine?

Dr. Philippart: Yes, it does.

Dr. Wherrett: I have been interested in lysobisphosphatidic acid because we found it in patients with what is probably the Nova Scotia form of Niemann-Pick disease, which is rather similar in some ways to Batten's disease.   About the only thing that anybody has ever found is an increase in lysobisphosphatidic acid, as far as I know.   We didn't really think that this was the primary substrate for the deficient enzyme. We tried incubating abnormal and normal tissues in a medium that I think Dr. Tappel described, and just studied the breakdown of lipids in a homogenate incubated at a pH of 4.5 or so. Of course, the lipids break down very rapidly, but under those circumstances, we found that the amount of lysobisphosphatidic acid seemed to increase, at least the material that ran at that point in the chromatogram.   I have no idea how to interpret that.

Dr. Philippart: We use the bidimensional TLC system described by Rouser[64] in his first paper on lysobisphosphatidic acid accumulation in Niemann-Pick.   We can separate not only all the phospholipids that were mentioned in Rouser's paper, but also most glycolipids.

But the system, however, does not separate lysobisphosphatidic acid from the ceramide dihexoside (Fig. 24).   The turnover of lysobisphosphatidic acid seems to be active. Maximum label incorporation is found after 2 days in cultured fibroblasts.   The radioactivity goes down very quickly, even in Niemann-Pick patients where you would expect an impaired degradation because you find a net accumulation.

Dr. Wherrett: That's very interesting.   We completed a study some time ago[65] in which we examined the subcellular distribution of lysobisphosphatidic acid in rat livers, using the Trouet procedure to purify lysosomes, and we find that it's very highly concentrated in the lysosomes produced in that way, and I wonder if it doesn't play some specific role in the lysosome.

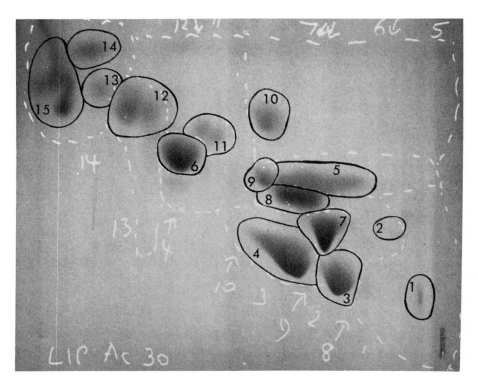

Figure 24. Separation of phospholipids. Lipids were applied as a 1-cm
            streak in lower right corner. Carrier lipids consisted of
            glycolipids isolated from erythrocytes and neutral lipids and
            phospholipids extracted from spinal cord. This mixture was
            added to an aliquot of the cell lipid fraction. The plate
            (silica gel G) was first developed in chloroform-methanol-
            water (65:25:4) in the horizontal direction. After air
            drying for 10 min, the plate was developed in 1-butanol-
            acetic acid-water (3:1:1). Lipid areas were revealed by
            exposure to iodine vapor. Circled areas (black figures)
            correspond to: (1) GM_1 ganglioside; (2) GM_3 ganglioside;
            (3) sphingomyelin; (4) lecithin; (5) phosphatidyl serine;
            (6) ethanolamine phosphoglyceride; (7) globoside; (8)
            phosphatidyl inositol; (9) trihexosyl ceramide; (10) sulfa-
            tide; (11) lactosyl ceramide; (12) galactosyl and glucosyl
            ceramide;(13) unknown; (14) free fatty acids; (15) neutral
            lipids.

     Dr. Zeman: Dr. Wherrett, did you say that the lysobi-
sphosphatidic acid is highest in the lysosome fraction of
the liver?

     Dr. Wherrett: In rat liver. It parallels acid phosphatase
very closely.

180

Dr. Zeman: What ratio of total phospholipids did you find there--about 1%?

Dr. Wherrett: It's less than 1% in the whole liver; in the lysosome it's as high as 10% or better.

Dr. Zeman: Does an increase in the number of lysosomes per unit volume of cytoplasm always imply an increase in lyso-bisphosphatidic acid?

Dr. Wherrett: That's our hypothesis at the moment. The literature doesn't support it, but we wonder how well it's been examined.

Dr. Philippart: I would not support it. As Rouser has shown[64] there is a striking accumulation in Niemann-Pick disease type A characterized by a sphingomyelinase deficiency. Since then we have been able to confirm that in seven cases of Niemann-Pick type C without sphingomyelinase deficiency. We have occasionally found a small increase, as indicated by Rouser, in all other known types of lipid storage diseases. In Tay-Sachs there is a small increase, but certainly nothing to be compared with what is found in two forms of Niemann-Pick with which I am familiar. Possibly you could show that there is a significant increase, but it's not as large as what is found in Niemann-Pick. You are probably familiar with the Yamamoto publication[66] showing that a drug which is used in Japan to control artherosclerosis includes lysobi-sphosphatidic acid storage in the liver.

Dr. Wherrett: It's true apparently of Triparanol, and of 2,2-diethylaminoethoxyhexestrol, as well.

Dr. Philippart: So it may have something to do with the lysosomal metabolism, but in Niemann-Pick disease it's not a direct reflection of the number of lysosomes.

Dr. Witting: Don't you also get an increase in the lysobis compound in the carbon tetrachloride-treated liver?

Dr. Philippart: I have never analyzed any such case.

Dr. Witting: I think there are one or two reports on that.[67]

Dr. Rider: Do we know very much about what the lipids do; I mean, is this an end product which should be gotten rid of, or is it supposed to serve some useful function? Is it part of a chain of reactions? What is the function of these various lipids that they find in the cells?

181

Dr. Zeman: I will try to answer the question as to the significance of the various lipids which Dr. Philippart has studied in his tissue cultures, though I am not a lipid chemist. There are structural lipids which form integral parts of membranes; for example, several of the gangliosides are essential in providing physiochemical characteristics to neuronal membranes, that is, membranes of neuronal somata and membranes of the synaptic vesicles, such as, for instance, disialo- and trisialo-gangliosides with the latter and monosialogangliosides in the former. Other lipids are simple precursors, and yet others are products of metabolic degradation.   It is by no means true that in lysosomal disease only structural lipids are involved. This is the case in GM_1 gangliosidosis; but, for instance, ganglioside GM_2 is probably not a structural lipid, but an intermediary. It's probably a breakdown product such as trihexoside ceramide. The lipids we are speaking about may belong to generally three classes: structural lipids, precursors, and metabolic intermediaries in the breakdown chain.

Dr. Desnick pointed out that we should make material available to Dr. Philippart for his studies. Just to reconfirm, did you say you had studied one case of Batten's disease with curvilinear bodies, but did not make the same observations as you did on the two other patients? Is that correct?

Dr. Philippart: Yes, but unfortunately we were not too successful with that specific case. We had not much material available, but fibroblasts seemed to have a normal lipid turnover. We had had ten different fibroblast lines from curvilinear patients, and we didn't find any definite abnormalities using eight different labeled precursors.

Dr. Zeman: While this is, I believe, as good a circumstantial evidence for the genetic heterogeneity of this disorder, which we have proposed for some time,[68][69] it does not absolve us from making material available to you, and perhaps you could very briefly outline in which form you wish to receive it. Would you perhaps address yourself to the possibility of the use of postmortem tissue and, if so, under what conditions? Can you utilize any biopsy tissues, and how does it have to be shipped, and how does it have to be treated before shipment, and so forth?

Dr. Philippart: To grow a brain explant successfully you have to have your technician in the operating room. We have tried a few times to ship brain biopsies, but it doesn't work as well. Regarding biopsy material, I have a large collection of small specimens which I plan to study later when it will become possible to develop a reasonable working hypothesis. Right now I concentrate on dynamic studies on brain explants. I would love to study dog cell lines. Perhaps you could ship a puppy so that we could grow brain explants under the best conditions. When we will reach a better understanding of the basic defect, when we study a few key enzymes we will take better advantage of brain biopsy or even autopsy material.

Dr. Zeman: Since Dr. Philippart mentioned the dogs, I should say that we do have a good supply of them, and we are certainly prepared to make animals available to anyone here in the audience and perhaps also to other qualified investigators.   I must point out that I have no exclusive franchise on those dogs, although we do use them according to our experimental protocol.   These dogs have been bred by Dr. Koppang at great expense, both in time and money.   It is for this reason that I ask those of you who are interested in obtaining dogs to write a letter to me for transmittal to Dr. Koppang himself who is in our laboratory, and tell him what you have in mind and ask him if you could have one of those dogs. I must emphasize that these dogs represent a considerable financial investment.

Dr. Nair: It's interesting that there is a certain amount of accumulation of lipids in these studies.   The question is: what is the total effect on the physical properties of the membranes into which they are being incorporated?   The second question is: what are the results in the increase in the different types of lipids which might alter the half-life of the membrane itself, and also the integrity of the various membranes?   Is there anything known about it in terms of physical properties and things of that sort?

Dr. Philippart: First of all, I want to emphasize that the lipid turnover which we are exploring might represent only a small pool of total activity.   If we determine the total lipid distribution in a biopsy, for example, we don't find any striking accumulation in total lipids.   Of course, there is some variation, but it is possible to get very precise figures, and we do not find any significant difference.[70] This suggests that only a small pool is involved.   The defect is compatible with a long survival.   Deleterious effects take several years to become apparent; then the neurons die one day, choked with lipids and granules which cannot be recycled.

Dr. Zeman: One of our efforts, with respect to unraveling the pathogenesis of these disorders is to devise some rational treatment.   Out of the previous symposia emerged an approach devised by Dr. Tappel, and I will briefly report on our observations.   For 21 months we have treated two siblings with the Spielmeyer-Sjögren type, giving them daily doses of 1 g of vitamin E, 0.5 g of vitamin C, 200 mg of butylated hydroxytoluene, and 1 g of DL-methionine.   I see these patients at regular intervals, and I personally have not noticed any

183

change with respect to the neurological status, the electro-
encephalographic tracings, and the general state of health.
To me it appears that these children have been relatively
stable during the entire period of treatment. I realize that
repeated neurological and neuropsychological studies and EEG
tracings do not tell you a great deal about the progression
of the disease, especially of a disease that is as disabling
as this one. On the other hand, the parents who have to cope
daily with their children are in a somewhat better position
to evaluate the evolution of the disease over a long period
of time, because they can more readily assess functionality.
They notice whether control of bowel and bladder function
become less regular and they observe the children when they
feed themselves. They assess their ability to enter into
social intercourse (other than speech, because these children
could not speak at the time we started them on treatment).
So, the only yardstick which we have so far for the efficacy
of the treatment is that the parents religiously come every
four weeks to pick up a new supply of the drugs, because we
dish them out in small quantities. Of course, this is dangerous
reasoning and I don't think it would pass the editorial board
of any journal, yet it's the only evidence we have. On the
other hand, the same type of treatment of the dogs--and these
setters, for all we know, have probably a different type of
disease which produces a phenocopy--has as yet not produced
any increase in longevity. The only statement we can make
at the present time is that there is an inverse relationship
between the age at which the treatment has been initiated
and the occurrence of clinical signs of the disease. In other
words, a dog that has been started on the treatment at 4 months
seems to come down with the disease at 16 months, whereas
a dog which has been treated beginning at age 7 months would
show first signs of the disease at about 1 year of age. These
data are preliminary and certainly not very encouraging.
We have not gone to the very high doses which Dr. Miquel has
used in his flies.

We hope that the treatment will produce better results
if started before the patients develop symptoms, or even
before pigment formation has begun. Serial brain biopsies
in dogs have conclusively shown that pigment formation begins
at or before birth as seen with the electron microscope.
At the age of 2 1/2 months pigmentation is so massive that
the pigments can be visualized by light microscopy. Inasmuch
as there seems to be some indication that once the pigments
have formed in large quantities, lipid peroxidation becomes
a self-perpetuating process, we must push for very early treatment. Therefore we have initiated experiments in which we
breed homozygous affected dogs by mating homozygous males
and females and we treat the bitches already during pregnancy.
This is one possibility, and I notice that Dr. Tappel is
going to address himself to that problem.

Dr. Rider: I'd like to ask one question. Is the female dog heterozygous?

Dr. Zeman: No, it is homozygous.

Dr. Rider: No, but I'm not talking about the puppy; I'm talking about the mother.

Dr. Zeman: Yes, the mother is homozygous.

Dr. Rider: She actually has the disease too.

Dr. Zeman: Yes.

Dr. Rider: I see, because in humans you don't have that, of course.

Dr. Zeman: No, of course not. I am not aware that the patients with Spielmeyer-Sjögren type bear children, and I have no information as to the sexual potency of the patients. What have been your personal observations? Are there erections or not?

Dr. Rider: Yes, that's true, but a child who gets the disease at 8 or 9 years of age is not going to get married.

Dr. Zeman: Well, they don't get married, but we can mate the affected dogs.

Dr. Rider: The reason I brought that up was because I thought you could postulate that there might be some protective mechanism from the mother. In humans, for example, the disease does not manifest itself until age 7 or 8 or 9 years, and presumably the brain is of normal size at birth. In other words, if there were a defect from the time of conception, maybe there is some protective mechanism from the mother that protects this brain until such time that the child is born, and then slowly the degeneration begins. However, if your dogs come from homozygotes this wouldn't fit; but then again, that doesn't mean that the dog has the same disease. The other thing is I wonder whether you really will get anywhere starting treatment when the disease is far advanced. If you started treatment before the disease began, perhaps you could prevent its beginning at all.

Dr. Zeman: This is precisely what we are now trying to find out. We do know one thing. Dr. Tappel's treatment has not produced encouraging results in the dogs, but we have not done the crucial experiment, namely, to treat the animals at a time at which lipid peroxidation is minimal or absent. He is now going to make a few remarks about this.

Dr. Rider: Well, you might decrease its production;
perhaps there is a period in which the massive production
occurs.

Dr. Zeman: That's possible. There might be a slight
retardation or slowing down in the rate of progression, but
certainly no definite arrest, let alone improvement, with
respect to the functionality of the cells.

Dr. Philippart: The question of early diagnosis would
certainly be important in such patients, especially if we
have a treatment one of these days. I wonder, Dr. Zeman,
if you have any experience with early diagnosis using electro-
retinograms. We ourselves have studied some such patients,
but it is hard to know how long in advance we would be successful. I wonder if you have any personal experience about
that.

Dr. Zeman: Early diagnosis is, of course, a relative
thing. If you have one affected child in a sibship the diagnosis in the other affected siblings could be made early during the disease, not with the help of the electroretinogram
perhaps, because that is less sensitive than visual acuity
of central vision. In the Scandinavian countries, where soc-
ialized medicine works to the benefit of the people with
genetically controlled disorders, they pick up homozygous
affecteds at a time when no physician would find anything
wrong with these children. They do this by a very careful
check of visual acuity and by a variety of neuropsychological
tests, such as have been developed here in this country by
Halstead at the University of Chicago. They uncover abnormalities which would be missed even by the most experienced
pediatric neurologist. This, in my opinion, is the only
way to ascertain homozygosity by clinical means. We have
not been able to develop convincing evidence for dosage compensation of either lymphocytic vacuolization or neutrophilic
hypergranulation, but if the enzyme data should pan out--
the ones which Öckerman reported, and which seem to be confirmed by Dr. Kolodny--I think that we must try to do needle
biopsies of livers of infants at risk with the aim to ascertain
homozygosity by enzyme determinations. Then if our dog data
would support early treatment, we will treat the homozygous
siblings at a time when they are asymptomatic.

Dr. Tappel: I'd like to indicate the rationale for
the use of this type of a mixture in humans, and then show
some models which can be used for animal experimentation which
might add to the various models that have already been presented. First of all, the mixture being used consists of
vitamin E, the main biological antioxidant which would inhibit
lipid peroxidation by a chain-breaking mechanism, and then
a food antioxidant, BHT. BHT is really homosynergistic with

186

vitamin E, and that seems to be very important in terms of
adding to it. Then there is quite a bit of nutritional evidence
that vitamin C would form a good synergist with vitamin E;
and then, further, if peroxides are formed, it seems that the
best-known reduction mechanism is via glutathione peroxidase.
This might be affected by building up the level of glutathione
from the metabolic pathway of methionine--methionine to cysteine
incorporation in glutathione. Methionine might have other
advantageous effects, and it is known nutritionally to support
this type of inhibition in some way. It is utilization of multiple
inhibitors, in effect, built around vitamin E as the primary
one. I'd like to show some models now. Although they don't
relate directly to brain, they're more easily manipulated.

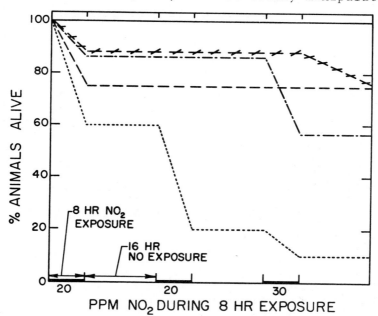

Figure 25. Effect of dietary α-tocopherol acetate on the survival of
            rats during acute toxic NO₂ exposure: diets contained (···)
            0, (-·-) 10.5, (--) 45, (-/-) 150, and (——) 1500 mg α-
            tocopherol acetate/kg diet. The last diet contained in addi-
            tion 1500mg Vit E/kg diet each of DL-methionine and ascorbic acid
            and 45 mg BHT/kg diet.

Figure 25 is for animals that are exposed to nitrogen dioxide,
a major air pollutant. We used rats as an experimental animal.
They received a vitamin E-deficient basal diet, and there
were increasing amounts of vitamin E fed, varying from zero
through 1500 mg/ kg. The number of animals that were alive
after this exposure is indicative of the protection afforded
by vitamin E; there were about 8 animals per group. We got

a very nice correlation between protection and the amount
of vitamin E and other antioxidants that were present in these
animals. The turn-around time for this kind of experiment
is about a month; starting with the fresh animals and getting
the results in other words, it's a fast turn-around time.

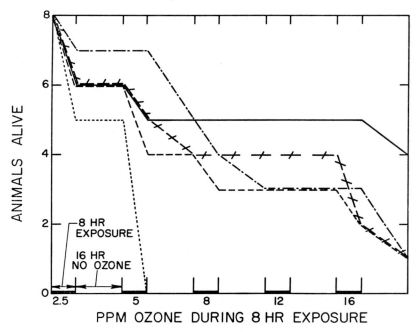

Figure 26. Effect of dietary α-tocopherol acetate on the survival of rats
during acute O_3 exposure. Symbols are described in Figure 25.

A very similar experiment is shown in Figure 26, however
a little differently. In this one we used the same kinds
of vitamin E mixtures and exposed the animals to an increasing
gradient of ozone--an acute toxicity test. The number of
animals here is eight, and they dropped off until all of them
were dead, when they did not get added vitamin E, by the second
day at 5 ppm ozone. Those that were fed vitamin E in the
range of 11 to 1500 mg/kg of diet had a different death pattern, showing increased survival over those receiving no
vitamin E. Again, this is a very steep gradient of ozone;
the LD_{50} for ozone is 8 ppm. Of those animals fed the highly
protective diets--or what should have been highly protective
in the biochemical sense--50% survived two times the LD_{50}
of ozone, so they really withstood a high level of oxidants.
So in this "quicky" type of experiment we imposed a tremendous
oxidant challenge. Granted it was all through the lungs,
but we were able to test different antioxidant mixtures, and
one was a very powerful protective mixture.

188

Dr. Desnick: Are these again vitamin E-deficient animals?

Dr. Tappel: Yes, the basal diet is vitamin E-deficient, the animals receiving a Draper-type diet. Vitamin E is the only thing missing from the diet and, of course, what it shows is that vitamin E-deficient animals are very susceptible to air pollutant oxidants like ozone and nitrogen dioxide, so this is a very important practical protector in the population; the animal experiments tend to implicate that. This has been done in about four different laboratories.[42]

Dr. Desnick: Can you show any protection in animals that are not vitamin E-deficient, but receive your cocktail as a supplement?

Dr. Tappel: In fact, the normal requirement for vitamin E for the rats, in other words, the dose equivalent to the recommended dose for humans, would be 45 mg, so then these would be the normal. High levels of antioxidants are, in fact, protective above that.

Dr. Nair: How long do you have to give this supplemented diet before putting the animals on the experiment?

Dr. Tappel: Within 3 weeks on the diet they become vitamin E-deficient, and so the animals are normally kept 3 to 5 weeks, depending upon when we can get the ozone chambers ready. The minimum turn-around time would be about a month for this kind of experiment. Incidentally, the biochemical studies show that in the animals dying--or more susceptible, let us say, even when they don't die--there is lipid peroxidation with formation of malonaldehyde, and also a response of the glutathione peroxidase system directly related to the amount of vitamin E in the animals, so we have quite a bit of evidence for lipid peroxidation in the lung.

Table 9 shows another type of model, and the aim of this experiment is to develop fluorescent products in vivo. We were following some of the earlier work which has been reviewed by Porta and Hartroft,[71] particularly, and feeding very high levels of polyunsaturated lipids in the diet. The values shown in Table 9 are the amounts of fluorescence, and the spectra are of the same type that I showed before (Fig. 13). These are the biochemical measurements of these pigments formed in fat at different levels of vitamin E. We obtained very good regression coefficients for fluorescence versus 1/log vitamin E, and the values are all statistically significant. The highest development of fluorescence happened to be in the renal fat, but all of these fat tissues fluoresced very brightly in the animal. When the tissues were extracted, all of the extracts lit up very brightly with a tremendous amount of fluorescence under ultraviolet light. These animals

189

Dr. Witting: Kayden[72] reported on a number of patients who had been taking 3-5 g/day for two to three years at the New York Academy of Science Symposium on vitamin E.

Dr. Tappel: Yes, that was self-administration and un-controlled.

191

are very highly damaged, also, of course, they have a poorer growth performance.

Fluorescence at various vitamin E levels

Dr. Witting: Yes, unfortunately.

Dr. Zeman: Who was that?

Dr. Witting: Herbert S. Kayden, Department of Medicine, School of Medicine, New York University Medical Center, 550 First Avenue, New York, New York 10016.

Dr. Wherrett: I've just forgotten how you assay fluorescence. Your material is a lipid extract?

Dr. Tappel: Yes. The fluorescent material forms both in the lipid-soluble phase--this is mainly crosslinked phosphatidyl ethanolamine--and in the water-soluble material-- this would involve enzymes, amino acids, nucleic acids, and so forth. The water-soluble fluorescence is much more difficult to get at because of interference, so we do primarily lipid solubles at this time. It's a very simple method: just chloroform-ethanol extract in a spectrophotofluorometer.

Dr. Wherrett: This hasn't been done on white cells or fibroblasts in Batten's disease?

Dr. Tappel: No, but we've analyzed some of the pigment that Dr. Siakotos has separated, and in various cases there is quite a bit of polyene, like vitamin A, in the pigment; otherwise, it looks like this type of lipid peroxidation damage of the pigment.

Dr. Kolodny: The finding of very high levels of fluorescence in the bone marrows of vitamin E-deficient rats treated with the cod liver oil diet raises the possibility that bone marrow aspirates of patients with Batten's disease might also contain high levels of fluorescence. If so, then the degree of bone marrow fluorescence might serve as both an adjunct to diagnosis and a measure of the effectiveness of therapeutic trials in the disease.

Dr. Tappel: Yes, I think that Dr. Nair would confirm the fact that it's known that bone marrow is very susceptible to vitamin E deficiency, and peroxidation has been implicated there as well as decrease in heme biosynthesis, so this would be a good suggestion.

Dr. Zeman: That's quite correct, because the first case from which Dr. Siakotos isolated ceroid was clinically diagnosed as a ceroid storage disease on the basis of bone marrow study.[4] Since the mechanism of causative pathogenesis and etiology of lipid peroxidation in Batten's disease still remains enigmatic, the following proposition may be entirely premature, or even unwarranted. Nevertheless, the fact that these diseases are inherited would suggest that they are due

192

to a single mutation, although different mutations presumably account for the spectrum of disorders. Since these enzyme disorders seem to yield to supplementation of normal enzymes by transplanted tissues and organs, we may consider such a therapeutic approach even though we have no evidence for the nature of the defective enzyme. We have designed a number of experiments on dogs whereby we use heterozygous donors and homozygous recipients. First we will transplant kidneys, with the idea of supplying a hypothetical defective enzyme protein. Kidneys are well supplied with blood, so if there should be any release of enzyme into blood the kidney would offer a source of such missing or defective enzyme. The second possibility is to produce chimera. The difficulty here is not so much with rejection as in the case of kidney transplant, but the other way around: the graft versus host reaction. However, modern immunological engineering seems to have overcome this impasse; at least, there are people who know how to do it, and I am very much interested to hear from Dr. Desnick. He could contribute to this particular question.

Dr. Rider: Could you explain what you meant about the latter transplant?

Dr. Zeman: Another source of enzyme would be white blood cells. The great advantage of white blood cell transplantation is the easy accessibility because we can get white blood cells from any donor. Moreover, we don't do any damage to the donor, whereas if we take a kidney out we deprive a person of one kidney, which is a very serious type of proposition.

Dr. Rider: Wouldn't that be very transient though? If you just injected some white cells, you wouldn't expect the enzymes to last very long, would you?

Dr. Zeman: No, because repeated injection of white blood cells stimulate antibody formation and the white blood cells are very rapidly destroyed, and over a period of time you get into a situation where you can elicit any type of immunologic catastrophe.

Dr. Rider: That's what I meant. If you could supply some missing enzyme, it seems to me that you would have to supply this repeatedly.

Dr. Zeman: The point is that we supply a population of cells which settle permanently in the recipient, either in the form of an organ transplant or in the form of a bone marrow exchange, where the donor cells are genetically competent in comparison to the recipient's incompetent cells. That is the idea. With the organ transplant, we face the possibility of graft rejection; with the bone marrow transplant we are troubled by a graft versus host rejection. In other words, we are talking about two different situations, both of which should produce the same effect, but they carry different implications with respect to availability, method of procedure, and reactivity. Is that clear now?

Dr. Rider: Yes, I understand now.

Dr. Desnick: Perhaps I can make a few comments about therapeutic approaches to this disease, in particular methods which could be derived from the previous experiences of Dr. Philippart and other workers, and our work, means of approaching genetic diseases that are due to specific enzymatic deficiencies. Initially, enzyme replacement therapy by providing an exogenous source of enzymatic activity in patients with inherited enzymatic deficiencies was attempted. Early attempts by various workers utilized a preparation of fungal enzyme in the glycogenoses. Hug et al[73] and Baudhuin et al[74] have tried using concentrated fungal enzyme preparations for the treatment of Pompe's disease, type II glycogenosis. Huijing[75] has tried similar concentrates in type IV glycogenosis, and Greene et al[76] and Austin[77] have attempted to use a similar preparation intrathecally and intravenously in patients with metachromatic leukodystrophy. These early studies with the use of non-human enzyme indicated that the continuous administration of exogenous enzyme resulted in the uptake of enzymatic activity in various tissues and, most interestingly, in brain tissue in Pompe's disease and in type IV glycogenosis. These findings were of significant importance because they suggest that a large enzyme protein intravenously administered can cross the blood-brain barrier to cope with the neuronal accumulation of the accumulated substrate.

Subsequently, various workers have tried using human enzyme preparations. In Fabry's disease, together with Sweeley's group at Michigan State University, we have intravenously administered plasma from normal individuals to hemizygous patients with Fabry's disease. We were able to show (1) that the enzyme could be introduced into the plasma of the Fabry recipient in an active form, (2) that it was metabolically active, and (3) that it would break down the accumulated Fabry glycolipid trihexosyl ceramide.[78][79]

In the mucopolysaccharidoses, for which we do not know the specific enzymatic deficiencies or the specific accumulated substrates, DiFerrante et al and Knudson et al and now many others, have utilized serial fresh and frozen plasma infusions and white cell infusions into patients with mucopolysaccaridoses, Type I and II (Hurler's and Hunter's diseases) in order to attempt to provide the missing enzyme, i.e., the corrective factor. Following the plasma or white cell infusions, they demonstrated an increase in the short-chain mucopolysaccharide in urine, which they suggest are the catabolic products resulting from the mucopolysaccharide accumulation. Others attempting enzyme replacement in the mucopolysaccharide disorders have demonstrated some morphological changes in the hepatic accumulation of mucopolysaccharide by electron microscopy, and some subtle subjective clinical improvement.

Dr. Philippart's group was the first to utilize a transplanted organ for enzyme replacement[82] with the rationale that the major difficulty in enzyme replacement therapy is that of providing a continuous supply of active enzyme. Thus, if you could give the patient a tissue which would act as a "factory" and continuously administer the active enzyme to that patient or provide a site where the substrate could come for catabolic breakdown, you might be able to deplete the substrate accumulation.

We have also accomplished two successful renal transplants in patients with Fabry's disease.[83-85] The work of Dr. Philippart's group and our group suggests that this is a rational and feasible approach, particularly for this glycosphingolipidosis. Following transplantation, the accumulated glycosphingolipid in the plasma decreases from a level of five to ten times normal to the normal range. Concurrently, there is an increase in the plasma α-galactosidase activity, which is low in Fabry's disease. Furthermore, the level of this glycosphingolipid in urinary sediment decreased to normal range.

In one recipient, we purposely left the patient's two kidneys in place, and transplanted a third kidney. Subsequently there has been a continual decrease in the accumulated material in the urinary sediment which is an indirect biopsy of renal cells. As expected, the transplanted normal kidney contributed to normal levels of urinary enzyme.

We have also approached another disease--Gaucher's disease-- utilizing the third kidney transplant approach,[86] and we are now about 4 months past transplantation. The patient was severely affected, and the parents were looking for any approach which might provide some information in the treatment of that disease, realizing that their child most likely would not gain anything from it. This study is in collaboration with Dr. R. O. Brady, NIH, who is measuring the enzymatic activity, utilizing the natural substrate, and there is an indication that the enzymatic activity has increased in the serum. The spleen was taken out at the time of transplantation, and the glucocerebroside levels (the accumulating substrate) in the plasma initially increased, as one might expect following splenectomy, since the spleen was providing the depot or warehouse of the Gaucher lipid in the patient.

Subjectively, the neurologists note that the patient has stabilized and has not regressed since the transplantation. The parents also feel that the patient's condition has not changed; in fact, they have noticed that the patient is able to perform some new tasks--for instance, holding her bottle and showing certain motor and language skills--better than prior to transplantation. These are subjective evaluations: the subsequent biochemical data will indicate whether transplanted kidney enzyme can reach brain tissue and, in fact, catabolize the accumulated brain glycosphingolipid.

We are also studying enzyme replacement by organ transplantation in an animal model. A colony of dogs with Krabbe's disease is maintained at the University of Minnesota by Dr. T. Fletcher. The enzymatic deficiency in these dogs is analogous to the human Krabbe's disease and is similar to the dog model for Batten's disease. Our approach is to exchange kidneys between a normal sibling (heterozygous) and a homozygous affected dog. By reciprocal kidney transplantation, enzyme replacement can be studied in the affected dog, and the effect of an abnormal kidney in the unaffected dog can be evaluated. We do tissue matching by mixed lymphocyte cultures on our dogs in order to choose appropriate matches for transplantation. These dogs are genotyped by Dr. Suzuki, and therefore, we can make an early diagnosis of the homozygous state. What we are trying to do is actually to exchange from a normal dog and a homozygous dog a single kidney, so that we can observe the effects of a normal kidney in a Krabbe dog, and the effects of a Krabbe kidney in a normal dog, and then after an appropriate time analyze the results clinically, morphologically, and biochemically.

To date, these studies have not been technically successful; the dogs are small cairn terriers and cause some difficulty in transplantation. It is important to transplant the kidney into a site away from the other kidneys so that renograms will accurately indicate profusion in the allografts. Transplantation into the neck of those dogs has been attempted. Furthermore, a separate os for the ureter will allow monitoring of urinary enzyme and substrate levels of the allografts. However, with larger dogs--the Batten's dog model for example-- these technical difficulties should not occur. If we could diagnose the affected Batten's dogs at one month by electron microscopy of the tissue from brain biopsy and choose appropriate dogs by exchanging kidneys, we might be able to study the long-term effects and see if we can delay the onset of the abnormal accumulation by periodic morphologic evaluation.

We might approach parents of patients who are willing to allow us to either do white cell or plasma infusions on a serial basis, particularly in patients who have the lymphocytic vacuoles. It might be interesting to see if we can reverse them. Dr. Zeman indicated earlier that there were patients available with these hematological abnormalities. The other approach would be to do a renal allograft into a

196

patient. I choose a cadaver transplant because we like to have normal enzymatic activity--whatever the enzyme is--in the transplanted tissue, since the patient should have maximal enzymatic activity from the grafted tissue. Evaluation of the effectiveness of transplantation would be both clinical and morphological. If a patient that had the white cell changes was transplanted, another abnormal parameter could be monitored.

These approaches are now being utilized by workers to replace the deficiencies in other inherited diseases. Preliminary work indicates that they are effective, particularly, in Fabry's disease, where we now have at least four patients doing quite well biochemically and clinically, post transplantation. I think this approach is aggressive, but at this point in time, since we don't have a handle, it may give us some very helpful information about the nature of the primary defect and about therapy in this particular entity.

Dr. Zeman: Thank you. I would like to ask Dr. Desnick two questions. Do these dogs have galactosyl ceramide galactosidase deficiency?

Dr. Desnick: Yes.

Dr. Zeman: Secondly, there is only one place I know of where bone marrow exchange transfusion has been successfully achieved and that is the University of Minnesota. Have you considered the possibility of bone marrow transplant rather than kidney transplant for the reasons you have outlined?

Dr. Desnick: Yes. The bone marrow transplantation experience has been successful only in combined immunodeficiency. The experience of bone marrow transplantation in diseases which were not of an immunological nature has been unsuccessful to date, but some encouraging results have recently been reported for aplastic anemia. The concept, however, of transplanting hematopoietic tissue that would produce enzymes in the white cells or platelets and subsequently release them into the plasma for distribution to other tissues is an excellent one. Hopefully, the future work in bone marrow transplantation will overcome some of these limitations, particularly the inability to successfully transplant bone marrow into immunologically competent patients.

Dr. Zeman: One further question. Inasmuch as many of those diseases can be diagnosed in utero, the aspect of prevention, of course, will deprive us of future patients; but those who are presently alive and those who are born without benefit of early recognition of the disease will be with us. Therefore, the question comes up--and I think it would be an interesting problem also from the theoretical point of

view--that we can perform either organ transplants or bone
marrow grafts during the neonatal period, hoping to exploit
the possibility of immune tolerance in these immature individuals. Have you given any thought to that with respect
to our dogs?

Dr. Desnick: The Krabbe dog model is not suitable technically for early transplantation since the animals are very
small. However, I might point out that in affected patients
that have been diagnosed at an early postnatal state, tissue
transplantation, particularly kidney transplantation, can
be accomplished. Renal transplantation in the newborn period
has been successful at the University of Minnesota.

Dr. Zeman: Do you require immunosuppression in those
individuals?

Dr. Desnick: I believe so.

Dr. Zeman: Dr. Philippart, who pioneered these studies,
is going to tell us a little bit before we start the general
discussion.

Dr. Philippart: We started playing with the idea of
organ transplant in 1965 when Austin first presented his
results[87] on enzyme replacement in metachromatic leukodystrophy.
At that time it became clear that if we were not able to
supply an enzyme which would not be treated as a foreign
antigen we would not be successful. There are wide variations
in the amino acid composition of a few proteins like ribonuclease
and insulin in mammals.[88] The best approach in these conditions
was to try to purify human enzymes to the point where they
would not elicit antigenic reactions. This has been exceedingly
difficult. It is now technically feasible to purify a variety
of lysosomal hydrolases, but the yields are extremely low
and it would be prohibitively expensive to treat patients
on such a basis.

In the future, hopefully, it should become possible to
map all of these different human enzymes. I want to emphasize
that in man one given enzyme might have a slightly different
amino acid composition from one individual to another, and
histocompatibility antigens indicate that different people
have different proteins, although we don't know to what extent. There will therefore be many problems to be solved
before we are able to prepare a pure enzyme which will be
tolerated by a patient with a deficiency.

One first approach would be to map the enzyme precisely
and then start industrial production. That probably could
be accomplished now. A great deal of progress is being made
in automating protein synthesis, but of course it may be 10

years or more before we will become able to do it routinely and cheaply. Since this is not yet practical, I played with the idea of organ transplantation. Transplanting an organ means several things. An organ may trap some products which circulate in the blood, for example. This is the case in mucopolysaccharide storage disorders. We were recently able to demonstrate traces of sulfatides in the blood from patients with metachromatic leukodystrophy. Since there is not much accumulation of sulfatide outside of the nervous system, it is unlikely that trapping circulating sulfatide would be of much help. In Gaucher's disease, however, which was the first direction of our efforts, the spleen appeared to trap efficiently most of the glucosyl ceramide carried by erythrocytes and leukocytes. If a normal spleen could be grafted, the bulk of the circulating cerebroside would normally be taken up and digested protecting the other organs.

Another function of a transplanted organ, which had not been clear at first, was its ability to secrete some of its enzymes and furnish them on a stable and permanent basis to the recipient. The key work to substantiate such a function was that of Fratantoni and Neufeld[89] showing that cultured fibroblasts from different types of mucopolysaccharide storage could correct each other. Of course, it had been known for a long time that lysosomal hydrolases could be found in body fluids like serum and urine, but nobody had seen the potential of such an excretion. The next step was to see whether a transplanted organ would excrete some of its enzymes and how efficient this would be in people with deficiencies. We started transplanting spleen in dogs with Dr. Fonkalsrude. It turned out to be exceedingly difficult; we had sharp rejection even when inbred dogs, very closely related antigenically, were used. Although in theory it would have been a good organ for transplant, the immunlogical reaction made it impractical. We have also investigated bone marrow transplantation, but, as Dr. Desnick has just indicated, only people with severe immune deficiences will tolerate these transplants.

Serum or white blood cell infusion might be of benefit if we could use it only infrequently. Indeed, experience with people who require repeated transfusions has shown that intolerance is bound to occur. For chronic inborn metabolic disorders in which you would have to infuse for decades, this approach would be self-limiting. It might relieve an occasional crisis in a patient; but I don't think that on a long-term basis it would be of any benefit unless we find a better way to control immune reactions. The only organ that has been transplanted with some success has been the kidney. The kidney is a good organ to transplant because most surgeons know how to handle it, all the technical problems have been worked out well, and the rate of success is quite high. When you transplant an organ, you transplant a very complex mixture

of tissue, blood vessels, reticuloendothelial system, and
a multiplicity of specialized cells as well. We don't know
yet which cells could supply enzymes to the recipients, but
we have some indication that it might be the reticuloendothelial
system. Hydrolase activities are very high in these cells
which have a scavenger function and can be induced to proliferate
actively. Such functions are severely impaired in lysosomal
storage disorders. Fabry's and Gaucher's disease as well
as mucopolysaccharide storage disorders are all characterized
by a significant amount of undigestible substances circulating
in the blood. Transplanted reticuloendothelial cells might
help in clearing the blood of substances which might be taken
up by the blood vessels and possibly diffuse from there into
other tissues. Of course in kidney transplantation we also
have to face the problem of immunosuppression.

Our results with our first patient with Fabry's disease,
transplanted[82] in 1969, were outstanding for the first 18
months. Glycolipid levels in the plasma and urine returned
to normal levels, and the patient had up to 25% of the normal
α-galactosidase activity in the plasma. Then we had a rejection
episode. By increasing Prednisone from 15 mg to 60 mg per
day, we were able to control the rejection episode successfully,
but we entirely upset the benefit of the transplant. Plasma
glycolipid went up again--not as high as before the transplantation, but still in the range of most patients with Fabry's.
Enzyme activity both in the plasma and urine decreased markedly.

Dr. Zeman: May I just ask one question: how was the
kidney functioning radiologically at that time?

Dr. Philippart: Very well. We biopsied the kidney at
that time and found signs of chronic rejection as expected,
but there was no lipid accumulation. We also checked the
liver with a needle biopsy, and there we were able to document
an actual reversal. We could not find any evidence of Fabry's
disease in that specimen, while before transplantation lipid
storage was conspicuous. So it means that some of the substance
which had been stored there for years had been actually metabolized and that the liver was able to take up circulating
enzymes. The pathology in Fabry's disease is centered around
the blood vessels where lipids accumulate. Dawson and Sweeley[90]
have shown that in the pig, complex glycolipids from aged
erythrocytes are shed into the plasma. Then they may be metabolized in situ or taken up by blood vessels or reticuloendothelial cells. In Fabry's disease lipid accumulates in the
plasma and blood vessels, realizing a kind of atherosclerosis.
Primary involvement of most organs is discrete with the exception
of the kidney. These patients develop severe kidney insufficiency, most of them by the third decade of life.

Brain damage may occur following strokes since brain

vessels are choked up by lipids, but there is little or no primary involvement in the brain.

A transplanted kidney can thus supply relatively small amounts of the deficient enzyme. It seems that blood enzymes can reach most of the organs, including the liver. Patients with Fabry's disease are unable to sweat to any extent; however, two years after transplantation, sweat secretion recurred.

Immunosuppressive drugs may have some undesirable effects. Prednisone depresses the inflammatory reaction by acting on the cells which are among the most active in producing lysosomal hydrolases. It is possible that the part of the kidney which is the most active in secreting enzymes is the reticuloendothelial system of that kidney. If this happens to be the case, a mild chronic rejection may be of help by increasing enzyme secretion, while a too rigid control might depress enzyme excretion defeating the purpose of the transplantation.

Another major problem is that most of the storage disorders involve the brain, which is well protected by the blood brain barrier. We just don't know how we are going to get such proteins across the barrier. Maybe we could get them in the brain blood vessels, but brain cells will remain out of reach; the solution would be to transplant something in the skull cavity. We are exploring the feasibility of transplanting there a source of enzyme such as a benign tumor which might excrete hydrolases into the cerebrospinal fluid. Although no part of the brain is more than 3 or 4 cm away from the spinal fluid, large enzyme molecules are unlikely to diffuse very far.

Dr. Rider: I have a quick question. I remember from medical school that it was said that you could transfuse a mongrel dog with blood from another mongrel dog and you never had to worry about reaction. I presume that doesn't hold true if they're thoroughbred dogs or closely related dogs. On the other hand, what about organs? Can you transplant an organ from one mongrel to another without worrying about typing?

Dr. Zeman: I have no idea.

Dr. Rider: Do you, Dr. Desnick?

Dr. Desnick: Dogs undergo the same kind of immunological rejection that humans do, and you have to immunosuppress them in the same manner.

Dr. Rider: But is it still true that, for example, in blood transfusing one mongrel you can take the blood from another mongrel without much trouble?

Dr. Desnick: I don't know.

Dr. Rider: I know when I was in Physiology we would transfuse one dog with another, and they'd say you didn't have to worry about the dogs but in humans you have the blood typing to do.

Dr. Desnick: We're quite careful about the dogs we select for transplantation, and we tissue type them. We try and choose siblings for these studies.

Dr. Zeman: So you use heterozygous donors?

Dr. Desnick: Yes. However, we would like to use normal dogs. There are two other comments that I might make with respect to the problem of getting across the blood brain barrier. Again, we don't really know whether or not enzymes can successfully enter brain cells after transplanting a kidney. However, the studies that have been done in fibroblasts-- particularly those in Porter's group[91] and Weismann's group[92] in metachromatic leukodystrophy--indicate that you can put exogenous enzyme into the medium of cultured fibroblasts, and it can cross the membranes into the cytoplasm. In fact, the enzyme becomes stablized in the lysosome. Secondly, one of the appraoches that we are now pursuing is the isolation and purification of lysosomal hydrolases, and in our laboratory with Dr. Robert Bernlohr, a biochemist at the University of Minnesota, we are pursuing methods to obtain these hydrolases in significant quantities so that we can begin preliminary studies. We are now able to obtain these hydrolases in large amounts from human tissue. Our approach, in association with Dr. Finn Wold, University of Minnesota, will be to stabilize these hydrolases by using bifunctional reagents, as has been done for various bacterial enzymes. Then we will utilize the stabilized derivatives, for decreasing the substrate accumulation in these diseases. We are in the early stages of developing these methods, but hopefully we'll have large quantities of α-galactosidase, hexosaminidases, and arylsulfatases available for subsequent stabliziation and therapeutic study. Since our enzyme fractions contain a number of lysosomal enzymes, we may have a source of other lysosomal enzymes in this preparation; as we proceed to analyze our various fractions we may have a whole host of lysosomal enzymes in various fraction tubes that we would make available for study.

Dr. Rider: What is your source of material again?

Dr. Desnick: We use human placenta. We found that the placenta has very high activity per gram of tissue for various lysosomal enzymes compared to other tissues. Also we are attempting to automate the procedure so that we can obtain large amounts of purified enzyme more conveniently. We feel

that the experience with hemophiliacs and others who have
received multiple transfusions of blood indicates that the
immunological problems of giving a human protein similar to
the one that they have will be less antigenic, if at all.
Since hemophiliacs have received multiple transfusions, and
now specific human globulin--in each of these transfusions
they're probably getting hundreds of isozymes that are incompatible with their genotype but which they do not react to
clinically--we think it will be feasible to administer these
modified enzymes, providing an insulin-like therapy for the
replacement of specific hydrolases.

Dr. Rider: Well, at least on theoretical grounds you'd
expect that an absolutely pure enzyme, which presumably these
patients have anyway but may have much less of, would not
be a foreign substance for them, especially if it's pure.
Then you shouldn't have any reaction.

Dr. Desnick: It may be foreign substance to them. If
they have a mutant enzyme which has a single base substitution
responsible for a single amino acid change, and if our immunologic system fails to recognize that active enzyme as foreign,
the antigenic problem may be minimal or negligible.

Dr. Rider: Would you anticipate that purified enzyme
preparations could probably be given intramuscularly rather
than intravenously? I cite that example because it's much
easier and simpler to do that than to give multiple intravenous
injections.

Dr. Desnick: I think initially we'll begin by doing
intravenous studies, because we can then monitor the half-
life of the enzyme and...

Dr. Rider: The exact time of the uptake.

Dr. Desnick: Yes, and be able to characterize its effect
in plasma and then its subsequent tissue distribution.

Dr. Rider: Dr. Zeman, in the light of this information
on different enzymes, I wonder how much we really know about
what influences the rate of turnover of the various lipid
fractions which you are starting to find in ceroid deposits?

Dr. Zeman: The only evidence for an enzyme defect is
really given by the genetics, and that is not conclusive evidence
because we might just as well assume that the genetic defect
produces a faulty structural protein which does not afford
the protection of the oxidizable hydrophobic groups of the
structural lipids and therefore triggers peroxidation; we
do not know that, you see.

Dr. Rider: What I meant was, do you know that some lipids accumulate, at least in your ceroid deposit or in your lipofuscin?

Dr. Zeman: Oh, yes, but this is much farther down the chain of events. I think we would all agree that the pigments which accumulate are the end product of something that is way up metabolically which we don't know.

Dr. Rider: Let me go back to some theories we had before: is it a matter of making too much of a certain substance, or is it a matter of making the proper amount but not being able to get rid of it? In other words, is it clogging up the carburetor, so to speak? If you think in terms of clogging, then if you know what is clogging it up maybe you can discover, on theoretical ground, the kind of enzyme which ought to degrade this.

Dr. Zeman: If we could show a beneficial effect of kidney transplant, the assumption that a lysosomal hydrolase is missing or deficient would be strengthened. So far the only good evidence for a possible lysosomal enzyme deficiency is in the findings of deDuve.[93] He tells me that his observations suggest that there must be dehydrogenases in lysosomes.

Dr. Rider: Well, wouldn't this be another ideal place for your dogs? For example, just take one of your dogs and if you could do a kidney transplant....

Dr. Zeman: Well, that's the way I started the discussion; this is what we are going to do, you see.

Dr. Desnick: We would be happy to collaborate in any way; say to transplant two of the Batten's dogs.

Dr. Rider: I think that would be something you ought to do very quickly, because it's a relatively simple thing, and in a very short time you would know whether you're getting someplace or not.

Dr. Philippart: The critical issue here is to know if there is any exogenous factor which may have an influence on the process. Ideally, if we could use the Neufeld model[89] to mix normal fibroblasts with fibroblasts from the patient and show a corrective effect, then we would know whether the transplant has a chance to help or not. However, fibroblasts are not strikingly involved, and it may be very difficult to show that the mixture of normal fibroblasts will correct this very subtle defect. This might be better tested by using a brain explant from your dogs, to be grown in combination with a normal brain explant. The problem may well be entirely different. Lysosomal disorders are a special kind of problem,

204

and as far as we know we could not really qualify Batten's disease as a lysosomal disorder, in the sense of a specific deficiency of a given hydrolase which is accompanied by an increase in the corresponding substrate. We are still looking for a primary substrate. We know that lipid turnover is abnormal, but there is no specific storage. This indicates we are dealing with a different mechanism.

Dr. Desnick: I'd like to reinforce Dr. Philippart's point. I agree, and believe that the dog model will provide us with this basis. However, we have to be cautious in extrapolating from the dog model to the human disease, because we may be dealing with genetic heterogeneity and we may not find the same primary defect.

Dr. Philippart: Yes, but of course this would give us a handle, to study a different type of mechanism that we might then start to explore more rationally.

Dr. Rider: Dr. Desnick, what about a cross-circulation experiment, where you could just connect one dog to another, in the event that their blood was compatible and yet the blood streams were mixed; so that you'd have the completely normal circumstance of one dog possibly supplying enzymes, and washing out the abnormal products in the sick dog.

Dr. Philippart: You have to realize that this is a very slow-going process which takes years to develop, so that you don't have much chance to see differences over a few hours or even days.

Dr. Zeman: The dogs take 12 to 15 months to develop signs of the disease.

Dr. Rider: Yes, but from brain biopsy, progression of the pigment in the brain could be seen very quickly.

Dr. Zeman: Yes, but then we would have to start on a cross-transfusion in the infant dog. It might be possible, I don't know.

Dr. Desnick: Transplantation is a simpler approach. We should also do the Neufeld-like experiments[94] [95] and see if there is a corrective factor that might alter the fibroblasts or brain accumulation of ceroid.

Dr. Rider: I don't suppose it would get you anywhere, but you could also consider taking the "bad" kidney and putting it into a "good" dog.

Dr. Desnick: Yes, I suggested a reciprocal exchange.

Dr. Wherrett: It seems to me though, that we still need a chemical index of the disease, an estimate of a substrate-- be it primary or secondary--and this is why I'm sort of interested in the assay that Dr. Tappel was talking about earlier.

Dr. Zeman: You mean, to measure fluorescence in absolute units? This can be done on tissue biopsies, and I think bone marrow would be the tissue of choice because of the high degree of fluorescent material and the easy accessibility. I must confess that we haven't looked at the bone marrow in those dogs, but there is no reason why we shouldn't.

Dr. Philippart: What about in humans? Did you look at bone marrow in your tissues?

Dr. Zeman: I mentioned that case from Minnesota in which the diagnosis emerged from a bone marrow study.

Dr. Philippart: Yes, but did you find clean vacuoles or lipofuscin or ceroid accumulation?

Dr. Zeman: They called it ceroid because they looked at it with fluorescence microscopy and noticed a very low solubility.

Dr. Rider: What's the status of the rectal biopsy? You know rectal biopsy is one of the simplest things one can do. First of all you put a small scope into the anus, then you take a biopsy forceps and pick off a piece of mucosa. There's absolutely no pain to it, because there are no nerves there to transmit pain. The very worst thing that could happen is if we get a little bleeding we can use a little cautery. The risk would be one in a million, perhaps, and no discomfort, and the question is, what is the status of this? We did a biopsy, for example, on Chuck, and there was no fat in the ganglion cells, but again this was relatively early in the condition. This is something that could be done very easily. I think this is much simpler to do than a bone marrow.

Dr. Zeman: The difficulty, of course, with the rectal biopsy is the paucity of nerve cells in relation to supporting tissues, such as mesenchyma and epithelial cells. The ratio of these various elements is highly variable and cannot be predetermined, even if the utmost caution is used for selection. You may obtain 100 mm^3 of tissue, which is a lot for rectal biopsy, and yet find only one nerve cell or none.

Dr. Rider: But, assuming you have nerve cells, I would agree that maybe you don't have enough to analyze, but at least you could look at them.

Dr. Zeman: Oh, yes, you can look at them, and it's a diagnostic tool in an advanced case. It's a very good procedure, but it has not been very helpful in early cases, as you yourself experienced. Because of the limited amount of nerve tissue, the biopsy sample does not lend itself to biochemical studies which you would like to do.

Dr. Desnick: I'd like to make one point, and that is that at our present state of knowledge we understand only that this is an autosomal recessive defect, the majority of which are due to inherited enzymatic deficiences. There are, however, autosomal recessive defects that do result in gross morphologic changes, for instance, Kartagener's syndrome, which is a straightforward Mendelian recessive characterized by situs inversus, bronchiectasis, and sinusitis. I think it would be important to understand the primary etiology of this disorder. A year from now when we get together we might be able to have a little more firm basis for our therapeutic approach to this disorder. If we were able to study the dogs, one involved and one uninvolved, and do the reciprocal exchange kidney transplantation, we may obtain some morphological indication of the effect of transplantation. This might provide us with in vivo corrective factor information. We could do this simultaneously along with the other studies of fibroblasts and cultured brain tissue, the vitamin E studies, etc. These studies might provide a firmer understanding of the biochemical etiology of this disease.

Dr. Rider: I am really intrigued with the placenta. I just somehow have the feeling that these children with Batten's disease have been protected by their mothers, and that when they're born if you did a biopsy of the brain you'd probably find no abnormality. As time goes on, protection has been lost, and they're making say, only 10% of an enzyme they need, so gradually something goes wrong. From my clinical experience however, I'd say they have been protected up to the time of birth, and that's where the enzyme of the placenta comes into the picture.

Dr. Zeman: The dog model, at least, indicates that the accumulation of pigments is continuous and proceeds at least for 10 months, but the average time lapse is 12 months for the development of the overt neurological defect. Incidentally, I should say that this strain which develops this disease has been bred specifically for its excellence as a duck-hunting animal, and the better the qualities for the hunting, the higher the risk for the genetic defect.

In response to Dr. Desnick's observation, I think the Neufeld experiment in the dog is quite feasible because the dogs, unlike the human cases, display enormous accumulation of lipopigments in the lymph nodes, and it is relatively

207

simple to culture reticulum cells from lymph nodes.

Dr. Philippart: By the way, it is also easy to grow bone marrow.

Dr. Desnick: Do the dogs from homozygous mothers have the disease at day one? Are their brains abnormal?

Dr. Zeman: We have seen electron microscopic evidence of pigment in brain biopsies from newborn animals examined with the electron microscope.

Dr. Desnick: From homozygous mothers?

Dr. Zeman: Homozygous affected dogs, because we produce them by mating homozygous bitches with homozygous dogs.

Dr. Philippart: You have never examined any homozygous fetus to see if there is already something?

Dr. Zeman: No, not yet.

Dr. Rider: How long does it take for your dogs to develop this disease?

Dr. Zeman: Twelve to fifteen months.

Dr. Rider: When do you mate them?

Dr. Zeman: We mate them as early as possible after the second heat, which is at about 12-15 months or so.

Dr. Rider: So they've already begun to manifest some signs of the disease?

Dr. Zeman: They might or might not manifest signs of the disease at that time.

Dr. Philippart: Is there any difference between a homozygous dog which results from the mating of two heterozygous dogs, and another one resulting from the mating of two homozygous dogs?

Dr. Zeman: No, there is no difference. The disease in the dog is exceedingly homotypical and homochronical; that is to say from a statistical point of view you can almost say that by age 14 months the disease is clinically established, and we have not seen a single dog which has survived age 25 months. Conversely, we have not had any premature deaths, that is, before age 22 months.

In closing, I thank Dr. Desnick for giving us a very concise summary as to what has to be done. We will collaborate with him and hope that at least some of the hypotheses developed here, will be tested by the time we reconvene. Thank you very much for your valued contributions to this conference.

REFERENCES

1. Zeman, W., S. Donahue, P. Dyken, and J. Green. The neuronal ceroid-lipofuscinoses (Batten-Vogt syndrome). In: Handbook of Clinical Neurology, Vol. 10, P. J. Vinken and G. W. Bruyn, eds., North-Holland, Amsterdam, 1970, pp 588-679.

2. Zeman, W. Historical development of the nosological concept of amaurotic familial idiocy. In: Handbook of Clinical Neurology, Vol. 10, P. J. Vinken and G. W. Bruyn, eds., North-Holland, Amsterdam, 1970, pp. 212-232.

3. Koppang, N. Canine ceroid-lipofuscinosis. A model for human neuronal ceroid-lipofuscinosis and aging. Mech. Age. Dev. 2, 421-445 (1973/74).

4. Levine, A. S., B. Lemieux, R. Brunning, J. G. White, H. L. Sharp, E. Stadlan, and W. Krivit. Ceroid accumulation in a patient with progressive neurological disease. Pediatrics 42, 483-491 (1968).

5. Öckerman, P. A. Lysosomal enzymes in juvenile amaurotic idiocy. Acta Paediat. Scand. 57, 537-539 (1968).

6. Desnick, R. J., P. D. Snyder, S. J. Desnick, W. Krivit, and H. L. Sharp. Sandhoff's disease: ultrastructural and biochemical studies. In: Sphingolipids, Sphingolipidoses, and Allied Disorders (Advan. Exp. Med. Biol., Vol. 19), B. W. Volk and S. M. Aronson, eds., Plenum Press, New York, 1972, pp. 351-371.

7. Patel, V., A. L. Tappel and J. S. O'Brien. Hyaluronidase and sulfatase deficiency in Hurler's syndrome. Biochem. Med., 3, 447-457 (1970).

8. Strouth, J. C., W. Zeman, and A. D. Merritt. Leukocyte abnormalities in familial amaurotic idiocy. N. Engl. J. Med. 274, 36-38 (1966).

9. Roels, O. A. In: The Vitamins, W. H. Sebrell, Jr., and R. S. Harris, eds., Academic Press, New York, 1967, pp. 196-200.

10. Philippart, M. Glycolipid, mucopolysaccharide and carbohydrate distribution in tissues, plasma and urine from glycolipidoses and other disorders. Adv. Exp. Med. Biol. 25, 237-254 (1972).

11. Sharp, H. L., and R. J. Desnick. Sandhoff's disease: diagnosis and evaluation by percutaneous liver biopsy. Gastroenterology 60, 752 (1971).

12. Hartroft, W. S., and E. A. Porta. Ceroid. Am. J. Med. Sci. 250, 324-345 (1965).

13. Dinning, J. S., and P. L. Day. Vitamin E deficiency in the monkey. I. Muscular dystrophy, hematologic changes, and the excretion of urinary nitrogenous constituents. J. Exp. Med. 105, 395-402 (1957).

14. Porter, F. S., C. D. Fitch, and J. S. Dinning. Vitamin E deficiency in the monkey. IV. Further studies of the anemia with emphasis on bone marrow morphology. Blood 20, 471-477 (1962).

15. Majaj, A. S., J. S. Dinning, S. A. Azzam, and W. J. Darby. Vitamin E responsive megaloblastic anemia in infants with protein-calorie malnutrition. Am. J. Clin. Nutr. 12, 374-379 (1963).

16. Poston, H. A. Effect of dietary vitamin E on microhematocrit, mortality and growth of immature brown trout. Fisheries Res. Bull. No. 28, Cortland Hatchery Report No. 33, p. 6 (1964).

17. Nafstad, I. Studies of hematology and bone marrow morphology in vitamin E-deficient pigs. Pathol. Vet. (Basel) 2, 277 (1965).

18. Bencze, V. B., F. Gerloczy, E. Ugrai, and F. Kneiszl. Über die Wirkung des Tocopherols auf die Synthese des Hämoglobins bei eiweissarmer Ernährung. Intern. Z. Vitaminforsch. 36, 24-38 (1966).

19. Oski, F. A., and L. A. Barness. Vitamin E deficiency: a previously unrecognized cause of hemolytic anemia in the premature infant. J. Pediat. 70, 211-220 (1967).

20. Weglicki, W. B., W. Reichel, and P. P. Nair. Accumulation of lipofuscin-like pigment in the rat adrenal gland as a function of vitamin E deficiency. J. Gerontol. 23, 469-475 (1968).

21. Murty, H. S., P. I. Caasi, S. K. Brooks, and P. P. Nair. Biosynthesis of heme in the E-deficient rat. J. Biol. Chem.

245, 5498-5504 (1968).

22. Caasi, P. I., J. W. Hauswirth, and P. P. Nair. Bio-
     synthesis of heme in Vitamin E deficiency. Ann. N. Y.
     Acad. Sci. 203, 93-102 (1972).

23. Granick, S. The induction in vitro of the synthesis of
     δ-aminolevulinic acid synthetase in chemical porphyria:
     A response to certain drugs and foreign chemicals. J.
     Biol. Chem. 241, 1359-1375 (1966).

24. Murty, H. S., and P. P. Nair. Prevention of allyliso-
     propylacetamide-induced experimental porphyria in the
     rat by vitamin E. Nature 223, 200-201 (1969).

25. Murty, H. S., A. Pinelli, P. P. Nair and A. I. Mendeloff.
     Porphyria cutanea tarda: therapeutic response to vitamin
     E. Clin Res. 173, 474 (1969).

26. Nair, P. P., E. Mezey, H. S. Murty, J. Quartner, and A.
     I. Mendeloff. Vitamin E and porphyrin metabolism in man.
     Arch. Int. Med. 128, 411-415 (1971).

27. Nair, P. P., H. S. Murty, and N. Grossman. The in
     vivo effect of vitamin E in experimental porphyria. Bio-
     chim. Biophys. Acta 215, 112-118 (1970).

28. Nair, P. P., H. S. Murty, P. I. Caasi, S. K. Brooks, and
     J. Quartner. Vitamin E regulation of the biosynthesis
     of porphyrins and heme. J. Agr. Food Chem. 20, 416 (1972).

29. Emerie, A., and C. Engel. Colorimetric determination of
     α-tocopherol (vitamin E). Rec. Trav. Chim. 57, 1351 (1968).

30. Nair, P. O., and Z. Luna. Identification of α-tocopherol
     from tissues by combined gas-liquid chromatography, mass
     spectrometry and infrared spectroscopy. Arch. Biochem.
     Biophys. 127, 413-418 (1968).

31. Binder, H. J., and H. M. Spiro. Tocopherol deficiency in
     man. Am. J. Clin. Nutr. 20, 594-601 (1967).

32. Hirsch, J., J. W. Farqhuar, E. H. Ahrens, Jr., M. L. Peterson,
     and W. Stoffel. Studies of adipose tissue in man. A
     microtechnic for sampling and analysis. Am. J. Clin. Nutr.
     8, 499-511 (1960).

33. Nair, P. P. Vitamin E and metabolic regulation. Ann. N.Y.
     Acad. Sci. 203, 53-61 (1972).

34. Rao, K. S., and R. O. Recknagel. Early incorporation of

carbon-labeled carbon tetrachloride into rat liver particulate lipids and proteins. Exp. Mol. Pathol. 10, 219-228 (1969).

35. Zeman, W. The neuronal ceroid-lipofuscinosis. A model for human aging? Adv. Geront. Res. 3, 147-170 (1971).

36. Tam, B. K., and P. B. McCay. Reduced triphosphophyridine nucleotide oxidase-catalyzed alterations of membrane phospholipids. III. Transient formation of phospholipid peroxides. J. Biol. Chem. 245, 2295-2300 (1970).

37. McCay, P. B., J. L. Poyer, P. M. Pfeifer, H. E. May, and J. M. Gilliam. A function for α-tocopherol: stablization of the microsomal membrane from radical attack during TPNH dependent oxidations. Lipids 6, 297-306 (1971).

38. Miquel, J., K. G. Bensch, D. E. Philpott, and H. Atlan. Natural aging and radiation-induced life shortening in Drosophila Melanogaster. Mech. Age. Dev. 1, 71-97 (1972).

39. Miquel, J. Aging in insects. In: The Physiology of Insecta, M. Rockstein, ed., Academic Press, New York, 1973, pp. 371-478.

40. Harman, D. Free radical theory of aging: effect of free radical reaction inhibitors on the mortality rate of Male LAF$_1$ mice. J. Gerontol. 23, 476-482 (1968).

41. Tappel, A. L. Will antioxidant nutrients slow aging processes? Geriatrics 23 (10), 97-105 (1968).

42. Tappel, A. L. Lipid peroxidation and fluorescent molecular damage to membranes. In: Pathological Aspects of Cell Membranes, B. F. Trump and A. Arstila, eds, Vol. 1, Academic Press, New York, in press.

43. Fletcher, B. L., C. J. Dillard, and A. L. Tappel. Measurement of fluorescent lipid peroxidation products in biological systems and tissues. Analyt. Biochem. 52, 1-9 (1973).

44. Recknagel, R. O., and A. K. Ghofhal. New data on the question of lipoperoxidation in carbon tetrachloride poisoning. Exp. Mol. Pathol. 5, 108-117 (1966).

45. Smith, L., and L. Packer. Aldehyde oxidation in rat liver mitochondria. Arch. Biochem. 148, 270-276 (1972).

46. Ingold, K. Third Round Table Conference on Batten's Disease, San Francisco, January 23-24, 1971.

47. Tappel, A. L. Lipid peroxidation damage to cell components, Fed. Proc. 32, 1870-1874 (1973).

48. Barber, A. Unrecorded discussion of paper by A. L. Tappel, Ann. N. Y. Acad. Sci. 203, 12-28 (1972).

49. Tarladgis, B. G., B. M. Watts, M. T. Younathan, and L. Dugan. A distillation method for the quantitative determination of malonaldehyde in rancid foods. J. Am. Oil Chemists' Soc. 37, 44 (1960).

50. Hagberg, B., P. Sourander, and L. Svennerholm. Late infantile progressive encephalopathy with disturbed polyunsaturated fat metabolism. Acta Paediat. Scand. 57, 495-499 (1968).

51. Berra, B. and C. Galli. Abnormal fatty acid pattern in brain gangliosides in a case of Kufs' disease. Life Sci. 10, (part 2), 213-216 (1971).

52. Bailey, J. M. Lipid metabolism in cultured cells. IV. Lipid biosynthesis in serum and synthetic growth media. Biochim. Biophys. Acta 125, 226-236 (1966).

53. Philippart, M. ^{14}C incorporation into brain explants from lipofuscinosis and sulfatidosis. In: 3rd International Meeting of the International Society for Neurochemistry, Budapest 1971, J. Domonkos et al., eds., Akademia Kiado, Budapest, 1971, p. 343.

54. Menkes, J. H., D. R. Harris, and N. Stein. Biochemical studies on brain explants and fibroblast cultures in Batten's disease. In: Sphingolipids, Sphingolipidoses and Allied Disorders (Advan. Exp. Med. Biol., Vol. 19), B. W. Volk and S. M. Aronson, eds., Plenum Press, New York, 1972, pp. 549-560.

55. Dhopeshwarkar, G. A., C. Subramanian, and J. F. Mead. Fatty acid uptake by the brain. IV. Incorporation of $(1-^{14}C)$ linoleic acid into the adult rat brain. Biochim. Biophys. Acta 231, 8-14 (1971).

56. Hers, H. G. Inborn lysosomal diseases. Gastroenterology 48, 625-633 (1965).

57. Cristofalo, V. J. Metabolic aspects of aging in diploid human cells. In: Aging in Cell and Tissue Culture, E. Holeckova and V. J. Cristofalo, eds., Plenum Press, New York, 1970, pp 83-119.

58. Kritchevsky, D., and B. V. Howard. Lipid metabolism in human diploid cells. In: Aging in Cell and Tissue

Culture, E. Holeckova and V. J. Cristofalo, eds., Plenum Press, New York, 1970, pp. 57-82.

59. Warren, L., and M. C. Glick. Membranes of animal cells. II. The metabolism and turnover of the surface membrane. J. Cell Biol. 37, 729-745 (1968).

60. Sharma, C. B. Selective inhibition of α-galactosidases by myoinositol. Biochem. Biophys. Res. Commun. 43, 572-579 (1971).

61. Van Hoof, F., and H. G. Hers. The abnormalities of lysosomal enzymes in mucopolysaccharidoses. Europ. J. Biochem. 7, 34-44 (1968).

62. Aronson, N. N., Jr., and E. A. Davidson. Lysosomal hyaluronidase from rat liver. J. Biol. Chem. 242, 441-444 (1967).

63. Samuels, S., N. K. Gonatas, and M. Weiss. Formation of membranous cytoplasmic bodies in Tay-Sachs disease: an in vitro study. J. Neuropath. Exp. Neurol. 24, 256-264 (1965).

64. Rouser, G., G. Kritchevsky, A. Yamamoto, A. Knudson, and G. Simon. Accumulation of glycerolphospholipid in classical Niemann-Pick disease. Lipids 3, 287-290 (1968).

65. Wherrett, J. R., and S. Huterer. Enrichment of bis-(monoacylglyceryl) phosphate in lysosomes from rat liver. J. Biol. Chem. 247, 4114-4120 (1972).

66. Yamamoto, A. K., S. Adachi, K. Ishikawa, T. Yokomura, T. Kitani, T. Nasu, T. Imoto, and M. Nishikawa. Studies on drug-induced lipidosis. III. Lipid composition of the liver and some other tissues in clinical cases of "Niemann-Pick-like syndrome" induced by 4,4'-diethylamino-ethoxyhexestrol. J. Biochem. 70, 774-784 (1971).

67. Sgoutas, D. S. Phospholipid changes during hepatic injury caused by carbon tetrachloride. Metabolism 16, 382-391 (1967).

68. Boehme, D. H., J. C. Cottrell, S. C. Leonberg, and W. Zeman. A dominant form of neuronal ceroid-lipofuscinosis. Brain 94, 745-760 (1971).

69. Zeman, W., and P. Dyken. Neuronal ceroid-lipofuscinosis (Batten's disease): relationship to amaurotic familial idiocy? Pediatrics 44, 570-583 (1969).

70. Philippart, M. Glycolipid, mucopolysaccharide and carbo-
hydrate distribution in tissues, plasma and urine from
glycolipidoses and other disorders. In: Glycolipids,
Glycoproteins and Mucopolysaccharides of the Nervous
System (Advan. Exp. Med. Biol. Vol. 25), V. Zambotti,
G. Tettamanti, and M. Arrigoni, eds., Plenum Press,
New York, 1972, pp. 231-254.

71. Porta, E. A., and W. S. Hartroft. In: Pigments in
Pathology, M. Wolman, ed., Academic Press, New York,
1969.

72. Kayden, H. J. and L. Bjornson. The dynamics of vitamin
E transport in the human erythrocyte. Ann. N. Y. Acad.
Sci. 203, 127-140 (1972).

73. Hug, G., W. K. Schubert, and G. Chuck. Type II glycogenosis: treatment with extract of Aspergillus niger.
Clin. Res. 16, 345 (1968).

74. Baudhuin, P., H. G. Hers, and H. Loeb. An electron
microcsopic and biochemical study of type II glycogenosis.
Lab. Invest. 13, 1139-1152 (1964).

75. Fernandes, J., and F. Huijing. Branching enzyme-deficiency
glycogenosis: studies in therapy. Arch. Dis. Child. 43,
347-352 (1968).

76. Greene, H. L., G. Hug, and W. K. Schubert. Metachromatic
leukodystrophy: treatment with arylsulfatase-A. Arch.
Neurol. 20, 147-153 (1969).

77. Austin, J. Studies in metachromatic leukodystrophy.
XII. Therapeutic considerations. In: Enzyme Therapy in
Genetic Diseases. Birth Defects: Original Article Series,
New York, IX 2, 125-129 (1973).

78. Mapes, C. A., R. L. Anderson, C. C. Sweeley, R. J. Desnick,
and W. Krivit. Enzyme replacement as a possible therapy
for Fabry's disease, an inborn error of metabolism. Science
169, 987-989 (1970).

79. Sweeley, C. C., C. A. Mapes, W. Krivit, and R. J. Desnick.
Chemistry and metabolism of glycosphingolipids in Fabry's
disease. In: Sphingolipids, Sphingolipidoses and Allied
Disorders (Advan. Exp. Med. Biol., Vol. 19), B. W. Volk
and S. M. Aronson, eds., Plenum Press, New York, 1972,
pp. 287-304.

80. DiFerrante, N., B. L. Nichols, P. V. Donnelly, G. Neri, R.
Hrgovcic, and R. K. Berglund. Induced degradation of
glycosaminoglycans in Hurler's and Hunter's syndromes by

plasma infusion. Proc. Nat. Acad. Sci. U. S. <u>68</u>, 303-307 (1971).

81. Knudson, A. G., Jr., N. DiFerrante, and J. E. Curtis.
     Effect of leukocyte transfusion in a child with Type II
     mucopolysaccharidosis. Proc. Nat. Acad. Sci. U. S. <u>68</u>,
     1738 (1971).

82. Philippart, M., S. S. Franklin, A. Gordon, D. Leeber, and
     A. R. Hull. Studies on the metabolic control of Fabry's
     disease through kidney transplantation. In: Sphingolipids,
     Sphingolipidoses and Allied Disorders (Advan. Exp. Med.
     Biol., Vol. 19), B. W. Volk and S. M. Aronson, eds.,
     Plenum Press, New York, 1972, pp. 641-649.

83. Desnick, R. J., K. Y. Allen, R. L. Simmons, J. S. Najarian,
     and W. Krivit. Treatment of Fabry's disease: correction
     of the enzymatic deficiency by renal transplantation.
     J. Lab. Clin. Med. <u>78</u>, 989 (1971).

84. Desnick, R. J., R. L. Simmons, K. Y. Allen, J. E. Woods,
     C. F. Anderson, J. S. Najarian, and W. Krivit. Correction
     of enzymatic deficiencies by renal transplantation: Fabry's
     disease. Surgery, <u>72</u>, 203-211 (1972).

85. Desnick, R. J., K. Y. Allen, R. L. Simmons, J. E. Woods,
     C. F. Anderson, J. S. Najarian, and W. Krivit. Fabry's
     Disease. Correction of the enzyme deficiency by renal
     transplantation. Birth Defects: Original Article Series
     ix 12, (New York), 88-96 (1972).

86. Desnick, S. J., R. J. Desnick, R. O. Brady, P. Pentshev,
     R. L. Simmons, J. S. Najarian, K. Swaiman, H. L. Sharp,
     and W. Krivit. Renal transplantation in Type II Gaucher
     Disease. Birth Defects: Original Article Series (New York)
     <u>72</u>, 109-119 (1972).

87. Austin, J. H. Some recent findings in leukodystrophies
     and in gargoylism. In: Inborn Disorders of Sphingolipid
     Metabolism, S. M. Aronson and B. W. Volk, eds., Pergamon
     Press, New York, 1967, pp 359-387.

88. King, J. L. and T. H. Jukes. Non-Darwinian evolution.
     Science <u>164</u>, 788-798 (1969).

89. Fratantoni, J. C., C. W. Hall, and E. F. Neufeld. The
     defect in Hurler and Hunter syndromes. II. Deficiency
     of specific factors involved in mucopolysaccharide degrada-
     tion. Proc. Nat. Acad. Sci. U. S. <u>64</u>, 360-366 (1969).

90. Dawson, G. and C. C. Sweeley. In vivo studies on glyco-
     sphingolipid metabolism in porcine blood. J. Biol. Chem.
     <u>245</u>, 410-416 (1970).

91. Porter, M. T., A. L. Fluharty, and H. Kihara. Correction of abnormal cerebroside sulfate metabolism in cultured metachromatic leukodystrophy fibroblasts. Science 172, 1263-1265 (1971).

92. Weismann, U. N., E. E. Rossi, and N. N. Herschkowitz. Treatment of metachromatic leukodystrophy in fibroblasts by enzyme replacement. N. Engl. J. Med. 284, 672-673 1971).

93. de Duve, C., personal communication.

94. Neufeld, E. F., and M. H. Cantz. Corrective factors from inborn errors of mucopolysaccharide metabolism. Ann. N. Y. Acad. Sci. 179, 580 (1971).

95. Neufeld, E. F., and J. C. Fratantoni. Inborn errors of mucopolysaccharide metabolism. Science 169, 141-146 (1970).

Dr. Donald Armstrong
Assistant Professor of Neurology
University of Colorado Medical School
Denver, Colorado

Dr. James H. Austin
Professor of Neurology
Department of Neurology
University of Colorado Medical School
Denver, Colorado

Dr. Glyn Dawson
Assistant Professor
Departments of Pediatrics and Biochemistry
University of Chicago
Chicago, Illinois

Dr. W. Stanley Hartroft
Professor of Pathology
University of Hawaii School of Medicine
Honolulu, Hawaii

Dr. Paul Hochstein
Professor of Pharmacology
University of Southern California School of Medicine
Los Angeles, California

Dr. John H. Menkes
Professor of Pediatrics, Neurology & Psychiatry
University of California
Los Angeles, California

Dr. John S. O'Brien
Chairman, Department of Neurosciences
University of California
San Diego, California

Dr. Vimalkumar Patel
Assistant Professor
Indiana University Medical Center
Indianapolis, Indiana

Dr. Alan Percy
Director of Pediatric Neurology
Charles R. Drew Postgraduate Medical School
Los Angeles, California

Dr. Michel Philippart
Associate Professor of Pediatrics Neurology &
  Psychiatry
University of California
Los Angeles, California

Dr. J. Alfred Rider
President
Children's Brain Diseases Foundation
San Francisco, California

Mr. Mark Ruddick
Student, School of Medicine
University of California
San Diego, California

Dr. A. N. Siakotos
Associate Professor of Pathology
Indiana University Medical Center
Indianapolis, Indiana

Dr. Frank Yatsu
Associate Professor of Neurology
University of California School of Medicine
San Francisco, California

Dr. Wolfgang Zeman
Professor of Neuropathology
Indiana University Medical Center
Indianapolis, Indiana

FIFTH ROUND TABLE CONFERENCE ON BATTEN'S DISEASE

<u>Dr. Wolfgang Zeman</u>: I will introduce this conference
by giving you a thumbnail sketch on a group of diseases which
we have come to name neuronal ceroid-lipofuscinoses or, in
deference to the early authors, the Batten-Vogt syndrome.
This is a group of diseases in which the clinical manifestations
are a progressive deterioration of mental and motor functions,
blindness, and, during the later stages, generalized convulsions
and a host of vegetative disturbances. From a morphological
point of view, the condition is characterized by the accumulation
of autofluorescent lipopigments in the nerve cells to the
point that they first suffer a reduction of an enormous proportion of their dendritic apparatus and eventually the neuronal
perikarya disintegrate and disappear. Thus, the disease is
associated with gross brain atrophy which, in certain forms
of this condition, may reach staggering proportions--down
to about 250 g. Originally, these conditions have all been
described as amaurotic idiocy with the specific implication
that the nerve cell perikarya become distended by the accumulation of lipid matter such as is the case in Tay-Sachs disease;
and, accordingly, this group of disorders--neuronal ceroid-
lipofuscinoses--has formed the so-called noninfantile forms
of amaurotic idiocy such as the late infantile form, the
juvenile form, and certain instances of the adult form. We
have coined the term neuronal ceroid-lipofuscinosis in an
effort to distinguish this group of conditions pathogenetically,
morphologically, and biochemically from disturbances of sphingolipid metabolism, in particular those lysosomal diseases which
are associated with an accumulation of gangliosides and, in
the case of Niemann-Pick disease, also with sphingomyelin.

The pathogenesis of the neuronal ceroid-lipofuscinoses
is reasonably well established; however, the biochemical defect
is as yet unknown. For several years we have entertained
the hypothesis that the formation of intracellular autofluorescent lipopigments is a result of a disturbance of lipid
peroxidation, more specifically in the peroxidation of unsaturated fatty acids, which from all we know is a nonenzymatic
process, and that the peroxidized unsaturated fatty acids
by scission and formation of peroxy radicals produce lipid
polymers which accumulate in the cytoplasm. In the wake of
repetitive focal cell lysis, they become progressively incorporated into tertiary lysosomes. We have also assumed that
these polymers cannot be broken down by enzymatic cleavage

221

and, therefore, rest presumably as inert bodies within the
cell. However, in the process of lipid peroxidation, formation
of carbonyl compounds as well as lipid peroxide occurs. All
these species are highly reactive and, as shown by Tappel
and others,[1] are capable of binding biological species such
as proteins and nucleic acid bases. Thus, the process of
lipid peroxidation is not entirely innocuous, inasmuch as
there is a possibility that biological species become inactivated
and incorporated into the crosslinks and polymerized mixture
of biological constituents. As a follow-up of this hypothesis
we have begun to treat patients who have neuronal ceroid-
lipofuscinosis with high doses of antioxidants such as vitamin
E, Santoquin, and butylated hydroxytoluene, adding ascorbic
acid as a hydrogen donor, and DL-methionine as a radical scavenger. This, as far as I can see, has been the status of
our knowledge of this disease until recently.

On the basis of the strong evidence for lipid peroxidation as a significant aspect of the chemical pathogenesis,
several of us have been looking at the activities of various
types of peroxidases. In addition, we have begun the antioxidant
treatment with relatively gratifying results, especially if
practiced in children with the so-called Spielmeyer-Sjögren
type of disease (a relatively slowly progressive disorder)
and if instituted during the early stages of the disease.[2]
Quite recently, Armstrong and Austin reported[3] a significant
decrease in the activity of myeloperoxidase in patients presumably suffering from the Spielmeyer-Sjögren type and lesser
reduction of the activity of this enzyme in ascertained heterozygotes. In addition, Dr. Patel in our laboratory has been
looking at another peroxidase system--glutathione peroxidase--
which, according to Tappel,[1] is probably the most important
and crucial enzyme system that detoxifies aliphatic acid peroxides, and he will report certain observations in this area.
Nevertheless, it appears from the data currently available
that we can now really come fully to grips with the possible
underlying enzyme defects which would produce an accelerated
peroxidation of unsaturated fatty acids and hence result
in the manifestation of this disease. This is the reason
why Dr. Rider and I felt it would be the time to get together
and discuss some of the pending aspects of the peroxidase
systems as they relate to the human and animal body.

I should mention before I yield the floor to general
discussion that Dr. Hartroft about ten years ago, on the basis
of a series of ingenious experiments, came to the conclusion[4]
that formation of these autofluorescent lipopigments is actually
governed according to thermodynamic principles in the following
fashion. High concentrations of polyunsaturated fatty acids
generally facilitate lipid peroxidation, as do high concentrations of oxidants such as, for instance, bivalent metal

ions; on the other hand, high concentrations of saturated
fatty acids and high concentrations of antioxidants will slow
down lipid peroxidation. There are thus at least four groups
of variables which would have to be considered as possible
pathogens. With respect to the high concentration of polyunsaturated fatty acids, there is some spotty evidence that
this per se may either be responsible for the disease, as
suggested by Svennerholm,[5] or may explain certain manifestations
of these disorders of lipid peroxidation--for example the
rapid and, unfortunately not yet treatable, degeneration of
the receptor part of the optic epithelium, the rods and cones.
It has been shown by Svennerholm[6] that during a certain stage
of human development the rods and cones contain a rather high
concentration of a polyenic acid, dodecosahexaneic acid, and
from what we know about lipid peroxidation this is a type
of fatty acid which lends itself very readily to spontaneous
peroxidation if not properly protected.

These are some of the aspects which form the background
of this meeting. I think we should first try to have some
understanding as to the molecular and subcellular aspects
of peroxidative mechanisms, and I just wonder who's going
to volunteer. Dr. Hochstein, could you address yourself to
that problem?

Dr. Paul Hochstein: You've indicated quite properly
what the problems are in terms of initiation, in terms of
the substrate available for peroxidation, and in terms of
the chain-breaking or antioxidant mechanisms. I'd like to
take issue with one of your statements and perhaps provide
a basis for further discussion. You indicated that the initiators
for lipid peroxidation were nonenzymatic in nature--and there
are many nonenzymatic initiators of peroxidation, for example,
certain metals--but in addition there is an enzymatic mechanism
for forming lipid peroxides which might possibly be relevant
in Batten's disease.

A few years ago we described[7] in the liver a system which
peroxidizes endogenous lipid in the hepatic tissue. This
system is very interesting in that it uses the electron transport
system that the liver normally uses for drug hydroxylation.
These reactions convert phenobarbital, for example, to its
hydroxylated or demethylated products. Normally this peroxidation system, which requires NADPH and pyrophosphate, is
suppressed in the liver. It is not functioning because drugs,
steroids, and other complex molecules compete for electrons
and prevent that kind of enzymatic peroxidation, which one
can demonstrate in vitro but with only great difficulty in
vivo. Anything that happens to remove the substrates for
drug hydroxylation, be they endogenous steroids or exogenous
drugs, will release the lipid peroxidizing system and permit

damage to occur in the liver in the form of peroxidation or
the accumulation of malonaldehyde in these fluorescent pigments.
This system occurs in liver and kidney. Its activity in
brain tissue is very, very weak--at least when you deal with
brain as a tissue as opposed to a heterogeneous organ. This
might be very relevant to the problem of lipid peroxidation
in brain if this system is active in brain tissue in localized
areas and suppressed normally by endogenous agents. In disease,
the mechanism might be released and might permit lipid peroxidation to take place. This is now another way in which lipid
peroxides might be formed and I think highly relevant, so
I think you have to add enzymatic initiaton to the things
that we are going to talk about. I was also a little puzzled
about the antioxidant mechanisms you mentioned. You say ascorbic
acid is currently used in treatment of Batten's disease. To
my knowledge, ascorbic acid is not really an antioxidant in
lipid compartments; it's highly water-soluble and functions
in water compartments in the cell. As a matter of fact, in
vitro ascorbic acid can act as a pro-oxidant because it auto-
oxidizes; it reacts with oxygen to produce hydrogen peroxide,
which can induce lipid peroxidation. I would like to ask
the question: what is the evidence that ascorbic acid is really
of value in the treatment of this disease as an antioxidant?
Is there good evidence that that's the case?

Dr. Zeman: Well, our treatment has been given to seven
patients thus far, and I must admit that we never felt we
could evaluate it in double-blind studies, simply because
the disease is so exceedingly rare. The evidence for using
ascorbic acid in addition to vitamin E is obtained only from
in vitro observations, which indicate that in the presence
of antioxidants such as vitamin E, the ascorbic acid acts
as a hydrogen donor and thus complements the antioxidant action
of vitamin E.

Dr. Hochstein: I know there are models for ascorbic
acid acting as a hydrogen donor. I'm just questioning how
effective they are in a heterogeneous system where you have
no mixing of fat and water.

Dr. Zeman: I must say we do not know.

Dr. Hochstein: Also with regard to the antioxidants
problem, I'd like to reinforce what you said about glutathione
peroxidase being a key enzyme involved in chain terminating
or preventing accumulation of lipid peroxides. Along with
Dr. Tappel, I agree that this is an essential enzyme for this
step, and it's an interesting enzyme for this reason: the
substrates for glutathione peroxidase are lipid peroxides
and reduced glutathione, a tripeptide. In order for glutathione
peroxidase to continue to function, glutathione has to be
maintained in the reduced form in the cell; and this is done

through a sequence of reactions ultimately depending on glucose metabolism. In other words, if a cell is going to maintain glutathione or glutathione peroxidase activity, the cell has to be using glucose normally and generating reduced nucleotides to maintain glutathione in the reduced form. We have shown, for example, that red cells can be sensitized to peroxidation reactions by depriving the cell of glucose. Lipids will then peroxidize very rapidly, even though vitamin E is present, because this reduced glutathione is not being maintained in the cell. For this reason, I think it would be highly relevant to know something about glucose metabolism in Batten's disease. Is there a normal glucose tolerance curve, for example? My point is that the problem may involve not only lipids but carbohydrate metabolism as well. Removing hydrogen donors, such as reduced glutathione, would expose the cell to oxidant damage. I think this would be an important area to consider this afternoon.

Dr. Zeman: I might give you an answer to this particular problem. The rate of oxidative phosphorylation which in this respect would be some indication for glucose metabolism, was measured by Korey and his associates[8] many years ago and was found to be normal. The glucose tolerance curve in these patients is usually normal during the early stages of the disease, but as soon as there is hypothalamic involvement, of course, a secondary disturbance in the glucose metabolism becomes manifest. We do know, that the accumulation of the pigments is a process which, at least in the dog model, begins before birth and continues throughout the life span of the animals, seems homozygous for the trait, although clinical manifestations of the disease do not show up until about age 15 to 18 months. From observations in humans, especially with respect to the accumulation of these autofluorescent lipopigments in such tissues as the intestines and vegetative ganglia which are functionally normal, it appears that the presence and the formation of pigment is not directly related to a disturbance of function. That's all I can say to this subject.

Dr. Hochstein: Dr. Zeman, I'd like to stop now and perhaps resume our discussion of mechanisms later.

Dr. Zeman: I think we should have someone talk to us a little bit about the precise molecular and subcellular mechanism by which peroxidation is occurring in the cells and by which its products become detoxified. Does this take place inside peroxisomes, for example, or is this a cytoplasmic process? Could you tell us about that?

Dr. Hochstein: For those of you who know more about this than I do, please bear with me; and for those of you who know less, I hope I can shed some light on what we mean by peroxidation

in cells. I can state the biological problem very clearly.
The problem that all cells have to solve in living with oxygen
concerns the fact that they also live with unsaturated fatty
acids. If I were to take pure unsaturated fatty acids and
put them in a glass on this table, within minutes they would
begin to go rancid. Rancidity, for the present discussion,
may be considered simply the addition of oxygen to unsaturated
fatty acids. The reaction is initiated by the abstraction
of hydrogen from a carbon atom in the chain adjacent to a
double bond; the initiator may be a metal, an organic compound,
or an enzyme. The initiator abstracts the hydrogen and creates
a free radical, i.e., a carbon with an unshared electron.
This unshared electron is now highly reactive to molecular
oxygen and can form a peroxy radical. This is also an unstable
chemical species which can undergo a variety of reactions.
For example, this species may react with substances known
as chain breakers. The peroxy radical may also react in vivo
with a hydrogen atom donated by glutathione to form a hydroperoxide; vitamin E may also donate a hydrogen to terminate
this reaction. If there is no vitamin E around and if there
is no glutathione around--in other words, if you have only
pure unsaturated fatty acid sitting in the beaker--the peroxy
free radical could react with a second molecule of an unsaturated
fatty acid to abstract a proton from it, forming a hydroperoxide
and another free radical; this is what is referred to as a
chain reaction. Once initiation takes place, once the first
molecule of a peroxy fatty acid is formed, the second molecule
will likely be formed through interaction of these two fatty
acid molecules unless a chain breaker is present. The chain
breakers then permit formation of only the first molecule
of peroxy fatty acid and not the second. This is why substances
like vitamin E are so essential if cells are going to live
with unsaturated fatty acids in the presence of oxygen. The
formation of the hydroperoxide may lead to formation of various
other breakdown products of the unsaturated fatty acid. Once
breaking of this carbon chain takes place, it is possible
to get what Dr. Zeman referred to as carbonyl compounds; the
most common compound formed as a result of peroxidation reactions
is malonyl dialdehyde. This three-carbon dialdehyde is formed
as a result of spontaneous breakdown of hydroperoxides, perhaps
through epoxides once they're formed. It is malonyl dialdehyde
which reacts with proteins--with nucleic acids perhaps, but
certainly with proteins--to give the fluorescent pigments
with which you are all familiar. The malonyl dialdehyde reacts
with amino groups in proteins and crosslinks proteins to make
fluorescent compounds, and this is what Dr. Tappel has demonstrated so clearly.

    To summarize: whether malonyl dialdehyde is formed depends
on what initiators are present, what chain breakers are present
and how much unsaturated fatty acid is present and in what
sites. Once these lipid peroxides are formed, malonyl dialdehyde

is formed; tissue damage follows. You can see it--depending on the tissue--in a variety of ways: for example, in vitamin E deficiency which occurs in premature infants, one often sees the formation of lipid peroxides and a consequent anemia. In the liver, for example, lipid peroxidation is accompanied by damage to the endoplasmic reticulum and altered liver function.

Dr. Zeman: Could you perhaps put this into perspective with respect to the cellular and subcellular anatomy?

Dr. Hochstein: Certainly. What one is usually dealing with in lipid peroxidation is unsaturated fatty acid associated with membranes. Depending on the cells, various membranes may be involved. In the cell I know best of all--the red cell--all the lipid is associated with the outer membrane of the cell. In that case it's the outer membrane of the erythrocyte in which peroxidation takes place, not in any aqueous compartment. In more complex cells, the lipid is usually associated with membranes in the reticulum, mitochondria, and nuclear membranes, and it is in these areas where one sees the formation of these products. The peroxisome, to my knowledge, is not thought to be involved in the initiation process, but the peroxisome is loaded with an enzyme called catalase, which is very efficient in destroying peroxide, and the peroxide level is quite low in the peroxisome. I do not know of any demonstration that the peroxisome has a greater tendency to undergo lipid peroxidation than does a mitochondrial membrane, for example.

Dr. Zeman: Is the glutathione peroxidase, glutathione reductase, and glutamate dehydrogenase system located in the peroxisome, or where do we place this glutathione shuttle system?

Dr. Hochstein: The glutathione peroxidase system is by and large an aqueous system which interacts with lipid structures, although one can isolate mitochondria which contain glutathione peroxidase. Presumably they contain the enzyme in the inner mitochondrial space but in intimate association with lipids. The ways in which glutathione peroxidase interacts with lipids is very unclear at present, but it certainly may occur in association with lipid structures. The enzymes involved in maintaining reduced glutathione, which is the other substrate for glutathione peroxidase, are by and large cytosol enzymes i.e., water-soluble enzymes, and glutathione itself is water-soluble, but through its reaction with glutathione peroxidase the glutathione does interact with lipid compartments.

Dr. Zeman: One final question, Dr. Hochstein. The myeloperoxidase, about which we will talk later, is this a peroxisomal enzyme?

Dr. Hochstein: My understanding is that the myeloperoxidase of the white cell, for example, is not a peroxisomal enzyme. It occurs in granules distinct from the peroxisome, and the granule also contains hydrolytic enzymes, nonperoxisomal enzymes, and more of the lysosomal type.

Dr. John H. Menkes: One question, Dr. Hochstein. In addition to the polyunsaturated fatty acids which can initiate peroxidation or lose a proton, are there any major or minor physiological substances that can do the same thing; that is, should we look at something else besides polyunsaturated fatty acids?

Dr. Hochstein: Yes, as a matter of fact, it is possible to form peroxides with a variety of biological materials, including nucleic acid. It has been postulated, for example, that one of the consequences of radiation damage is the oxidation or peroxidation of nucleic acids. Usually the energies involved in peroxidizing substances other than fat are much higher, and so when one thinks of peroxidation one thinks of unsaturated fats.

Dr. Menkes: I was thinking of one of my experiments where I found that cholesterol or steroids will actually do the same thing. Can you comment on that?

Dr. Hochstein: I'm not familiar with that reaction, but it doesn't surprise me that a steroid molecule will form, rather than a hydroxylated product, a peroxidized metabolite-- it's not a surprising thing.

Dr. Menkes: The most obvious one that most steroid chemists know about is that cholesterol, under the presence of light, will go to ketocholesterol rather readily.

Dr. Hochstein: There are lots of reactions of this kind which are enhanced, and some of them are really not peroxidation reactions. For example, the well-known reaction in which adrenalin reacts with oxygen to form adrenochrome, is not really a peroxidation but is an auto-oxidation involving the uptake of molecular oxygen to form a very reactive species which can initiate peroxidation in other molecules. Numerous biologically important compounds will undergo these auto-oxidation or peroxidation reactions; the unsaturated lipid system is simply the most highly reactive. The unsaturated bonds and the carbons adjacent to them are extraordinarily reactive in a biological system. It's one of the miracles of evolution on this planet that we have made our peace with oxygen and learned to live with oxygen and unsaturated fatty acids which require a membrane through development of antioxidant systems. In an evolutionary sense we have developed systems to handle the formation of these radicals which lead to cell deterioration and pathology.

Dr. Alex V. Nichols: Would you put into context again the subcellular distribution of these enzymes. Are they specifically in mitochondrial and peroxisome locations? Are there any other sites that are potential sites of peroxidation?

Dr. Hochstein: Yes, any site that is membranatious in nature...

Dr. Nichols: No, I meant in terms of the location of the enzymes themselves.

Dr. Hochstein: Oh, I see. Well, we have to decide which enzymes we're going to talk about. The enzyme that I mentioned initially--TPNH, lipid peroxide-inducing enzyme-- is located in the endoplasmic reticulum of the cell. Glutathione peroxidase, the enzyme which is involved in free-radical chain breaking and breaking down of these lipid peroxides, is primarily a soluble enzyme, but it may also be associated with the endo- plasmic reticulum, some of it with mitochondria. The other enzymes involved in maintenance of glutathione or glutathione peroxidase activity are water-soluble enzymes. Because of our feeling that carbohydrate metabolism is so important in maintaining glutathione peroxidase activity, one has to include in the antioxidant system all the mechanisms by which glucose is transported to the cells, by which it is phosphorylated through the hexokinase reaction and passed down the appropriate pathway. All of those enzymes, in that they generate reduced nucleotides which are involved in glutathione reduction, are important in evaluation of the total antioxidant capacity of the cell. They tend to be water-soluble, by and large, except for the transport mechanisms involving glucose.

Dr. James H. Austin: As a follow-up on what Dr. Hochstein was saying, I think we all know it's possible to cut down on the levels of polyunsaturated fatty acids in tissues by putting patients or animals on a diet free of polyunsaturated compounds or, conversely, to increase the levels of saturated fatty acids by putting the animals or people on a diet rich in saturated fatty acids. Considering the vulnerability of tissues that have a high degree of polyunsaturation, I wonder if we might not consider adding a diet low in polyunsaturated fatty acids to the regimen our patients are on.

Dr. Zeman: As a rule of thumb, I believe, it is assumed that 0.02 wt-% of artificial oxidant or synthetic antioxidants are sufficient to prevent auto-oxidation in vitro. This is about the concentration of the various additives to diets, to rubber, to gasoline, and so forth, to prevent either rancidity or autocatalytic oxidation. The doses which we give in our treatment are several orders of magnitude above this level. So, while we basically agree that we should be cautious with the ingestion of unsaturated fatty acids, in our ordinary daily diet it does not make that much of a difference.

There is, as you know, the yellow fat disease in cats, which Dr. Hartroft among others has studied extensively.[9] This is a disease in which the ingestion of high quantities of polyunsaturated fatty acids does produce auto-oxidation, particularly in storage fats. However, I'm afraid this may lead us off on a tangent which we do not want to follow at the moment, and I wonder if there are any further remarks or questions with respect to the various mechanisms of per-oxidation of unsaturated fatty acids in cells and in tissue.

I would like to ask one question of Dr. Hochstein. You mentioned, and I agree, that catalase is very efficient as a peroxisomal enzyme to break down hydrogen peroxides. However, how about peroxide which is bound to other biological species in the form of either a peroxide radical or a hydroperoxy radical? Catalase doesn't deal with these compounds, and this requires a peroxidation reaction. My question therefore is this--would you consider it possible that in the presence of normal catalase activity some other peroxidation reaction may proceed so slowly or at such a reduced level that there is a build-up of peroxide or peroxy or hydroperoxy radicals?

Dr. Hochstein: Yes, Dr. Zeman, you have touched upon a sensitive topic, because I am continually involved in a controversy on the role of catalase in destroying hydrogen peroxide in cells. We were able to demonstrate some years ago[10] that glutathione peroxidase, before we knew that it reacted to lipid peroxides, was more efficient than catalase in handling hydrogen peroxide. The evidence that glutathione peroxidase is the key enzyme, at least in certain cells, is overwhelming. For example, there are acatalasic individuals in the world; there are some 100 individuals now known and 20 families who have no catalase in their red cells, for example, and they are able to handle hydrogen peroxide in a very satis-factory manner. They have no clinical problems, because gluta-thione peroxidase takes over this function that we all thought catalase performed in the red cells. For example, while birds have no catalase in their red cells, they don't need it as long as they have glutathione peroxidase present and glucose to maintain the reduced glutathione and hence glutathione peroxidase activity. So, at least in certain cells glutathione peroxidase is the enzyme involved. In the brain and liver or in tissues in which you have peroxisome, the situation is a little more complex There catalase probably does have the function of destroying peroxide in the peroxisome, and

glutathione peroxidase plays a lesser role. What other enzymes
might be involved I don't know. Certainly in the white cells
myeloperoxidase is very important, not so much in destroying
peroxides but in using peroxides to help kill bacteria. In
these cells the myeloperoxidase competes with the catalase
and the glutathione peroxidase for peroxides. I think you'd
have to ask this question in each tissue in a different way.

   Dr. Austin: Could you say a word about how myeloperoxidase uses peroxides to kill bacteria?

   Dr. Hochstein: The role of myeloperoxidase in bacterial
killing has been defined in a very elegant way in recent years[11]
in patients with chronic granulomatous disease. Apparently
hydrogen peroxide is necessary for a reaction that may involve
the fusion of lysosomal membranes with the phagosomes containing
bacteria. The best evidence right now is that the reaction
involves inorganic iodide ion. The reaction involves the
oxidation of iodide by hydrogen peroxides in the presence
of myeloperoxidase to somehow open up the lysosomal membrane
for fusion with the phagosomal vacuole, and this permits "dumping"
of the hydrolytic enzymes of the lysosome into the phagosome
containing the bacteria. A second concept is that after
"dumping" and the fusion of lysosomal and phagosomal membranes
take place, the myeloperoxidase comes in contact with the
bacterial cell itself. There the hydrogen peroxide and iodide
are involved in a reaction to destroy the lipid envelope around
the bacteria. The details of this reaction are obscure. It
is possible that the myeloperoxidase oxidizes the iodide into
something called triiodide which then reacts with phospholipids
with fixed positive charges--choline, for example--in phospholipids and causes opening of membranes. That membrane may
be the lysosomal membrane or it may be a bacterial membrane.
The amounts of peroxide in cells--the amounts of iodide in
cells--are not sufficient per se to kill bacteria; they will
not permit "dumping"; myeloperoxidase is necessary for "dumping"
and/or killing.

   Dr. Frank Yatsu: I'd like to ask Dr. Hochstein a question
about enzymatic suppression of lipoperoxidation. Pritchard
and Singh studied formation of peroxide in rat brains by
assessing malonaldehyde. From infancy to adulthood, the amount
of polyunsaturated fatty acid increased so that polyunsaturates
constituted fully a third or so of the total fatty acid content.
Pritchard and Singh reasoned that if these tissues were incubated, increased amounts of malonaldehyde formation would
be observed. Contrary to expectation, however, the amount
decreased. They therefore reasoned something within the brain
of a mature animal must protect against lipoperoxidation.
Apparently there was a dialysable protein which contained
iron, and was heat labile. I don't know if this was pursued
further and I was wondering if you thought this had merit

and whether it has in fact been pursued.

Dr. Austin: A protein which was nondialysable?

Dr. Yatsu: I think it was dialysable; it was a small protein. A similar protein was also found in serum which, when added to the incubation medium, protected the system against lipoperoxidation.

Dr. Hochstein: I've always been impressed whenever we work with brain tissue. It seems to me that the brain has very little reservoir of reducing capacity. As a biochemist, I see brain as a tissue that is really exposed to oxidizing agents in unique ways. The liver has a reducing capacity, in terms of its ability to reduce oxidizing agents, that is ten to one hundred times that of the brain. Certainly brain belongs in a category by itself in terms of sensitivity to oxidation. It certainly has intrinsic interest to those concerned with peroxidation reactions.

Dr. Zeman: We may add that not only is the brain in a very special position, but different regions of the brain are very different in their capability of providing reducing activity.

Dr. J. Alfred Rider: Could I ask a question? Is the process of peroxidation damaging, or is it the peroxide itself that's damaging? In either case, how are they damaging?

Dr. Zeman: Peroxidation of unsaturated fatty acid, of course, changes the physio-chemical property of the lipid molecule per se, so the peroxidation of a lipid molecule essentially destroys its biological activity. However, the process is significant as a damaging one not because of inactivation of the lipid molecule, but rather because of the chain reaction which has been pointed out by Dr. Hochstein. That is, once a lipid molecule has been peroxidized, the next unsaturated fatty acid molecule will be subject to the same process by a proton radical. The peroxidation reaction involves a relatively large portion of adjacent molecules. This in itself is still only lipid inactivation, but once these chain scission reactions take place, the aliphatic chain becomes broken down and transformed into carbonyls. The carbonyls-- dialdehydes essentially--are excellent fixatives (as a matter of fact for electron microscopy we use dialdehyde as a fixative), and the aldehyde groups in these carbonyl compounds strongly interact with amino and amide groups (with lysine, for example, or with the amine group in complex lipids such as ethanolamine). Furthermore, the peroxy radicals of free fatty acid may engage in covalent binding with any kind of biological molecule. So the answer to your question is that while lipid peroxidation per se is relatively harmless, the secondary and tertiary

232

reactions which are a consequence of the lipid peroxidation are the ones which are severely damaging.

Dr. Rider: And how are they damaging--by destroying the essential molecules?

Dr. Zeman: By inactivating biological molecules, by crosslinking them, by fracturing them, by peroxidizing them. These peroxides can jump over to another biological molecule, and so forth; so this is a chemical in situ fixation and fracturing of biological molecules.

Dr. Rider: It's a molecular disruption then?

Dr. Zeman: That's right.

Dr. Hochstein: To add to what Dr. Zeman said, once these carbonyls are formed, they can crosslink any protein, and that reaction is nonspecific. The proteins they crosslink may be enzymes which are essential in carbohydrate metabolism or nucleic metabolism, so it is possible to get a very generalized kind of damage: crosslinking of enzymes which are essential to cell function.

Dr. W. Stanley Hartroft: My comment is relevant to yours concerning chain breakers. By use of a simple model in which the epididymal fat pad is mechanically crushed at operation, ceroid is formed within a few days. It was unexpected to find that the pigment continued to accumulate once we set up the initial reaction by the one simple traumatic event at time zero. We are continuing to study this phenomenon to obtain better quantitation than originally available. In any case, it appears that in this model, a sort of chain reaction is triggered by crushing of the tissue in which more and more pigment continues to form, even for months.

I believe you suggested that malonyl aldehyde reacts with protein, and this may be responsible for production of fluorescent compounds. Even with the simplest in vitro system in which one produces ceroid by oxidation of unsaturated fats, that product is autofluorescent even in the absence of protein in the test tube. In this situation, at least, protein is not necessary for the phenomenon of autofluorescence.[14][15][16]

Your remarks about cholesterol are of great interest because by electron microscopy of the Kupffer cells of the liver, cholesterol crystals can sometimes be demonstrated within masses of ceroid pigment held within lysosomes.[17] I had interpreted this finding to indicate that probably unsaturated fat had become disassociated from bound cholesterol and had become converted to ceroid around the residual free

crystals of cholesterol. But this hypothesis would not hold
if cholesterol itself--not cholesterol esters--can undergo
conversion to ceroid.

Dr. Hochstein: Well, if I can respond in order to your
queries, it is possible to obtain fluorescent products in
the absence of protein. However, the product is not the same,
that is, with same fluorescence of either excitation or emission
spectrum, as that product obtained in the presence of protein.
It's a different compound. In the first case you're making
malonaldehyde which fluoresces, and in the second case you're
making malonaldehyde complexes with something else which fluoresces
in a different way. Is that possible? Do you remember the
excitation or emission spectra?

Dr. Hartroft: We measured both the excitation and emission
in pigments produced in vivo in livers under a variety of
conditions.[4] The results corresponded to those previously
reported for ceroid pigment in tissues. We didn't measure
the bands in the pigment formed in vitro by simple oxidation
of corn oil and other unsaturated lipids, nor am I aware of
such reports. It should be done.

Dr. Hochstein: Well, if it is the same, it would be
very interesting.

With regard to your second point, I didn't really mean
to say that I thought there was a hierarchy of reacting organelles in the cell. What is peroxidized will obviously depend
on the nature and localization of the initiator, the unsaturated
fatty acid content of the various organelles of the cell at
a particular time, and the status and location of chain breakers
in the cell. I used the endoplasmic reticulum merely as an
example of an organelle with which we have worked which peroxidizes readily. I do not mean to imply that this is the
organelle which peroxidizes most readily. With regard to
the cholesterol question, perhaps someone here knows more
about this than I do. As a chemist I see this peroxidation
reaction as a possible one. I'm not familiar with the biological
order of events. Dr. Menkes, do you have a thought about
this?

Dr. Menkes: No, this is what I asked you: what is the
hierarchy of peroxidizability for say, something like chole-
calciferol, which obviously has conjugated double bonds, versus
some of the polyunsaturated fatty acids. I don't know the
answer to that.

Dr. Hartroft: The possibility of cholesterol as a starting
material for ceroid is surely more than a curiosity. Cholesterol
is ubiquitous and as everyone knows is in atheromatous plaques
of the aorta and coronary arteries. I had always assumed

that the ceroid, however, came from polyunsaturated acids deposited in these same areas. If the pigment could be formed from cholesterol alone through the reactions you've been discussing, it would help explain the quite large amounts of ceroid present in atheromatous lesions.

Dr. Menkes: Let me go back to the clinical problem, particularly one of the typical Spielmeyer-Vogt type, with late onset of visual problems followed by slow deterioration. We will assume two things: first of all, there is a very slow accumulation of this pigment within neurons--extremely slow; secondly, this is an autosomal recessive disorder, which means that we have a missing or nonfunctioning enzyme. What this indicates is that if the process is so slow and if the enzyme is really zero, we are not dealing with the inability to handle, say, arachidonic acid or linolenic acid; we must be dealing with the inability to handle a very small trace compound that gradually accumulates, whether this is derived from the diet, like phytanic acid, or whether this is derived from some intermediary metabolism. What I'm postulating, therefore, is the following: is there an inability, analogous to the inability to handle cholestanol--a trace substance--which produces cerebrotendinous xanthomatosis and takes about 15 years to develop symptoms, or the inability to handle trace amounts of copper, which produces Wilson's disease, or an inability to handle phytanic acid, which leads to Refsum's disease? A trace material, in all three instances, probably derived from the diet, eventually produces clinical disease. This is why I'm asking are these small amounts, a small trace material with a tremendous peroxidizability?

Dr. Hochstein: I'm not sure what you're talking about-- initiators or substrates?

Dr. Menkes: Substrates.

Dr. Hochstein: Well, we have the whole world of biology, you know, open to us. Frankly, I don't know. I was commenting before on the potentiality of peroxidizing steroids...

Dr. Menkes: I'm sorry, that is an initiator. It's an initiator that would have the polyunsaturation available.

Dr. Hochstein: Well, in Wilson's disease there is no question that copper deposited intracellularly may be an important initiator of peroxidative processes depending on the reducing capacity of the cell in which it's deposited. So there is a case where the potential initiator is present.

Dr. Menkes: Dr. Hochstein, you don't understand my question. I was using copper as an analogy--that's all--that this is a trace material that is in some way not handled ade-

quately, and the same with phytanic acid; I'm not saying these
are peroxidizable. Phytanic acid is probably not at all because
it's fully saturated. I'm just saying there must be some compound
that we have available with a high peroxidizability and yet
present in trace amounts.

Dr. Hochstein: The other criterion is that the compound
would have to accumulate and not be metabolized.

Dr. John S. O'Brien: Obviously, the rate of accumulation
is a function of the rate of synthesis and the degradation
rate. The rate of synthesis of a major component is very
low, but the rate of degradation is lower, that could account
for storage; the compound doesn't have to be a trace constituent.
For example, in Sanfilippo disease, we find that the activity
of the enzyme which breaks down heparin, sulfate-α-acetylgluco-
saminidase--is of very low specific activity. The disease
is a very slowly progressive disease, similar to Batten's
disease, but the molecule that accumulates, heparin sulfate,
is present in high concentrations in many tissues. That suggests
that the synthesis rate of that compound is slow. The molecule
that is being sought in Batten's disease may not be present
in trace amounts; it could be arachidonic acid or a peroxidizable
fatty acid which is a major constituent.

Dr. Michel Philippart: Excuse me, John, but the synthesis
of arachidonic acid is quite rapid.

Dr. O'Brien: That was just an example; there could be
another molecule having a slow synthesis rate and also a slow
degradation rate; it doesn't have to be a trace molecule.

Dr. Vimalkumar Patel: Another possibility is that the
enzyme is reduced, which leads to an increase in peroxide
level and thus more inhibition of the remaining enzyme. With
increasing age, the residual enzyme becomes progressively
less active, with finally clinical disease becoming manifest.

Dr. Menkes: This would be a good example for an autosomal
dominant gene. I do not know, but perhaps someone here knows
an example of an autosomal recessive disorder where the enzyme
is only reduced; autosomal dominant--this would be an excellent
idea.

Dr. Glyn Dawson: First, we're just dealing with a partial
enzyme deficiency in this late-onset form of the disease.
For instance, there have been cases of Tay-Sachs disease where
the onset was around 8 or 15 years of age and the hexosaminidase
A deficiency is only partial.[18][19] I guess we have to wait
until the detailed enzymatic studies are done to see if there
is a partial deficiency in the late-onset form of Spielmeyer-
Sjögren (Batten's) disease.

Dr. Zeman: Well, as a morphologist I'm trying to help

our biochemist friends out a little bit. I would maintain
that the process which is the result of an enzyme defect certainly begins at the very moment that the organism develops
into a metazoic system and has acquired the enzymatic endowment--
whatever it is--which is disturbed. There is a great difference
between the manifestation of the disease and the manifestation
of a genetically controlled defect, and I don't think that
we can very readily equate the onset of symptoms with the
manifestation of the metabolic defect. I would say that just
the opposite is true. These are two independent variables
which are governed by a great variety of factors, and many
people feel that in order to explain differences in the age
of manifestation you have to introduce as an auxiliary hypothesis
modifier genes, but this of course, as we all know, violates
the principle of Occam's razor of scientific parsimony. I
would say this: from our studies on a dog model with a disturbance of lipopigment accumulation--and this may apply to
Tay-Sachs disease also--the formation of the lipopigments,
at least in the brain tissue, takes place in the fetus, but
the manifestations of the disease are not apparent until 18
months later in our dog models. As a matter of fact, before
the manifestations of the disease, dogs that are homozygous
for this trait are particularly suitable for duck hunting,
and they have been especially bred for this purpose. It comes
as a surprise to most of the dog owners that after a glorious
career as a hunting dog these animals all of a sudden go
to pot; they lose their vision and hearing and sense of orient-
ation and everything over a relatively short period of time.
I think we have to separate this process from the biochemical
lesion and its dynamics.

Dr. O'Brien: I agree with Dr. Dawson's simple model
as being the one that explains most easily the difference
in rate of onset or time of onset for various similar diseases.
Certainly with the GM_2 gangliosidoses it is very pleasing
to sit down and calculate the rate of accumulation of ganglioside
GM_2. We have the fetal numbers, for instance, for a Tay-Sachs'
fetus after the fetus has been aborted. We know the concentration of GM_2 at the time that the child dies at age 3 years,
and one can make assumptions that a certain plateau has been
reached at some point in time, such as 2 years of age, and
set a rough number for GM_2 concentration. A straight line
can be drawn between those two points, and for a linear rate
of accumulation on a tissue concentration basis in the cortex
one can plot the point in time at which symptoms appear.
If you do that you get a number for Tay-Sachs disease. I
have done the same thing for the juvenile GM_2 gangliosidosis,
in which there is a partial deficiency of hexosaminidase A,
and the symptoms appear at age 18 to 24 months instead of
6 months. It is very interesting to note that in both diseases
the lines cross at about the same point with respect to symptoms,

237

that is after a certain tissue level is attained. This reasoning,
I think, leads to a good explanation of why the symptoms
appear at different times. Of course, it may be quite different
in any of the other storage diseases.

Dr. Philippart: When you are dealing with children
it is important not to neglect all the different parameters
introduced by development, such as myelination. In metachromatic
leukodystrophy the age of onset is widely variable. I have
seen 30-year-old patients who looked normal although they
had no arylsulfatase activity and increased amounts of sulfatide
in nerves and urine. No one would expect, without examining
them and working them up, that one day they are going to get
the symptoms.

Dr. Zeman: This would be in direct contradiction to
what Dr. Dawson and Dr. O'Brien have said; namely, that you
find differences in the age of onset under conditions of identical deficiency of the enzymes.

Dr. Philippart: No, because these observations stress
the importance of the synthesis mechanism, as indicated by
Dr. O'Brien. Of course, most of the sulfatide is being synthesized
during the myelination, and the bulk of it--probably about
90%--has been completed around 2 to 4 years of age. Later
on, myelin synthesis becomes much slower. You can demonstrate
sulfatide synthesis, however, in adult brain biopsy material,
but at a very low level.[20] It is conceivable that in some
people, as a result of a slight mutation decreasing the rate
of sulfatide synthesis, the need for degradation is less than
in those who develop early symptoms. Once myelination has
been completed, sulfatide turnover is probably much decreased.

Dr. Hochstein: Another model may be relevant to the
problem of variable onset. In the case of G-6-PD deficiency
in humans, there are many variants of this disorder. Those
individuals who have an absolute deficiency of the enzyme--
and they are few in number--have a chronic hemolytic anemia
of early onset. There is a larger group of G-6-PD-deficient
individuals who have no anemia, even though they have a 90%
deficiency of the enzyme, unless challenged by certain drugs--
the so-called oxidant drugs. In this instance, there is an
extraordinary variability of the disease depending on when
the initiator comes in contact with the patient. There could
be repeated episodes, as you know, of the same clinical picture,
and I wonder if this is not a model for what may be happening
in disorders under consideration now. There is a genetic
defect with a variable onset depending on what initiated lipid
peroxidation and what has accumulated over a period of time,
for whatever reasons, either biochemically or individually.
I don't know if that's a model that makes sense in terms of
what you know about this disorder.

Dr. Zeman: This, of course, would bring us back to the dietary factor that Dr. Austin brought up.   I don't know what the relationship is between the dietary intake of unsaturated fatty acids and their occurrence in the cytoplasmic pool of nerve cells. Can you enlighten us on that, Dr. Menkes?

Dr. Menkes: There is an effect, as Dr. Austin mentioned, of the diet on the polyunsaturated fatty acid composition of brain tissue; the effect is not marked apparently.   Paoletti's group[21] and Svennerholm's group[22] have published conflicting data as to whether a polyunsaturated fatty acid deficiency affects the fatty acid content composition of brain.   Everyone agrees, however, that there is an effect of the dietary polyunsaturated fatty acids on the liver composition of fatty acids in liver.

Dr. Hartroft: Is there a threat of ceroid formation everytime there are abundant amounts of unsaturated fats either in the diet or the tissues even when equally abundant amounts of antioxidants accompany the lipid?   In other words, can you protect the tissue against pigment formation even if the tissue is loaded with grossly abnormal amounts of unsaturated fat by elevating the usual antioxidant content of the tissue to a comparable or greater degree?   In experiments some years ago,[23][24]   with choline-deficient rats, we found that ceroid formation was abundant if the rats had been fed a choline-deficient diet containing generous amounts of unsaturated fat (corn oil).   Supplementing such a diet with massive doses of antioxidant reduced but did not prevent ceroid formation in the fatty livers.   Only by both supplementing the diet with large amounts of vitamin E and substituting dietary saturated fat (lard) for the corn oil was it possible to suppress completely the formation of pigment.   The results suggested that it was possible to greatly load the choline-deficient rats' livers with unsaturated fat derived from the diet, so that even large amounts of dietary vitamin E could not protect them.   Perhaps synthetic antioxidants would be more effective in this situation, but we did not try them.

Dr. Austin: Is it reasonable to think that a vitamin E intake will distribute itself closer to the lipid moieties in the membrane?

Dr. Hartroft: There is considerable support for that possibility.

Dr. Austin: Would you comment on some of the other ways in which different antioxidants might protect different portions of the cell?

Dr. Hartroft: The latter question I cannot answer.

239

Dr. Hochstein: BHT or BHA are highly lipid-soluble
also and localize in lipid compartments in the cell, which
is presumably why they are effective substitutes for vitamin E.

Dr. Hartroft: They are slightly water-soluble, unlike
tocopherol.

Dr. Hochstein: With regard to effective concentrations
of vitamin E necessary to suppress lipid peroxidation, the
amount of vitamin E required is a function of the unsaturated
fatty acid content of the diet. Vitamin E is destroyed in
the gut along with the unsaturated fatty acids in the course
of protecting the unsaturated fatty acid in transit through
the gut. When diets high in unsaturated fatty acid do not
show protection by vitamin E, the question always arises,
was the vitamin E level sufficient to protect the cell?

Dr. Hartroft: In other words, did we try to protect
by parenteral injection control? The answer is no. I'm sorry
we didn't; it should be done. The other thing following along
your line of thought is that when one prepares a diet high
in unsaturated fat but low in antioxidants a certain amount
of interceroid is formed in vitro before the animal receives
it. I still do not know whether interceroid can be absorbed
from the intestinal tract, although I do know that ceroid
cannot. [25]

Dr. Philippart: I think it is not safe to assume that
any type of component, be it water-soluble or lipid-soluble,
would ever be equally distributed in the different cell compartments. A very nice example of such a situation is Pompe's
disease--glycogen storage type II--in which cytoplasmic glycogen
is normally metabolized while glycogen accumulates inside
the lysosomes, because the lysosomes have only one way to
degrade the glycogen which is by cleaving it with the
α-glucosidase. In Batten's disease the cause of the lysosomal
storage is not obvious. Since lysosomes are equipped with
a number of lipolytic enzymes, they must contain a free fatty
acid pool. Whether these free fatty acids are further degraded
or released through the lysosomal membrane is not known.
Could it be that some peroxidative mechanism, which so far
has not been demonstrated in lysosomes might be a normal process
to start the degradation of an unsaturated fatty acid generated
by lysosomal hydrolysis. Some tissues, for example, liver,
contain a variety of oxidases which are perhaps involved in
such a mechanism. We know very little about the function
of the oxidases, but it would certainly be unreasonable to
assume that they have none. We may be dealing with an important
physiological mechanism, which in some cases may get out of
hand. Peroxidation is not necessarily a bad thing; it may
be a normal step in the degradation of unsaturated fatty acid.

Dr. Austin: I wonder if it's known, considering as we are the addition of dietary supplement, how much of the vitamin E that one gives orally actually winds up in the brain? I wonder if it's known how much of the BHT and BHA we give actually partitions itself in the brain. Within the brain are there any separate nuclei or any separate subcellular structures that have a greater affinity for these agents?

Dr. Hartroft: They do end up in the liver, but I can't answer for the brain.

Dr. Hochstein: I think the data are available. I'm not sure about the nature of partition; I don't think studies have been done on the heterogeneity of a partition within the brain. There is vitamin E in the brain, but I'm not sure if it's much less or much more than the other fatty tissues.

Dr. Menkes: I think you'll find that answer in one of the prior conferences here. I think Dr. Tappel gave us some data on that.

Dr. Hartroft: I have a question for Dr. Zeman.   I understand your dogs do not show much accumulation of pigment at the age of 18 or 20 months outside of the nervous system. Is that correct?

Dr. Zeman: No, that's not correct. There are certain parts of the body which show a rather magnificent accumulation, such as, for instance, the prostate and the thyroid.

Dr. Hartroft: And what about liver?

Dr. Zeman: The liver shows a fair amount of pigment. We can do a simple needle biopsy of the liver and see considerable quantities of pigment in the parenchyma, let alone the Kupffer cells. As a matter of fact, in this disease there is even accumulation of autofluorescent lipopigments in the epithelial cells of the nephron. That surprised me a little bit because these cells have relatively short half life and are readily turned over, and likewise the crypt cells of the gut also have these pigments. So there is considerable pigment formation throughout tissues other than the brain, whereas the functional disturbances are practically restricted to the central nervous tissue, not even to the peripheral nerve cells. This is, incidentally, also true for patients with the Spielmeyer-Sjögren type, as pointed out by people like Kristensson and Sourander.[26]

Dr. Hartroft: The question I am leading up to is if you were to produce fatty livers by choline deficiency in

your dogs and in control dogs for a standard period of time
would you have much more pigment formation in the livers of
your dogs than in the livers of the controls? Do your "Batten"
dogs have the proclivity of forming more ceroid in any tissue
including liver when conditions are favorable but standardized
when compared to normal dogs? Or is this proclivity more
or less limited to the nervous system?

Dr. Patel: I would like to make a comment on the role
of vitamin B_{12}. It has been shown recently that vitamin B_{12}
induces the peroxidase, both iodinating peroxidase and the
so-called true peroxidase measured with guaiacol, as much
as three to fivefold. I wonder if in this regimen we could
include vitamin B_{12} in the light of all that has been emphasized.
The fact that different individuals probably respond very
differently, and there may be as much as ten to hundredfold
differences should also be taken into consideration.

Dr. Zeman: Well, I think basically this is very true.
The idea is not too well entrenched in American medicine,
but certainly in Europe, under the leadership of people like
Wilder, there is very good appreciation of the individual
pattern of reaction to various pharmacologically active compounds.
I think when we will talk about the specific activities and
measured observations, this certainly will come up.

In summarizing our discussion, there seems to be little
doubt that the peroxidation of unsaturated fatty acids is
most likely to be the biochemical lesion involved in the neuronal
ceroid-lipofuscinosis. As pointed out by Dr. Hochstein, it
is indeed a remarkable fact that our fauna on this planet
has been able to exist under the extraordinary condition of
high oxygenation and the essential necessity of having unsaturated fatty acids present in the body as well. There are
natural protective mechanisms and some of those we have touched
upon or discussed. There is one question which we may still
discuss before we turn to Dr. Menkes and hear about his observations on the turnover of free unsaturated fatty acids
in brain cell cultures. Before we do this, however, we should
perhaps discuss the significance of selenium as an antioxidant,
and I wonder if we can call on you again, Dr. Hochstein.

Dr. Hochstein: For years people in the animal nutrition
field have known that the signs of selenium deficiency are
similar to those associated with vitamin E deficiency. It
is clear that there is some relationship between vitamin E
and selenium as an antioxidant. I can say very briefly that
it seems to me the picture has been cleared up in the last
year or two by the finding that selenium is an essential cofactor
of glutathione peroxidase. In other words, selenium occupies
an essential portion of the protein molecule glutathione peroxidase. In the absence of selenium, glutathione peroxidase

is inactive. We have some selenium-deficient animals at the present time and they have no glutathione peroxidase activity and, therefore, no way of handling lipid peroxides once they are formed in tissues. One may view vitamin E as protecting cells from lipid peroxides by preventing peroxide formation and selenium functioning through glutathione peroxidase as protecting cells from lipid peroxides by a detoxification mechanism.

Dr. Zeman: Thank you for this very succinct statement.

Dr. Hartroft: Can I just say one word about selenium? Ceroid pigment forms in large amounts in the Kupffer cells of livers of mice fed the hepatic necrogenic diet of Schwartz and Hinsworth.[27]   Supplements of vitamin E will suppress both formation of the pigment and the development of necrosis. Selenium supplements, however, will suppress only the necrosis but not the pigment production.   But it seems to me that if selenium is acting as a cofactor for glutathione peroxidase it should have prevented not only the necrosis but also the formation of pigment, which it did not.

Dr. Hochstein: Yes.

Dr. Zeman: Can you perhaps enlighten us as to the relationship between the time and the amount of pigment?

Dr. Hartroft: With a severe hepatonecrogenic diet fed to rats of 60-80 g body weight initially, the hepatic necrosis developed within 60 to 70 days.[27]   The pigment started to form within a few weeks.   Vitamin E supplements prevented both pigment formation and necrosis at any stage, but selenium suppressed only the latter.   We concluded from this that the pigment was not of pathogenic importance in producing necrosis.[24]

Dr. Austin: Could you maybe reconcile these observations by thinking of the selenium as working in the cell sap phase, and by the ceroid as being the accumulation of products that came from the membranous phase, so that your glutathione peroxidase could still be deficient?   You could still have a separation between the two, with the selenium taking care of the glutathione peroxidase, perhaps, but not covering the lipid peroxides produced in other portions of the cell by other peroxidase deficiencies.

Dr. Hochstein: No, I think the point is that the glutathione peroxidase must function in a lipid environment if it is to function at all, and it is the glutathione peroxidase in association with lipids with membranes in which we are interested.   That's what is absent in selenium deficiency.

Dr. Hartroft: My interpretation would be that selenium can be effective in maintaining membrane integrity but not be effective in preventing pigment formation.

Dr. Austin: Didn't I understand you to say earlier that glutathione peroxidase was primarily a supernatent type enzyme and not a membrane-bound enzyme?

Dr. Hochstein: It is primarily a soluble enzyme, and it's in that cell compartment in which it acts to destroy hydrogen peroxide. It also acts in lipid compartments to destroy lipid peroxides; it has to be present in both places. The selenium-deficient cell is thus a cell that is very sensitive to hydrogen peroxide, certainly, because it lacks the soluble enzyme. It is also a cell in which the lipid peroxides will accumulate more readily.

Dr. Hartroft: Dr. Austin, have you employed selenium in your therapeutic "cocktail" for the children with Batten's disease, although I am aware that in too large amounts it would be toxic?

Dr. Austin: Not yet. I think what you're saying is that it would be important not to have a selenium deficiency in these patients.

Dr. Hartroft: Is it possible that under conditions in which pigment is formed, that the requirement for selenium to protect membranes might be increased? Under these conditions could one postulate that the presence of the pigment is a necessary but not sufficient requirement for membrane damage of that type?

Dr. Hochstein: One has to go to rather heroic extremes to create a selenium deficiency.

Dr. Zeman: In other words, you are trying to separate the cofactor from another hitherto unknown protective mechanism.

Dr. Hartroft: In the liver we could never produce necrosis of parenchymal cells without accumulation of the pigment also.

Dr. Zeman: Did you measure glutathione peroxidase in these livers?

Dr. Hartroft: No.

Dr. Zeman: Well, I think this might be a crucial determinatio

Dr. Hartroft: In a hepatic model when we gave vitamin E we got both pigment and necrosis. When we gave selenium, we got the pigment but not the necrosis, and we've never seen the necrosis without the pigment. With your dogs, if you just gave as much selenium as possible without reaching doses that would produce liver damage, could you protect membranes of cells even though pigment would be abundant?

Dr. O'Brien: Your experiments suggest to me that, if we assume that selenium has as its only mode of action a cofactor for glutathione peroxidase, and if those animals are selenium deficient and the glutathione peroxidase activity is zero, and there is still pigment accumulation, then there may be another peroxidase or another enzyme there that we haven't found yet--that may be very important--that doesn't require selenium as a cofactor, and that may account for your findings. And I want to ask you about that, Dr. Hochstein, because I'm sure that people in the field have looked for all the peroxidases that exist. Are you convinced that we have found them all?

Dr. Hochstein: No, I'm sure we haven't, as a matter of fact. The problem is that peroxidase activity tends not to be very specific. In other words, any enzyme that contains iron will have peroxidase activity. Catalase itself can act as a peroxidase, and there is currently considerable controversy as to whether catalase functions in the metabolism of ethyl alcohol as a peroxidase. So there are many enzymes which we do not think of as peroxidases which may have peroxidatic activity in the cell. Peroxidatic activity simply means using hydrogen peroxide to oxidize some acceptor molecule. There are probably many nonspecific peroxidases which we don't begin to see as having specific functions.

Dr. O'Brien: The point I would make is that catalase and glutathione peroxidase are good examples of substrate specificity. Catalase doesn't take acyl peroxide and do anything to it, but the glutathione peroxidase does and seems to use hydrogen peroxide as well. So there's a very strict substrate specificity relationship between those two that wasn't known until just recently. I suggest that more specificities of that type which are still unknown may unravel the Batten's disease process; that's the kind of thing we have to look for.

Dr. Hochstein: I think it's an excellent idea.

Dr. Zeman: Dr. Menkes will now report on a long string of observations on the turnover of various types of fatty acids, saturated and unsaturated.

Dr. Menkes: Let me start by saying the interest in the polyunsaturated fatty acid metabolism in the brain was generated by the work of Hagberg, Sourander and Svennerholm[28] which is now nearly five years old, in which they showed that a

child, who undoubtedly had a form of Batten's disease, had
a defect in the metabolism or in the composition of polyunsaturated fatty acids in brain gray matter. We followed this
through using dissociated brain cells in culture.

I will just say a few brief words about our present method
to obtain cultured dissociated brain cells. Essentially,
both in experimental animals and in humans a small piece of
brain is obtained aseptically and is dissociated by a weak
trypsin solution and then is cultured in either Petri dishes
or plastic flasks. In a serum-supplemented medium, these
cells will soon reaggregate, form clusters which are very
shortly afterwards connected by neurites, and within a few
days in culture three different cell types can be distinguished
which are probably--and I must emphasize the probable--compatible
with neurons, glial cells, and ependyma.[29] Ultimately, by
the end of the first month, the ependymal cells will take
over, and glial or neuronal cells are no longer in evidence.

	CASE 2 Mixed Matter G/W	CONTROL (one 3 day old rat)
Total Radioactivity Uptake* . . .	42.6	-
Neutral Lipids.	51.2	92.2
Free Fatty Acids.	3.3	70.3
Cholesterol	3.7	3.0
Triglycerides	75.0	14.5
Cholesterol Esters	4.3	6.7
Diglycerides & Fatty Acid Esters .	11.3	1.2
Glycolipids.	3.2	1.6
Phospholipids.	45.6	6.1
PC.	24.1	49.2
PE	73.4	7.7
PS + PI	1.7	13.8
Sphingomyelin	0.8	2.8

* cpm x 10 -3/mg protein

Table 12. Incorporation of 1-C-[14] linoleic acid by brain explants.

Table 12 shows the composition of cultures from a patient
with Batten's disease at the time we are doing these metabolic
studies. The first thing which looked very encouraging was
a finding which we presented two or three years ago now[30]
on the metabolism of labelled linoleic acid by a patient with
Batten's disease (Table 13). A biopsy was obtained, of course,
and the disease was proven to be the curvilinear type of storage
disease. If you look at case 2--the radioactivity--you will
find that in contrast to controls, only some 2.8% of the
added linoleic acid is converted to 20:4, which is arachidonic
acid. The controls, however, converted about 19% of the radioactivity. This was very encouraging, and we initiated a more
thorough and systematic study of the cerebral metabolism of
the polyunsaturated fatty acids. It is very interesting that,

246

Carbon Chain Lengths	Control			Case 2		
	% Wt.	% R.A.	R.S.A.	% Wt.	% R.A.	R.S.A.
16:0	33.5	4.4	0.13	16.7	-	-
18:0	16.0	1.1	0.07	19.5	2.0	1.0
18:1	14.0	1.3	0.09	22.5	1.8	0.08
18:2	1.2	56.3	46.9	4.6	64.2	13.9
18:3 to 20:2	tr.	9.0	-	tr.	20.3	-
20:4	12.1	19.9	1.65	5.9	2.8	0.47
22:4	3.6	1.7	0.47	2.0	1.7	0.85
22:5	4.2	1.1	0.26	2.8	0.8	0.29
22:6	9.4	0.6	0.06	19.1	1.4	0.07

Table 13. Pattern of labelled fatty acids in brain tissue explants from patient with Batten's disease in presence of linoleic acid ($1-C^{14}$).

although a considerable amount is known about the fate of polyunsaturated fatty acids (PUFA) in the liver, very little study has been done on PUFA metabolism in brain. About 30% of fatty acids in the brain are derived from two polyunsaturated fatty acids, namely, linoleic and linolenic, both of which are derived exclusively from the diet or, in the case of the fetus, are derived from the mother.

I will summarize briefly the interconversion of PUFA in brain as we postulated it. The 18:2 acid, which is linoleic acid, is converted either to 18:3 ω6, which means that this is not linolenic acid but homolinolenic acid; or to 20:6, which in turn can go to 20:3, which in turn will go to 20:4 ω6 and this can go to 22:4 and 22:5.[31]

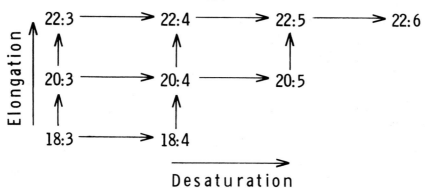

Figure 27. Metabolic interconversions of the linolenic acid (ω3) family.

Now, if you look at the linolenic acid metabolism (Fig. 27) there are also two types of metabolic mechanisms, a chain

247

elongation and a desaturation. It becomes quite evident that these two steps have different characteristics, and one way you can detect this is by lowering the environmental temperature of these cultures. We found that if you lower the temperature of the cultures from 37 to 30 C, you will find that the desaturation remains quite active, but chain elongation is reduced. It is only when you lower the temperature to 15 C that even desaturation will stop or become slowed down significantly.[31][32]

Fatty acid	Choline-PG		Ethanolamine-PG		Triglyceride	
	Mass	Radio-activity	Mass	Radio-activity	Mass	Radio-activity
16:0	26.0	17.5	6.3	1.2	18.0	18.6
16:1	9.3	-	2.0	-	5.9	-
18:0	8.4	8.1	20.9	1.7	10.2	7.0
18:1	42.1	0.9	16.5	-	22.7	0.9
18:3ω3	1.0	29.6	0.9	6.2	2.2	12.1
20:3ω3+20:4ω6	3.0	10.1	16.6	2.3	2.9	8.7
20:4ω3	0.1	4.8	0.2	4.8	2.6	11.2
20:5ω3	0.1	15.6	0.2	35.0	2.0	8.3
22:5ω3	0.3	13.3	1.7	37.0	0.9	29.3
22:6ω3	0.8	-	8.1	11.0	4.2	-

Table 14. Percentage distribution of radioactivity from (1-^{14}C) linolenic acid precursor into fatty acids of major labelled lipids.

Table 14 summarizes this. The ratio of 20:4 to 20:5 does not change markedly, while the ratio of 20:5 to 22:5, which indicates a chain-elongation step, drops precipitously, indicating this step becomes almost completely inhibited by reducing the temperature. So there are at least two different enzymatic reactions going on in these brain cells.

If you add a polyunsaturated fatty acid, into what fractions of the brain does it go? Essentially, you will find the first step is that the polyunsaturated fatty acid is bound to the cells as a free fatty acid and then converted to choline phosphoglycerides. If you plot the amount of radioactivity in choline phosphoglycerides (CPG), it will show a type of path, in which the maximum is about 6 to 8 hr and there is a gradual decrease over the incubation of 48 hr or more (Table 15). By contrast, ethanolamine phosphoglycerides (EPG) gradually increase in the course of incubation. If the cells are old--that is, far advanced in terms of culture--or if the subject from which we have derived the biopsy is older, a significant amount of radioactivity will enter the triglyceride fraction. The greater the demand of the cell for polyunsaturated fatty acids, the less activity in triglycerides. That is, if you have a cell that is very active in putting out processes, neurites, very little at that time goes into triglycerides. When the cultures have settled down and they're getting senile, so to speak, much more goes into the triglycerides. Now if we just look at the ratio of CPG to EPG--let's take a ratio at

Lipid Fraction	Incubation Time (in hours)				
	1/3	1	3	8	24
NEUTRAL LIPIDS	23.1	21.2	13.4	10.8	10.0
DG	4.0	3.3	3.5	2.5	1.9
TG	12.6	11.9	7.8	5.5	5.0
CE	0.1	1.7	1.4	1.6	1.5
FFA	4.5	3.4	0.4	0.8	1.0
PHOSPHOLIPIDS	76.9	78.8	86.6	89.2	90.0
SPG	11.0	11.9	10.5	12.5	16.2
CPG	56.9	53.8	53.6	38.8	19.9
EPG	8.2	12.1	21.7	34.1	48.9
Total Incorporation	158	323	502	528	637

Table 15. Distribution of radioactivity between lipid fractions after (1-^{14}C) linolenic acid incubation.

24 hr--we found, for instance, in rat embryos that the ratio is 0.4. Later on EPG will become more actively labile than CPG.[31] Let us apply this to the incorporation of linoleic acid in patients, and some normal controls. The kind of a control one can get in "normal" humans is, of course, very difficult. These included normal temporal lobe tissue gray matter from an 18-year-old girl with a tumor and brain tissue from two baboons. The ratios of the linoleic acid incorporation in 24 hr were 0.4 in a rat, 2.7 in the baboon, 4.7 in our control patient and 5.0 in our Batten's disease patient. What we see there is the rat being immature at this age. The baboon was 2 months old, which is apparently equivalent to a young child. The control and the Batten patient were all relatively of the same order. The more metabolically active the tissue is, the less linoleic acid goes into CPG. The less active metabolically the tissue, the more goes into CPG. That is, the more active the tissue is in developing new processes, new membranes, and so on, the more goes into the EPG, possibly into the EPG plasmalogens as we have recently shown.[31] We obtained essentially the same data when we used linolenic acid. Linolenic acid will also enter EPG, perhaps even more actively than linoleic acid.

The next question is: Is there an abnormality in the metabolism of linoleic acid to linolenic acid in children with Batten's disease? Table 16 shows the normal conversion of linolenic acid in the various lipid fractions in cultured brain tissue derived from rats. As you can see here, there is relatively active conversion of the 18:3 to 20:3 and further on to the higher polyunsaturated fatty acids. With the patients, we found that the conversion rate was indeed slower. In both the control and in the patient linolenic acid could not be converted to the higher PUFA; therefore, the conversion of

Fatty acids:	Incubation Temperature (C)					
	15°		22°		37°	
	Hours after pulse					
	0	4	0	4	0	4
16:0	-	-	-	-	5.0	5.0
18:0	-	-	-	-	2.0	2.0
18:3ω3	95.2	64.7	54.1	24.3	8.0	7.0
20:3ω3	1.8	3.4	1.8	1.2	1.5	1.2
20:4ω3	-	6.1	10.1	6.1	1.8	1.9
20:5ω3	2.9	25.7	33.9	46.8	27.0	24.0
22:5ω3	-	-	-	20.4	31.0	33.0
22:6ω3	-	-	-	1.1	23.6	25.8

Table 16. Distribution of radioactivity in fatty acid esters of the phospholipid fraction.

both linoleic acid and linolenic acid to the higher analogs is dependent on the age of the culture and on the age of the subject. If you look more carefully into the conversion of linoleic acid to arachidonic acid--that is, conversion of 18:2 to 20:4--you will find that this conversion is very active during the early days of normal brain culture, but subsequently becomes less and less active. During the early days of brain culture about 80% or so went to 20:4; later on, as the metabolic processes slowed down and no more new neurites were being formed, the conversion decreased. The explanation for our finding is that in Batten's cultures there was no elongation of the polyunsaturated fatty acid but that this was merely a function of the age and the cellular activity of these tissues.

The next problem is: could these polyunsaturated fatty acids go somewhere else? That is, while normally only about 1% to 2% of the radioactivity lies outside of the extractable lipids of the cells, could it be that in Batten's disease there is much more in some nonlipid material or material not appearing in the chloroform-methanol fraction? When this was checked out, the amount of radioactivity in this fraction was no more than in controls.

Dr. Hartroft: Is there any pigment (ceroid or interceroid) formation in your cultures, either those started from the normals or the pathologic?

Dr. Menkes: Yes, in the older cultures we are able to show that there are indeed lipid inclusions in the cells that we have in cultures. We tried to demonstrate on intracellular pigment, but it didn't work. Either there was not enough pigment to give any fluorescence, or our methods were not sensitive enough.

Dr. Hartroft: In your methods did you extract the ordinary lipids first? What did you extract with?

Dr. Menkes: We have described the preparation in detail in a recent paper.[29]   The cells are scraped off at the end, they are spun down, then methanol is added and the suspension allowed to stand a little bit; chloroform is added to give a final concentration of 1 to 2, again allowed to stand at room temperature for an hour or two, stirred very well, again allowed to stand, spun down; the residue is finally washed once more with chloroform-methanol. The supernatant, of course, is what we have been working with.

Dr. Hartroft: I admire the sophisticated biochemical approach. Have you attempted to demonstrate ceroid and inter-ceroid in the monolayers by histochemical means?

Dr. Menkes: Even though there were lipid inclusions, we looked for this. Either our method was not adequate--we're dealing with very little there--or our method was not sufficiently sensitive, or we didn't leave the cells in culture long enough.

Dr. Hartroft: I wouldn't predict much ceroid in the cultures because of the rather short periods of time with which you are dealing, but interceroid could form within these limitations of time.

Dr. Zeman: Dr. Philippart has been looking at cultured cells from the dogs with an electron microscope. Did you see pigments in there?

Dr. Philippart: We studied brain explants from Dr. Koppang's homozygote dogs. In these cells we found a granular pigment which appears quite different from pigments we have observed in human lines. There is a relatively small amount of the pigment, but without having seen your original material, I don't know if the ultrastructural appearance of our cultured cells is similar.

It is certainly very important to identify the type of cells you are dealing with. When you use a cell mixture which contains neurons, glial cells, and possibly ependymal cells, the rate of metabolism of these different cells may be quite different. It is essential to characterize them adequately, and there are many ways to do this. For example, when studying glycolipid synthesis, fibroblast-like cells incorporate galactose electively in ceramide trihexoside: this is an excellent marker. When we find a large amount of neutral lipid, I suspect we are dealing with a phagocytic type of cell which has a very active metabolism of neutral lipid. For oligodendroglial cells we might look for synthesis of galactosyl ceramides and es-

251

pecially sulfatides. Very few cells other than oligodendroglia
are able to synthesize sulfatide. The neurons might do it
to a small extent, but fibroblasts do not, and probably microglia
or astroglia do not either. You can also look for other markers,
such as specific enzymes or S-100 protein. Electron microscopy
is invaluable to define the morphology of the cells under
study.

Dr. O'Brien: We've done the experiment you suggested
using brain biopsies from children with a variety of diseases
as controls (including Tay-Sachs and undiagnosed neurodegenera-
tive disorders that we see on the ward) and the curvilinear
type of Batten's disease as our test subjects. We've taken
brain explants, growing them in tissue culture, and also done
the same thing with skin biopsies. We looked at them under
the ultraviolet microscope for fluorescent lipid products,
and at first there's no question in the Batten's explant,
as you would expect. The fluorescent pigment is easily visible.
After subculture, fibroblastic-like cells are obtained, and
if you subculture those and subculture the normals, no pigment
is visible in either of these by the fluorescent technique.
If you subculture again several weeks after subculture, again,
no pigment is observed. If you leave them stationary, without
subculturing them--(we've gone as long as 90 days in a confluent
monolayer maintained for three months), you see inclusions;
you see inclusions in the control, you see inclusions in the
Batten's. They're not fluorescent. If you do the histochemical
staining and you can demonstrate they're PAS-positive, they're
sudanophilic, and they look under the electron microscope
like neutral lipids, even though they are PAS-positive, which
is remarkable. They're not fluorescent. If you extract those
cells with lipid solvents and measure the fluorescence by
using the technique recently published[33] by Tappel, you
find no difference between Batten's and normals. We have been
unable to find any increase in fluorescence comparing the
Batten's cells with the control, and we cannot see by electron
microscopy anything that looks like curvilinear bodies or
lipofuscin. Now I don't completely understand the molecular
nature of all the ceroid forms you have described, and so
we've been very simple in our histochemistry.

Dr. Hartroft: I think you've answered my question, both
as to ceroid and interceroid. I know the publication to which
you're referring. I think it's a very nice paper, except
I don't think ceroid is being measured at all; I think it's
interceroid.

Dr. Dawson: Could it be, in effect, that the fetal calf
serum or the culture condition is somehow correcting this
peroxidase deficiency?

Dr. O'Brien: It certainly could. We've thought that the next thing we ought to do is to try the whole thing over and perhaps add a little cumene hydroperoxide to bring out the lesion (if it exists) without killing the cells, or take out the fetal calf serum, remove any antioxidants; these things will have to be tried, but it will take a very long time to do.

Dr. Austin: May I suggest something that might take a shorter length of time? That would be to add to this system some polyunsaturated fatty acids--grossly, not tracer amounts.

Dr. Menkes: We have done this and, as has been shown by Bailey and others,[34] if you add an excess of polyunsaturated fatty acids, you will find that these cells will develop lipid inclusions, but so will normal cells. What is happening is that the linoleic acid and linolenic acid begin to accumulate in the triglycerides, but this occurs normally too.

Dr. Hartroft: Have you tried any variations of your culture medium to try to prevent the inclusions in normal or other cells?

Dr. Menkes: No, we have not.

Dr. Austin: Have you looked for autofluorescent pigments having added more than tracer amounts of polyunsaturated fatty acids to the Batten's cultures?

Dr. Menkes: I see what you're driving at. No, we haven't. When we looked for autofluorescent pigments, it was not when there was an excess of linoleic acid in the culture.

Dr. O'Brien: No, but the amount of unsaturated fatty acids present in fetal calf serum is quite considerable. They're bound to albumin, but they're there just as you would expect they would be, and that's a pretty good dose for those cells. You would expect they would be getting a good supply of exogenous polyunsaturates. The critical question is the titratable level sufficient to bring out the lesion in the mutant and not swamp the control. We have tried it with the gangliosidoses, knowing that the enzyme defect was present in tissue culture in Tay-Sachs disease, and taking GM_2 G ganglioside and putting it into culture. There is no question you can produce cytoplasmic membranous bodies in the mutant, but we've never been able to find a level at which we can produce it in the mutant without producing it in the control strain as well, because we swamped the system. Dr. Dawson may talk about the same thing with Fabry's disease, and you may talk about it with Niemann-Pick disease. I think everybody's had a real problem trying to get a differential effect.

Dr. Hartroft: What about antioxidant in your situation?

Dr. O'Brien: We haven't tried antioxidant. I think we'd like to try something like cumene hydroperoxide or linoleic hydroperoxide in trace amounts so that it doesn't kill the cells and see if we can't bring out the lesion that way.

Dr. Austin: I wonder if perhaps the correct conclusion is that there is no direct linear relationship between polyunsaturated fatty acids and the autofluorescent lipopigments, at least in your cultures; if that's so, perhaps we ought to look for other mechanisms.

Dr. Zeman: Well, actually, if I understand Dr. Menkes' experiment and his interpretation correctly, he was concerned primarily with the possibility as to whether an abnormally high intracellular concentration of linoleic acid could occur, which in the long run, and over months and years perhaps, could lead to the type of picture as has been described by Hagberg, Sourander, and Svennerholm,[28] but I think the experiment was not primarily designed to observe pigment formation. As a matter of fact, if we consider that the sizable amount of pigments in these homozygous patients and dogs require several months of ideal conditions in situ rather than in tissue culture, it is perhaps not surprising that neither Dr. Menkes or Dr. O'Brien found these pigments in their cultured cells. There is only one system in which these pigments occur much more rapidly, and that is the system described by Dr. Hartroft, provided it is doped with a high concentration of bivalent iron or heme iron, and this is an entirely different situation. Here the pigments develop in macrophages and fat cells and all sorts of other things, but in these endogenous disorders which we are talking about, pigment formation is certainly an order of magnitude slower, you see, and that might very well explain the situation.

Dr. Armstrong and Dr. Austin are here representing a group of investigators who have recently shown[3] that in patients with the Spielmeyer-Sjögren type of neuronal ceroid-lipofuscinosis, a significant decrease not to 0.08% but to 8% of myeloperoxidase activity can be measured, and perhaps we can hear from Dr. Armstrong about these findings.

Dr. Armstrong: We've directed our studies[35] toward the identification and possible laboratory test for the Batten's disease either in the late infantile form or in the juvenile form. I will present results of five families. Figure 28 shows data for case 1, and it represents a late infantile form of the Bielschowsky-Jansky variety. When we first studied these patients for myeloperoxidase in the white blood cells, utilizing phenylenediamine as the secondary hydrogen donor, we found that this patient, an affected child age 3 1/2 who had all the classical signs of Bielschowsky-Jansky disease, fell well below the normal enzyme curve that we defined here

254

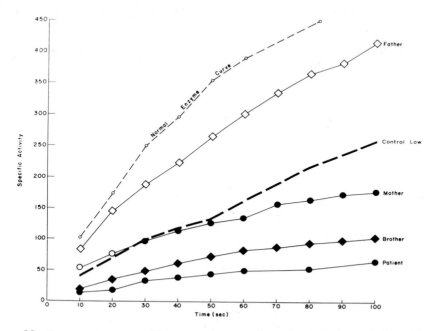

Figure 28. Leucocyte peroxidase activity. Case 1 with late infantile onset.

and well below the lowest normal control that we have found in some 80-odd patients. Some of the enzyme normally goes almost straight up in terms of activity as you increase the incubation time. As you can see, it's a very rapid reaction; even at 10 and 20 sec there is a lot of activity going on.

This patient, then, has a rather flat curve; the specific activity just never seems to get going as in a normal patient, and by 100 sec or even at 60 sec it is markedly deficient. This patient died a month ago at age 4, and we have autopsied the child and done some further studies on tissues. The younger brother, age 2 years and 9 months when we measured his peroxidase, was asymptomatic at the time, but there was a very low activity level. Two or three months after this analysis was made, the child had his first seizures. Examination of the eyegrounds showed marked retinal pigmentary changes. The neutrophils showed marked hypergranulation but there were no vacuolated lymphocytes, which you see much more frequently in the juvenile form than in the late infantile form. So we consider that this child now, the second of the two children in this family, also shows the peroxidase deficiency and has the late infantile onset of the disease. The father was per- fectly normal (the curve fell well within the normal range);

the mother started off with an apparently normal curve at the low incubation time, but with increasing incubation time, the activity became abnormal. This held true with a number of the mothers.

Dr. Zeman: Is the father the biological father of those children?

Dr. Armstrong: Yes.

Dr. O'Brien: Could you describe the assay for us?

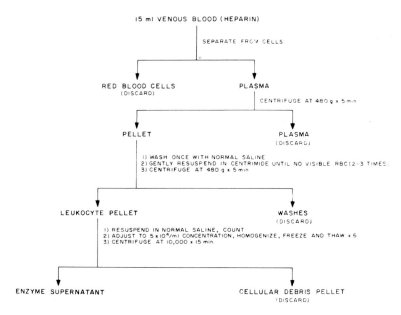

Figure 29. Procedure for obtaining solubilized leukocytic peroxidase.

Dr. Armstrong: Yes. The procedure is outlined in Figure 29. We just isolate white blood cells by gravity, letting the plasma separate in heparinized tubes and pipetting it off before the buffy coat forms. We wash it a couple of times with Cetrimide to lyse whatever red cells might be present in the preparation, and then spin down the pellet and count the number of cells we have, and we adjust our assays so that we have 5×10^4 cells per incubation mixture. We keep this routine with everybody we assay--controls or patients--and the importance of this has recently been reported. Then we rupture the cells by freezing and thawing six times and use that clear supernatant as our enzyme source. Dextran can be used, I'm sure, to isolate the white blood cells also, but I think it's important to get rid of any red cell contamination because there is a lot of peroxidase activity in a red cell, and it will really give you false answers, as we have already found out in one of our patients. Then we take the equivalent of 5 x 10^4 cells and incubate it with 0.15M phosphate buffer at pH 7.3, 0.28M phenylenadiamine, and 10^{-3}M hydrogen peroxide. The optical density is read in a 1cm light path cuvette against a blank at 485nm. This develops a purple color indicating conversion of the phenyldiamine which is brown, to the imine, which is purple.

Dr. O'Brien: How do you subtract for catalase?

Dr. Armstrong: Catalase really is very low in the white blood cell, and I don't believe it interferes yet. We're just getting ready to block it with aminotriazole. We've added a considerable amount of Sigma catalase to our incubation mixture--just the reagents without any other enzyme in it-- just water plus phenylenediamine plus peroxide and catalase. You don't get any color produced at all in quite sufficient amounts of this catalase, but we are going to block catalase very shortly with aminotriazole.

Dr. Hochstein: The relevant thing, it seems to me, is not whether catalase has peroxidase activity in this situation, but, rather, whether the catalase activity is high in the leukocytes of the patients, destroying peroxide and therefore decreasing activity?

Dr. Armstrong: We ran catalase as a control for that very reason (Table 17), and catalase levels do not appear to be elevated.

Dr. O'Brien: In the presence of excess quantities of catalase you still get the deficient activity in the patient; is that correct?

Dr. Armstrong: Yes. If you add catalase from any source to our incubation mixture, you get no color produced; therefore, it would take a very large amount of catalase from our patients to give us any color which would move them up into the normal range. On the other hand, we measured catalase along with the peroxidase; none of our patients--save one--had elevated catalase in their white blood cells, so that the hydrogen peroxide that we added to the incubation mixture was not being destroyed by excess catalase from the patient.

Dr. Philippart: De Duve's group[36] has shown that liver peroxisomes are quite stable to osmotic shock, providing a simple way to separate them from contaminating lysosomes. I wonder if you have tried a detergent to see if you get a better yield of enzymes.

PATIENT	DIAGNOSIS	AGE	PEROXIDASE[A)	CATALASE	ACID PHOS.	SOL. PROTEIN
RANGE	Normal (30)	Birth-89	172-795	1.7-5.2	9.2-110.0[B)	.36-1.1
	Abnormal (16)	4-54	162-673	1.6-4.2	4.6- 39.6	.23-1.1
MEAN			418	2.6	34.5	.64
(Case 1)	Late Infantile form	4	43	3.3	14.7	.70
	Late Infantile form	2	72	3.9	26.1	.51
Father		27	271	4.7	100.8	.43
Mother		25	126	2.4	111.1	.50
(Case 2)	Juvenile form	10	97	3.4	39.6	.64
Sister		8	201	3.9	7.1	.70
Mother		32	159	3.7	15.9	.61
Father		33	346	4.6	53.2	.83
(Case 3)	Juvenile form	11	129	3.7	85.0	.60
Sister		20	82+	6.6	22.1	.38
Father		50	130	3.0	33.7	.88
Sister		22	522	7.4	50.9	.27
Brother		16	257	4.4	156.0	.74
Mother		49	170	4.8	13.8	.54
(Case 4)	Juvenile form	14	46	2.1	20.0	.67
	Juvenile form	9	102	2.2	20.1	.67
Sister		8	67*	2.0	27.5	.78
Mother		36	201	2.0	40.0	1.20
Father		36	423	2.4	42.5	.77
(Case 5)	Juvenile form	12	40	3.0	35.0	.57
	Juvenile form	10	89	4.1	52.5	.61
Brother		9	239	4.2	67.5	.40
Brother		7	134	2.1	58.7	.72
Brother		13	286	1.7	36.3	.35
Sister		11	218	2.5	53.0	.80
Mother			137	2.3	32.5	.71

A = POD @ 60 seconds
B = Includes newborns and young children
+ = Average of 3 separate determinations (69-96)
* = Clinically normal

Table 17. Peroxidase and control enzymes in patients with Batten's diseases, family members and controls.

Dr. Armstrong: No, not yet.

The remaining four cases will go rather rapidly now; they all represent the juvenile form. Figure 30 represents

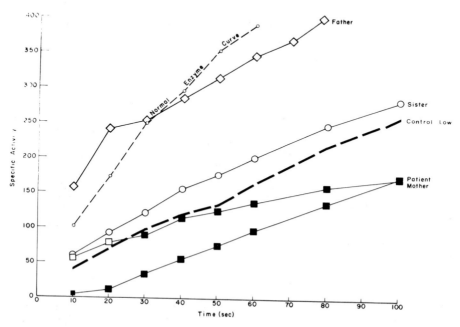

Figure 30. Leukocyte peroxidase activity. Case 2 with juvenile onset.

enzyme activity for a girl aged 10 now; the onset of her disease was about age 5. She is blind, mentally retarded, has seizures, hypergranulated neutrophils, and quite markedly vacuolated lymphocytes. The one sister and father are normal. The curve for the mother starts off normal again, and then deviates as the assay time is increased.

Dr. O'Brien: Could you comment on the possibility that you have two different rate constants?

Dr. Armstrong: Do you mean by the shape of those curves. No, I don't think I can comment on that.

Dr. O'Brien: The rate appears to be fast initially and then it slows down.

Dr. Armstrong: Well, you'll see as we go through that some of these cases do this; maybe we can explain this later.

259

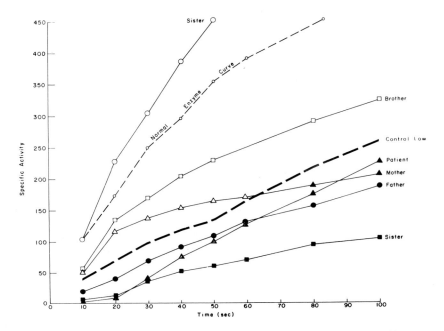

Figure 31. Leukocyte peroxidase activity. Case 3 with juvenile onset.

This third case (Fig. 31) is very interesting--another juvenile, which we have biopsied and for which we have electron micrographs of the thyroid. The father is low all the way too, and so is one sister; they even show a greater deficiency than he does. However, a brother and another sister fall within the normal range. The curve for the mother, again, true to form, starts out as normal, remains in the normal range at least for a while, but by 60 sec has fallen into the abnormal range.

Dr. O'Brien: How about the type of cell? Do you do a differential count too?

Dr. Armstrong: Yes, we've done all of that. There is no infection or excess number of cells. We have hematology on each of these patients and they are all perfectly normal in all parameters. Now this is the fourth family here, in which Mrs. Collum's children appear (Fig. 32). The oldest child died two years ago, I believe, with Spielmeyer-Vogt disease. Her older daughter is age 14 now; her son is age 9, and a young daughter has just turned 8. Specific activities of both the father and mother are in the normal range in this family, so Mrs. Collum is different from the previous three mothers. All three children have vacuolated lymphocytes, but

260

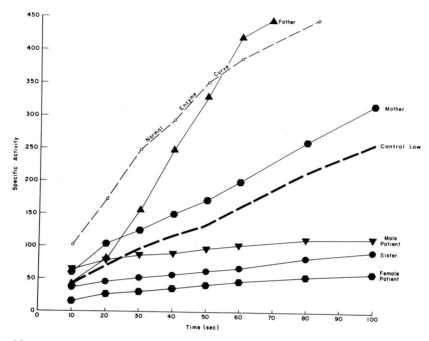

Figure 32.   Leukocyte peroxidase activity.   Case 4 with juvenile onset.

there is no hypergranulation in any patient in this family.
I think Dr. Zeman has reported this before: if the patients
do not have hypergranulation, then neither do any of the other
people in the family, and this seems to be true. One child
with low specific activity may be preclinical; we do not know,
even though she is 8 years old already. Yesterday a rectal
biopsy was done with the help of Dr. Diamond and Dr. Delorimer,
and perhaps we will be able to resolve the status of this
patient on the results of that biopsy.

The final family (Fig. 33) is one referred to us by Dr.
Wherrett from north of Toronto. This is a very large family.
The older patient is 12 years old, the other is 9; they both
have Batten's disease and are low in peroxidase. The specific
activity curve for the mother starts off normal, and then
with increased incubation time deviates from the normal enzyme
rate. A younger brother--about 7 years old, certainly is
below normal in activity, so he could be in the preclinical
range, or he could possibly be a heterozygote. A sister and
two brothers are all well within the normal range and never
fall outside of it, no matter how long you continue the incubation.

261

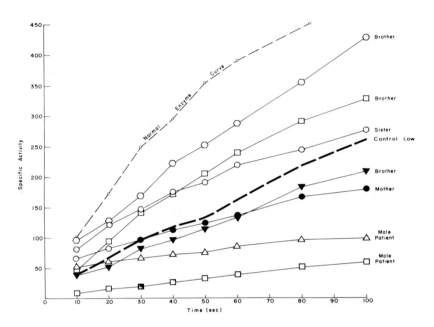

Figure 33. Leukocyte peroxidase activity. Case 5 with juvenile onset.

Now, some other things that we've been able to do besides assess the peroxidase deficiency is to measure hydrogen peroxide, or some peroxide-like material, from these leukocyte supernatants. Every patient in the five cases that I've shown you, whether they're the carrier or have the disease, has an elevation or some demonstrable level of peroxide or H_2O_2 (Table 18). We look at it in a very simple way: if the primary substrate for the peroxidase, which is H_2O_2, is absent, you don't get any color at all.

Dr. Austin: In normals?

Dr. Armstrong: In anybody. If you leave the H_2O_2 out, the reaction doesn't go. Now, if you then rely on the endogenous H_2O and peroxides from the enzyme supernatant on each patient to provide the H_2O_2 or peroxide then if any purple color is produced, this will be a measure of the H_2O_2 or peroxide. In every one of those patients we've discussed you can omit H_2O_2 and a very nice purple color will develop nevertheless, indicating the presence of a peroxide--hydrogen peroxide, which it probably is, or one of the other substrates acted on by peroxidase: peroxy acids, or something similar.

Dr. Hochstein: Is the color more intense than that observed

262

PATIENT	0-1+	2+	3+	VACUOLATED LYMPHOCYTES	H_2O_2*
Control	71	29	0	-	0
Control	62	38	0	-	0
Control	92	8	0	-	0
Late Inf. form (Case 1)	40	18	42	++	.095
Late Inf. form	52	20	28	+	.156
Father	94	7	0	-	0
Mother	52	18	30	±	0
Juvenile form (Case 2)	26	36	42	+++	.140
Sister	84	16	0	-	0
Mother	35	39	26	-	0
Father	77	21	2	-	0
Juvenile form (Case 3)	9	15	76	++++	.096
Sister	73	27	0	-	0
Brother	68	32	0	-	0
Father	40	32	28	+	.015
Sister	33	38	29	-	.050
Mother	70	15	15	-	.019
Juvenile form (Case 4)	66	33	1	+++	.062
Juvenile form	81	19	0	+++	.054
Sister	66	33	1	+++	.018
Mother	81	17	2	-	0
Father	79	25	1	-	0
Juvenile form (Case 5)	41	49	10	+++	.097
Juvenile form	50	47	3	+++	.086
Brother	84	16	0	-	0
Brother	79	21	0	-	0
Brother	67	24	0	+	.041
Sister	86	14	0	-	0
Mother	91	9	0	-	0
Newborn	50	50	0	+	.030
Newborn	53	47	1	+	.045
Newborn	47	53	0	+	.040

*Optical density after 5 minutes incubation at pH 7.3, with 1% phenylenediamine as hydrogen donor. H_2O_2 is omitted so that the color produced under these conditions is due to endogenous peroxide(s).

Table 18. Quantitation of hypergranulated neutrophils.

when you add hydrogen peroxide itself?

Dr. Armstrong: No.

Dr. Hochstein: It's of the same order of magnitude as that?

Dr. Armstrong: Yes.

Dr. Zeman: Have you any data on methemoglobin in these patients?

Dr. Armstrong: Yes, I did determinations on a couple of patients. There was no elevation of methemoglobin.

Dr. Zeman: What were the actual measurements? Do you recall?

Dr. Armstrong: No, I don't. We studied only a couple of patients.

Dr. Zeman: Did you try thiobarbiturate determination?

Dr. Armstrong: No. We haven't had time to do a lot of things yet; this is still fairly new. One other piece of evidence implicating perhaps hydrogen peroxide being elevated in the cells as a result of their peroxidase deficiency is the NBT test, which you all know is used for showing phago-cytizing properties of the neutrophil, and I think it's accepted now that H_2O_2 is what's reducing the nitro blue tetrazolium to the formazan. In every one of these patients who has a peroxidase abnormality and has the peroxide elevations, all of the NBT tests are at least greater than 20%.

Dr. Zeman: Can you describe that NBT test? How is it performed, and what is your endpoint?

Dr. Armstrong: You take some heparinized blood in a sterile syringe and collect it in a sterile test tube, and then you just incubate a small amount of that--I think it's about 3 drops of whole blood--with the NBT dye, nitro blue tetrazolium. If there is H_2O_2 present, by virtue of an increased hexose monophosphate shunt within the neutrophil, the dye is reduced to a black formazan material which shows up inside a neutrophil, and you just count 100 cells or 200 cells. You just find large, massive black deposits within the cytoplasm after you've counterstained with Wright's and just count them up. Probably up to around 10% or maybe 12% is normal out of 100 cells.

Dr. Rider: That test is elevated also in case of infection, isn't that true?

264

Dr. Armstrong: That is correct, but none of the patients had any otherwise abnormal hematologic findings.

Dr. Rider: How about in the case of malignancy or something like that? Has that been tested in that?

Dr. Armstrong: There is an elevated NBT in some of the lymphocytic leukemias and myelogenous leukemias which lack peroxidase. I don't know that anybody has done NBT on leukemia, but some of the forms of leukemia show a lack of peroxidase, so I would think that they would be probably NBT positive.

Dr. Hochstein: In addition to the NBT test, have studies of actual bacterial killings, phagocytic killings been done with these tests?

Unknown: I think Dr. Menkes has done that.

Dr. Menkes: I didn't; Dr. Schlegel did. He reported to me that they were normal in one family that was biopsied Batten's.

Dr. Zeman: Well, I think it's probably worthwhile to point out that there is no evidence that patients with these disorders show any greater susceptibility to infectious diseases than anybody with another type of disabling central nervous disease.

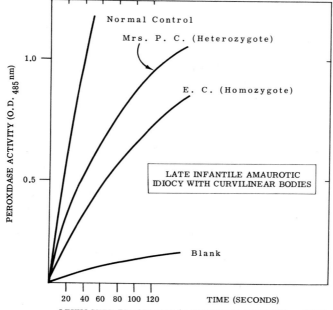

Figure 34. Leukocyte peroxidase activity at pH 7.3 with p-phenylenediamine.

265

Dr. Dawson: We were very intrigued on hearing Dr. Armstrong's presentation at the Columbus Neurochemistry meeting, and we thought we would try it ourselves, since we have a number of patients, and essentially we are in complete agreement with him, at least using the phenylenediamine substrate. Figure 34 shows tracings of the recording from a recording spectrophotometer for the younger brother of one of our patients who died a few years ago.[37] A brain biopsy had been carried out and the disease was the classic infantile form, with the first seizure at about the age of 3. Levels in normal subjects go shooting up, and this is very low. I think our findings are in good agreement with those of Dr. Armstrong. Figure 35

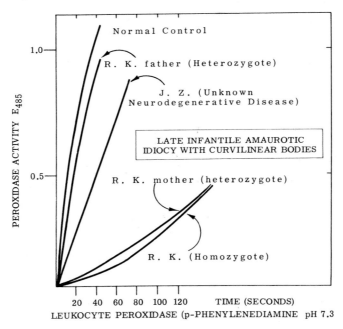

Figure 35. Leukocyte peroxidase activity at pH 7.3 with p-phenylenediamine.

shows results for another family; again the first seizure was about age 3. You can see the peroxidase activity in the homozygote is very low. Her mother was almost identical; we really couldn't distinguish the mother's leukocytes from the patient's, which I think is also what Dr. Armstrong pointed out a few minutes ago. The father, again as Dr. Armstrong found in one or two of his cases--or the putative father, perhaps I should say, was pretty much normal. So in a very crude way, in contrast to Dr. Armstrong's elegant work, it seems that one really can detect what we might call the Jansky-Bielshowsky or infantile form by this assay.

When we came back from the neurochemistry meetings we thought we would just try measuring peroxidase activity in leukocytes by the standard o-dianisidine or 3,3'-dimethoxy-benzedine procedure and were rather dismayed to find that our obvious Batten's disease patient had much greater activity than normal control (Fig. 36). However, on using these same extracts with the phenylenediamine substrate, the peroxidase deficiency showed up. Perhaps someone here can explain this finding to me.

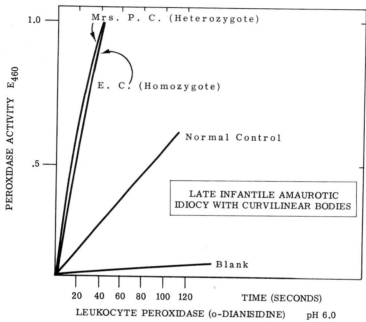

Figure 36. Leukocyte peroxidase activity at pH 6.0 with o-dianisidine.

Dr. Patel: We have been doing the same thing, and we had three families with Batten's disease. When we heard this report we also started out the same way you did. In our investigation we found that guaiacol was a far better hydrogen donor; in other words, the activity was about three or four times greater on the sensitivity scale. DMB was about ten times as sensitive as phenylenediamine, and we chose to use guaicol, but the difference was probably not detectable. I think Dr. Zeman might have communicated with you in that respect. Recently, only about a couple of weeks ago, I went down again to get the blood and measured the peroxidase activity by the technique Dr. Armstrong described. Although the deficiency was not as dramatic as before it did show a slower rate in one instance. I could not contact two of the families, however. Every time we made the determination either with DMB or guaiacol on our families, the specimens either showed higher activity or activity within normal range; in many cases the activity was much higher than in normal individuals.

Dr. Rider: When I first saw these slides I thought you were going to show that activity in all the mothers was decreased. I think actually that in all of them but maybe one that you've shown there was a greater decrease in activity in the mother than in the father. Would that imply possibly some kind of a sex linkage? Dr. Menkes stated earlier that you can tell whether you are dealing with a dominant or recessive gene by the activity of the enzyme. Here we see that some of the other children in the family have really a decreased enzyme activity, yet they don't show the disease. I was always under the impression that the dominant gene protected a recessive characteristic, yet actually you couldn't demonstrate this. In other words, if there was a dominant gene there, the activity and all functions of the body should be perfectly normal. However, your findings here would almost imply that some of the other types of functions might be abnormal in the person who is protected by a dominant gene. Yet we know that the parents who don't have the clinical disease to all intent and purpose are normal physically and mentally. Dr. Armstrong, from what you've shown, do you think it's more likely that the mother will show the defect than the father, for example?

Dr. Armstrong: I'll let Dr. Menkes comment on that one if it's all right with you, but I would like to indicate that peroxidase has multiple isozymes. Horseradish has 18 to 20 bands on electrophoresis, and in the white cell there are probably six or seven, with three major bands and three or four minor bands. We haven't perfected our procedure yet, but we do have some fragmentary data on one of the children with the disease; a couple of bands were missing. So I think probably one of the answers as to why the heterozygotes (if that's what they are--and I think they are, because at least they're hypergranulated) may have a low total enzyme is that they may have the correct isoenzyme still present which keeps them from getting the disease.

Dr. Hochstein: I'd like to comment if I may. These data are the most fascinating I've seen in quite a while. It's clear now that Dr. O'Brien may have put his finger on the problem earlier when he said there are many peroxidases in cells that we don't quite understand, which may account for differences in the activity observed with different substrates. These peroxidases may be isozymes of the same enzyme, or they may be peroxidases of which we know very little. There are some very provocative observations.

Dr. Rider: Let me ask Dr. Menkes if he would comment on the hereditary aspect.

Dr. Menkes: I don't know. I was wondering, seeing the changes here that in some aspects are the same in these four mothers--they all had a drop in activity--different in one mother. Is there any factor you can pinpoint--the age of those mothers, in the dietary intake, form of contraception, the presence of an infection in this one mother, or something like that--that might possibly change leukocytes? Is there any difference you could get between that one mother who was different and the other four?

Dr. Armstrong: No. Let me just respond to Dr. Menkes about some of the potential differences in these families. Three of the cases are from Oklahoma, the fourth one is from San Francisco, and the fifth one from Toronto, Canada. The fifth case is the mother who also acts just like the three cases that we have in Tulsa (Fig. 37). The age of the mothers range from about age 26 (in case 1 with the late infantile form) to age 49 (case 3), and the other mothers fall between. They come from different areas, they have different ages, and yet all except Mrs. Collum can be shown to be deficient if you increase the incubation time of the assay.

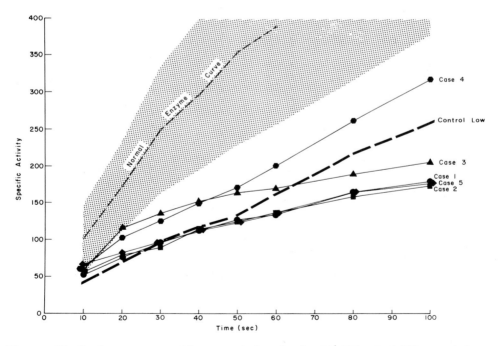

Figure 37. Leukocyte peroxidase activity in 5 mothers of children with Batten's disease.

Dr. Zeman: We found that there is an individual difference
of myeloperoxidase activity in normals, and if I look at Dr.
Armstrong's curves he has expressed the same situation by
a considerable spread and also by his control dose. In addition
to that, there is an individual difference of enzyme activity
as a response to dietary intake of vitamin E, and Dr. Patel
has accumulated considerable observations in this area.[38]

Dr. Rider: Dr. Armstrong, that could be a very interesting
thing though: take your heterozygous females and see if you
can change their enzyme activity with a large dose of vitamin E.
Dr. Zeman seems to think that his enzyme level has been increased
with intake.

Dr. Armstrong: I wouldn't think that their diets change
very much.

Dr. Rider: No, but I thought it would be interesting
to see whether you could now bring them up to normal by giving
them excess vitamin E.

Dr. Hartroft: Why should tocopherol increase the level
of the enzyme?

Dr. Patel: May I comment? This is perhaps premature,
but we have conducted a study with normal volunteers. We
give them vitamin E in increasing doses. The first observation
we made was that of 12 individuals--10 remained on the regimen
we prescribed--out of the 10, 8 responded with increased peroxidase activity with all three hydrogen donors; that is with
p-phenylendiamine, guaiacol and DMB. However, as we continued
the treatment, the activity dropped below normal with respect
to increasing the dose of vitamin E. We started out with
400 mg/day, and we went up to 1.2g/day. I am at a loss to
explain what really is going on. However, it is possible
that the peroxide levels in these individuals drop down considerably, and it may be speculated that the circulating peroxides perhaps reduce this enzyme. This is very hypothetical,
but that is the only possible explanation I can give.

Dr. Aristotle Siakotos: Is that change dose-dependent?

Dr. Patel: Perhaps so. You see, I also know that out
of these 12, one volunteer responded later than the others,
so it could be dose-dependent. That is why I thought the
vitamin B_{12}, which increases the peroxidase activity in animals
as much as three- to five fold (dose-dependent) should be evaluated.
In other words, it may not be as simple as we are thinking.

Dr. Zeman: I think we have reached our goal, namely,
to stimulate our thinking about these problems, so I take
the liberty as moderator of this meeting to authorize the
parting shot at this session to be given by Dr. O'Brien.

Dr. O'Brien: This is really fascinating. It seems to me the logical explanation is that this is an isozyme that you're pursuing. It's one of a number of isozymes that you're measuring when you measure with phenylenediamine. The other substrates have different substrate specificities, and the other isozymes are reflected in that measurement, so that you can't detect the defect with those. Those isozymes that are not defective are hormonally induced, or they are influenced by contraceptive medications, or they are dietarily changed by things that we really don't know much about. But if you had a specific measure for the isozymes, you would find that heterozygotes, both male and female, for that isozyme would run at half normal level, and you would have it all clinched. It is a formidable achievement, and I congratulate you.

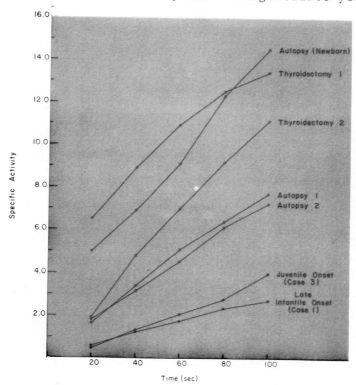

Figure 38. Thyroid peroxidase activity in cases 1 and 3 and in 5 controls.

Dr. Zeman: I would like to discuss the implications of Dr. Armstrong's findings with respect to further studies. But before we go to this point, we may perhaps ask a few more technical details of Dr. Armstrong. Then I think we should try to find some explanation as to how we can conceivably apply these data to the mechanism by which the disease becomes

manifest--or, at least, by which the biochemical lesion becomes
manifest. Dr. Armstrong, I wonder whether you could give
us your further observations on this peroxidase deficiency
with respect to tissues other than leukocytes.

Dr. Armstrong: Yes, Dr. Zeman. In one of the cases
that we showed yesterday--case 3--representing a juvenile
form of Batten's disease, we obtained a rectal biopsy and
a thyroid biopsy. The thyroid has very good peroxidase activity
and is used in the formation of thyroxin. Figure 38 clearly
shows specific activity of thyroid peroxidase in a patient
with the juvenile form. It also shows activity in another
patient that we've just added, one with the late infantile
form--this is the child who expired recently--and I've added
this to the chart with specific activities from two autopsy
thyroids, two thyroids from goiterous type adult patients
taken at surgery, and one newborn. Figure 38 clearly shows
that the thyroid tissue again reflects the deficiency of the
peroxidase with our assay system. The rectal ganglion biopsy
(Fig. 39) also showed cells which are markedly distended with PAS

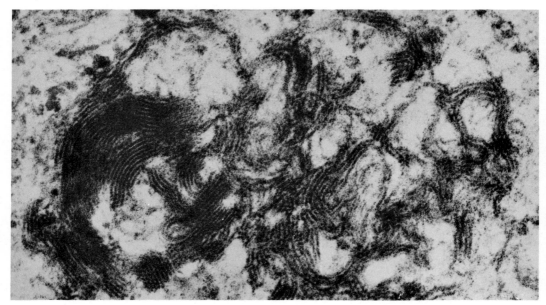

Figure 39. Neuron of Meissner's plexus with cytoplasmic pigment body of
           fingerprint type. X 68,000

positive and Sudan black B material, and I believe the pathologist told me this material also fluoresced. We've looked
at some of the tissues in the child who expired with the late
infantile form, and we have not run enough controls yet, but
in the data that we have available to us to date the deficiency
appears to be almost uniform in all of the other tissues.

Dr. Zeman: Thank you, Dr. Armstrong. Perhaps this would
be the time to enter into a more general discussion about
peroxidases. What I'm particularly concerned with is the following: there is no question that Dr. Armstrong has beautifully
demonstrated a peroxidase deficiency which appears to be restricted to either an enzyme component or an isozyme--or several
isozymes--and that this particular defective isozyme is, at
least in a test tube, particularly active towards the peroxidation of p-phenylenediamine. Now, would this then indicate
that the enzyme, which is in the literature described as myeloperoxidase, is actually part of a much larger system of tissue
peroxidases? If so, what do we know about other peroxidases
which are perhaps nonspecific and at least not comparable
to, for instance, "true" oxidase or to the peroxidases which
have been characterized as parts of peroxisomes by Müller[39]
and by DeDuve. [40] Can anyone enlighten us on this?

Dr. Austin: May I just make a suggestion here and express
a point of view? I think that we should get away from talking
about a myeloperoxidase deficiency in this disease and simply
restrict ourselves to talking about--if you will--a phenylenediamine peroxidase deficiency or, better still, deficient
phenylenediamine peroxidase activity. The sooner we do this,
I think the better off we'll be with respect to making conceptual
progress in our thinking. For example, the word myeloperoxidase
probably embraces many different peroxidases, each with different
substrate affinities. And really I think what Dr. Armstrong
has done is something rather specific and quite restricted
thus far, namely, focusing on deficient peroxidase activity
by use of phenylenediamine as a substrate, so I'm not sure
that the term myeloperoxidase will be helpful to us in proportion
to what it does to confuse us.

Dr. Zeman: Well, I agree with that statement completely.
Unfortunately, we all are subject to the influence of semantics,
and the reason I've used this term is because this is the
term which is being used in the literature in order to characterize or describe whatever information is available on this
particular enzyme as measured in leukocytes in the literature.
As we heard from Dr. Hochstein yesterday, there are rather
specific attributes given to the peroxidase that has been
demonstrated in leukocytes which, as Dr. Hochstein points
out, is instrumental in the membrane fusion between the primary
lysosome and the autophagic or heterophagic vacuole by the
intermediate of the iodate reaction. Let's rephrase the question, then, and let's ask: Is this peroxidase which has been
measured by Dr. Armstrong and found to be deficient in patients
and in heterozygotes for the gene of neuronal ceroid lipofuscinosis, is this particular enzyme a ubiquitous enzyme, and is
it part of a larger system of peroxidases which have different
substrate specificity?

Dr. Hochstein: I would like to concur with what Dr.

Austin has said in that I really think it's important to keep the terminology straightened out this early in the game, because one could create enormous confusion in the literature by referring at this time to this enzyme as leukocyte myeloperoxidase. It is, in fact, a peroxidase activity associated with one substrate, and this in terms of classical enzymology defines its activity in a very satisfactory way until one finds out what the real substrate is in the cell.

I don't know that I can make a contribution as to the nature of peroxidases in leukocytes or other tissues in the body, but there are many of them, each having specific functions. If I can just turn for a moment to the data here, I am most impressed, not by the differences in activity in the patients versus the newborn control, but rather the endogenous rate, the initial level of peroxidation without the addition of substrate; there is an enormous difference here. Dr. Armstrong, have you calculated what the per cent decrease in activity is? It doesn't look, frankly, like very much to me. It seems to me that the differences we're looking at here are not so much in enzyme activity but in endogenous substrate.

Dr. Armstrong: Well, as you can see from the units in Figure 38 it's about a fivefold difference perhaps--a five- or sixfold difference. These are just relative units here, so that thyroidectomy patient 1 is up at around 7 at 20 sec incubation; case 3 is less than 1.0--about 0.5. That's about a fifteenfold factor here; if you extend the incubation time out to around 100 sec, then the values are about 14 and 3.5, or about a three- or fourfold factor.

Dr. Hochstein: Are substrates and peroxide added at zero time?

Dr. Armstrong: Yes, this is the complete incubation mixture; everything is present there. We just add the tissue extract representing the enzyme, along with the phenylenediamine and the peroxide and start measuring. The reaction goes very rapidly, and we aren't able to measure less than 5 sec; it takes that much to mix it and get it into the cuvette and into the spectrophotometer. I don't know what's going on at those very, very short incubation times, but we have started at 10 sec; that's the first reading we take. Then we follow it with time.

Dr. Menkes: What do you add at zero time?

Dr. Armstrong: Everything--the entire incubation mixture-- just like in the leukocyte peroxidase assay. The system is exactly the same; it's just thyroid tissue supernatant versus white cell supernatant.

274

Dr. Hochstein: I see now; I really misunderstood these experiments. I think if you were able to do your mixing of your substrate very rapidly in the recording spectrophotometer, you'd pick up these rates in the first few seconds. I presume these are true initial rates, and what you're looking at really over this long time period are rates that result from enzyme activation with time. Are these done at 37 C?

Dr. Armstrong: No, they're done at 25 C.

Dr. Zeman: I had another question, Dr. Armstrong. If I understood you correctly, you have a 10^{-3} M concentration of hydrogen peroxide. Now, there are reports in the literature[41] that some peroxidase activity may be inhibited by as little as 0.4×10^{-3}M hydrogen peroxide, and I just wonder whether you have worked with various concentrations of hydrogen peroxide.

Dr. Armstrong: Yes, we start to see the inhibitory effects of excess substrate concentration, hydrogen peroxide, at somewhere between 10^{-2} and 10^{-3}M in our system.

Dr. Zeman: So you are below the threshold for inactivation; but the possibility, of course, which would exist is that at this concentration there is a differential inhibition of the isoenzyme which is defective in the disease, but still may not be inhibited in the normal.

Dr. Armstrong: Yes.

Dr. O'Brien: I wanted to ask a question about the mixing experiments with patients and controls. Soluble endogenous inhibitors might account for the enzyme inactivation if you haven't done mixing experiments that indicate that you get 50% kinetics.

Dr. Armstrong: Figure 40 shows results for a series of three patients where mixing experiments were done. The difference between any of these three patients--two juveniles and one with the late infantile form--plus one family in which both parents were apparent heterozygotes, plus one sister who had low activity. All showed there was no change greater than 11%.

Dr. O'Brien: It appears from this chart that your mixed homogenates give more activity than the...

Dr. Armstrong: No more than 11% difference.

Dr. O'Brien: Wouldn't you expect 50% kinetics in the mixed homogenate?

Dr. Armstrong: No. Those are equal aliquots; control and patient should be added together to equal the mixture.

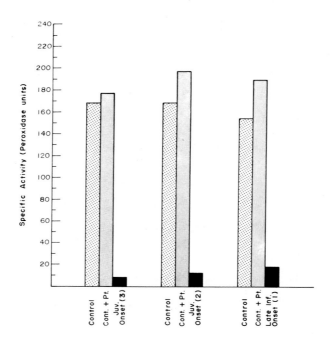

Figure 40. Peroxidase activity before and after mixing with appropriate controls.

Dr. O'Brien: Oh, I see. This is the sum of these two, so that if you divided by two you'd get 50%.

Dr. Armstrong: We didn't see any inhibition; we didn't see any stimulation either by the control for the patient.

Dr. Zeman: There is at least suggested evidence that there exist two forms: a so-called juvenile form, which we prefer to call the Spielmeyer-Sjögren type, and the so-called late infantile type, which we prefer to call the Jansky-Biel-schowsky type, which becomes manifest as late as age 20 years. Another question which is intriguing is whether a mixing of these two types of isozymes, or rather an isozyme hybridization, would correct the enzyme defect, at least in the test tube. This could be done by, say, fusion or by other hybridization techniques. I wonder whether any data are currently available on this aspect.

Dr. Armstrong: No, we don't have any, and I don't know if any exist.

Dr. Philippart: I think that is a very good point. There is also a distinct possibility that unrelated heterozygotes

276

may have a slightly different mutation which may account for some of the clinical variability from one family to another.

Dr. Austin: I'm not sure how many different kinds of peroxidase deficiencies there will turn out to be, but if there are, let's say, at least maybe 10 separate and distinct mechanisms by which one can arrive at a phenylenediamine peroxidase deficiency, then it may not be very long before it becomes difficult to squeeze into any clinical slot the cases we have seen and those that others have described in the past. What I'm saying is, rather than having to cope with the vagaries of classification--Bielschowsky-Jansky, Spielmeyer-Sjögren, Batten-Vogt, Kufs--perhaps we had better talk about some less specific and less charged kind of designation. If, as you point out, you think you have evidence that the Bielshowsky-Jansky form begins at 20 years of age, then one wonders how useful that eponym is. Are you really sure that you're now talking about the same Bielschowsky-Jansky form that was described many, many years ago?

Dr. Zeman: I think this is a point which can never be settled, because neither the cases of Jansky's four siblings, nor the three siblings of Bielschowsky, have been subject to enzymological, electron microscopic, and analytical chemical procedures, and you know very well that several cases of GM1 gangliosidosis, type 2, have been equated with the cases of Bielschowsky in the literature.

What we have done is simply to lump all these cases together and look at the dynamics, at the biology of the disease, and have termed those with a relatively short clinical evolution beginning with generalized convulsions and later on blindness as the Jansky-Bielschowsky type regardless of age of onset, and those in whom the clinical evolution is characterized by early visual failure and extremely slow mental and motor degeneration, with an average duration of the illness in the range of 11 years, as the Spielmeyer-Sjögren type because these were the definitions which these people originally gave. However, there is no Batten type; there is no Mayou type; there is no Vogt type; because these people described a whole spectrum of cases which fit very well the concept of neuronal ceroid-lipofuscinosis.[42] In other words, they described both patients with a very pernicious clinical course and with a very protracted clinical course. Batten's paper,[43] in 1914, pointed out that the characteristic of this disease is that its clinical course is highly variable. So this has been a guideline, by no means a classification, but simply a taxonomic approach. The interesting thing is that there is no evidence that in one and the same family even in collaterals, a pernicious one-year clinical course occurs together with the typical Spielmeyer-Sjögren picture of slow progression of mental deterioration and relatively late manifestations of motor disturbances.

Dr. Hartroft: It would be most helpful for those of us who are not clinicians to have a simple ABC of the different kinds of Batten's disease.

Dr. Zeman: We have lumped together a group of diseases, all of which are associated with a progressive deterioration of brain function and in which there are the pathomorphological findings of (1) a loss of nerve cells; (2) the presence, in the remaining nerve cells, of large quantities of an autofluorescent lipopigment, which has been isolated and identified as ceroid, a pigment which is yellow in the purified form, which has a density of above 1.25, and which is unstable to chelation, to ion exchange, and to exposure to salt solution. It differs from lipofuscin, which is stable under these conditions, and is black upon purification. Furthermore, ceroid contains approximately one-half its mass in the form of acidic lipid polymers, whereas lipofuscin has only 8% of acidic lipid polymers.[44]   We have included all the diseases of the brain in which we have been able to demonstrate the presence of ceroid in this group of neuronal ceroid-lipofuscinoses.   Now, if you use this definition, you will find that there is a variety of clinical diseases in which this chemical morphological correlation exists.   In other words, our clinical observations permit us to differentiate, but neither physico-chemical procedures, at least not to the extent to which they have been used, nor the morphology permits a clearcut differentiation. Some neuropathologists have tried to obtain further subclassifications on the basis of the ultrastructural appearance of the pigment bodies, and have delineated a type associated with curvilinear bodies; there is another type associated with fingerprint bodies, and yet another type associated with crystalloids, and so on.   But as soon as you have an opportunity to examine relatively large amounts of material from various parts of the body, you will find that the ultrastructural differentiation is doomed to failure.[45]   The best proof for this contention rests with a highly inbred strain of English setters with neuronal ceroid lipofuscinosis in which we find all these different types of pigment bodies and their respective ultrastructural characteristics.   This has encouraged us to place major emphasis on the biology of the disease in our efforts to break down this condition into different forms. It is almost a dictum that, if there are several affected siblings in one family, they all show the manifestations of the disease around the same age, (this is called homochronism), and they also show a fairly stereotyped evolution of the disease, whereby the first symptoms are the same in all siblings, and the evolution is very similar from one affected sibling to the next (this is called homotypism).   If you rely on those purely clinical, taxonomic, and descriptive criteria, then you find that there must be entirely different forms of this disorder which cannot be further differentiated by the pathologists.   There are other criteria: for example, we have examined a family with some 12 members affected in which a chronic brain disease with mental deterioration and a very spectacular cerebellar defect is inherited as a dominant principle.[46] Again, ceroids were isolated from the brain of one of the affected members of this family, but here we have clearly a different genetic defect. The rule of thumb which we have used is to define all those cases with a very short and stormy clinical course where the first symptom is usually some form of seizure and where within a span of less than one year the patient is completely immobilized, bedridden, and demented as Bielschowsky-Jansky type, because these were actually the clinical criteria proposed by these two men. (Actually, it's Jansky-Bielschowsky, because Jansky[47] preceded Bielschowsky[48] by some six years.) Unfortunately, Jansky's paper was written in Czech which few of us read, but his paper, in a sense, was much more lucid than Bielschowsky's.

On the other hand, the slowly progressive type of ceroid-lipofuscinosis, which begins invariably with visual disturbances at an age as early as 3 months and as late as 15 years, and then shows relatively mild but progressive mental deterioration has been termed the Spielmeyer-Sjögren type. Sjögren[49] reported on 115 cases from southern Sweden, involving about 50 different kindreds, which have been followed back to the 17th century, in which the disease is extremely stereotyped.

Finally, there is an adult form, which characteristically is never associated with any lesions of the retina. It is, of course, the adult form which is dominantly inherited. This is where our efforts at classification stand at the present time, which does not mean that these three differential clinical groups represent nosological entities or specific enzyme defects. However, for the needs of the physician who is faced with the tasks of diagnosis and prognosis, this classification has been helpful.

Dr. Rider: Dr. Austin suggested that we call this a phenylenediamine peroxidase insufficiency to make it more specific, and I think this is true--you have to get down to the basic enzyme defect present in all of these diseases. If this is so in the so-called Batten's disease, do you think that this defect is specific for this, or would you find it in others of these clinical classifications, different onsets, and so forth?

Dr. Austin: I would suggest, Dr. Rider, that phenylene-diamine peroxidase deficiency be used in a heuristic interim way just to keep our language straight before we get down to defining what the biological substrate is. That's the only way in which I would consider using the term. It's an awkward one, but one might even say deficient PDP or something like that.

Dr. Rider: But the point is you may be able to further define this. Perhaps this substrate is specific and perhaps not absolutely so; another peroxidase may react, for example. Acetylcholine esterase, for example, which is supposed to be very specific for degradation of acetylcholine, will react with some other things, but not nearly at the same level of efficiency as it will with acetylcholine.

Dr. Austin: Yes, many of our chromogenic substrates are by definition not biological substrates; they are not 100% specific, even though they're very helpful.

Dr. Rider: Could you isolate a peroxidase, for example, and see whether it would react with this phenylenediamine? Could you isolate different kinds of peroxidases and see whether they would react? Do you think you could crystalize or otherwise isolate some of these peroxidases to permit you to see whether there is a difference in how they react with a substrate?

Dr. Austin: You might be able to crystallize catalase; I don't know whether you could crystallize peroxidase or not. Yes, I think this would be an ultimate goal to isolate the peroxidases, perhaps not by crystallization but by column chromatography.

Dr. Rider: In other words, I suppose it's conceivable that one clinical entity could show a lack of one kind of peroxidase, and another condition perhaps a lack of another kind; or the defect could be the same but there might be a difference in the peroxidase degradation to account for the difference in the clinical picture. I think you have to get down to the basic enzyme chemistry.

Dr. Austin: A similar clinical situation has existed with regard to metachromatic leukodystrophy. Everybody has been perplexed by the disease because it can start anywhere from 12 months of age to the age of 60. I think as we look more and more at different families with this disease, it is becoming clear that there may be more than one route by which to disable an enzyme. An enzyme that is disabled by a certain kind of error, say, an error in its constituent amino acids, may express itself in a disease which begins at one age, has a certain velocity, and shows a certain char- acteristic pathological distribution of lesions; whereas an enzyme error, in this case a cerebroside sulfatase enzyme disabled by a different molecular error at a different part of the enzyme structure, may lead to a clinical entity which is different in terms of age of onset, tempo of the disease, and pathological expression. Even for one specific enzyme, I think there may be different ways to disable that enzyme. We should look here not only at subtly different differences

280

among different peroxidases, but at different ways to disable the same enzyme.

Dr. Rider: I guess the other thing I am interested in, of course, is what you can do in vitro to influence the enzyme activity. You have your system in a test tube, you've got your white cells, and you've isolated your peroxidase and so now you're going to measure its activity. Can you add something to that test tube to bring that activity up to normal? In other words, can you add another peroxidase? You could get some peroxidase from the normal white cell, but can you get it from some other source?

Dr. Zeman: Such as horseradish peroxidase?

Dr. Rider: That's right, something like that.

Dr. Menkes: More specifically, can you mix a Jansky-Bielschowsky with a Spielmeyer-Sjögren and get a normal?

Dr. Zeman: This hasn't been done yet.

Dr. Armstrong: I haven't tried that. They're both deficient, but I haven't mixed them. I've got both available; I'll do that when I get back.

Dr. Rider: What about extraneous enzyme?

Dr. Armstrong: The horseradish peroxidase reacts very well in the incubation mixture, and we use it as our standard for deriving specific activity.

Dr. Rider: When you say horseradish peroxidase, from what part of the horseradish is it derived?

Dr. Zeman: It is commercially available in crystalline form--horseradish peroxidase.

Dr. Hochstein: I'd like to ask Dr. Armstrong a more general question if we can go back just a little bit. We spoke yesterday about Batten's disease in terms of peroxidation reactions and excess of peroxidation in the cells, and now we're talking about a deficiency of an enzyme which peroxidates, so then what are we saying then about Batten's disease? Does the deficiency of this enzyme result in accumulation of substrate or peroxides in the cell--is that your view?--and is this why you get excess peroxidation?

Dr. Armstrong: Yes.

Dr. Hochstein: Are you thinking in terms of hydrogen peroxide or other peroxides?

281

Dr. Armstrong: We'll just call it "peroxide" right now, but very likely it is hydrogen peroxide; certainly you know that's produced in a lot of pathways. But there have been other reports involving other types of hydroperoxides, and various amines will work; peroxy acids can also be used as primary substrate. So whatever there is available in the cell endogenously, one or many may be reacting in vivo.

Dr. Hochstein: So in other words, the PPD peroxidase, then, is a detoxification enzyme in your view, and the failure to detoxify peroxides results then in excess peroxidation.

Dr. Armstrong: Right. Superimposed on that is the toxicity of H_2O_2 in terms of disrupting membranes and proteins.

Dr. Rider: Would you entertain the idea, for example, of using crystalline horseradish peroxidase, let's say clinically, and then retesting one of these patient's white cells to see what the peroxidase activity is after he's been on treatment for a day or a week or something like that? Could you predict by kinetics or mass of cells involved how much peroxidase it might take to do this?

Dr. Armstrong: What matters is, if you give one of the various isoenzymes of peroxidase--or all of them--the important thing is, can you get it into the nerve cells? If we gave it and just measured increasing peroxidase levels in the white cells, that might just mean that the white cells have taken it up.

Dr. Rider: At least that would be a step in the right direction; you at least would show that you could influence the peroxidase.

Dr. Armstrong: Peroxidase has been used for many years as a marker because it's a chromogenic type of a protein, in terms of measuring membrane transport: it does get absorbed across the gut, goes to the liver, and goes many other places after that. I think we eat lots of peroxidase in all types of food, and I'm sure it doesn't hurt you, and I think you could give it and see what would happen.

Dr. Rider: We can predict in diabetics how much insulin is needed. It is surprising, really, the small amount of insulin that a person needs to carry on his bodily functions. Is there any way that you know, Dr. Zeman, of predicting how much peroxidase would be required?

Dr. Zeman: The data on horseradish peroxidase are rather clear. The blood brain barrier does not permit a significant amount of horseradish peroxidase to enter the brain tissue.

The introduction of horseradish peroxidase into the ventricular system would be a major procedure, especially if you have to do it on a daily basis. It is also limited by the tight junction of the ependymal cells, and in fact horseradish peroxidase has been used in order to demonstrate the tightness of the junction in the ependyma. So in order to get the horseradish peroxidase into the interstitial spaces of the brain, you would have to produce brain damage, perhaps by way of anoxia or by radiation, and the question is whether, under the circumstances, the treatment is not worse than the disease. At the present time this is not possible. There are, however, suggestions that have been made, in particular by Karnovsky,[50] that you can slightly alter the configuration of the peroxidase molecule which has a relatively small molecular weight--about 28,000 or so--and by attaching some aliphatic moieties. Presumably this would make it slightly fat-soluble, and thus it could enter the brain. Along the same vein we might mention experiments on dogs in which we have transplanted the kidney from a nonaffected heterozygote to an affected homozygote, and conversely, the homozygotic kidney into the heterozygote; this experiment was performed about a year ago. It has not shown any modification of the disease, as we know it to evolve, in the dog with a life span limited to 25 months at the most, nor has it induced any changes in the heterozygous normal receptor. We have not as yet looked at the transplanted kidneys, but it seems that they are functioning normally just as before. We also have performed a set of experiments in which we have produced chimera--that is, animals who received bone marrow and/or splenic cells from matched litter mates, either recessive or heterozygous for the trait. These animals are still at an age (about 7 months) where you would not expect to find clinical abnormalities. One of the homozygous affected recipients has normal PPD peroxidase activity, but, not having broken the code, we do not know which treatment it had received.

Dr. Dawson: I think several people in this room have been probing the possibility of enzyme replacement therapy in many of these inherited diseases. There seems no doubt that in fibroblasts you can correct an α-galactosidase deficiency by adding this to the medium,[51] and Dr. Philippart and others have carried out renal transplantation in patients with Fabry's disease and shown some possible improvement.[52][53][54] I think that in all neurological disorders, enzyme replacement therapy has not been successful. Thus, in the mucopolysaccharidoses, the Hurler and Hunter syndromes, where plasma has been infused and the transitory improvement in neurological symptoms has usually not been sustained,[55][56] I don't think there's really any well documented case of neurological improvement by adding the missing enzyme, even though in many cases these missing enzymes can now be added in pure form. I think perhaps the most hopeful aspect of this disease is that there seems to be some residual phenylenediamine peroxidase activity, and

perhaps the thing to do would be to try to enhance that residual
activity, at least perhaps up to the heterozygote level.
I'm not sure, but perhaps some of the people who are interested
in working on peroxidases might give some clues as to how
one could perhaps stimulate this residual peroxidase activity
to get it up to slightly more normal levels, if indeed this
residual activity is genuine and not perhaps some artifact
of the system.

Dr. Zeman: Well, of course, one possibility, suggested
by results of loading experiments in heterozygotes with other
conditions, is to reduce the substrate concentration in order
to get along with whatever little residual enzyme is present.
This is a route that we have pursued in trying to reduce the
level of peroxides, hydroperoxy compounds, and hydrogen peroxide.
What you are talking about is the possible derepression of
enzyme induction of these things, and there are indeed reports
in the literature by which this has been possible with vitamin
B_{12}. Perhaps Dr. Hochstein or Dr. O'Brien can enlighten us
a little bit on these things.

Dr. Hochstein: The thought I have is that if this enzyme
is involved in the detoxification of hydrogen peroxide, and
if it's failing to do so in an adequate manner because one
of its substrates (other than hydrogen peroxide) is not present
at a level sufficient to allow it to act; perhaps one could
introduce, if one knew what that substrate was, the substrate
into the cells and therefore you would enhance detoxification
of peroxide, rather than inducing more enzyme.

Dr. Rider: What kind of substrate could it be?

Dr. Hochstein: Well, at this point one doesn't know.
The enzyme is now defined in terms of its artificial substrate.
What one will have to determine is the nature of the substrates
for this altered enzyme; if there is a naturally occurring
substrate for it--and I would hope that there is--that might
be the way to go with replacement therapy rather than try
to replace the enzyme. The problems with enzyme therapy are
enormous because the problem is not to get the enzyme into
the interstitial fluid but into the cell, and I'm not sure
that many enzymes are taken up in the cell. Given the immunological problems which accompany enzyme therapy, that
would be a poor route to go, I would think.

Dr. O'Brien: Yes, I think it's important to understand
in detail what this enzyme does. Here you have a situation
in which the evidence suggests a peroxidase deficiency, and
because there are peroxidized products accumulating you instantly
assume, and very rightly so, that this somehow relates to
the metabolic defect that accounts for the accumulation of

the peroxidized products. The question is, what does this peroxidase really do? You have in these same tissues--Mark Ruddick has demonstrated that the glutathione peroxidase activity is completely normal or increased in Batten's disease. In fact, the experiment that Mark did, and I can describe it for you, is to measure the activity of the glutathione peroxidase, according to the procedure of Little and O'Brien,[57] in autopsy tissues from patients with Jansky-Bielschowsky disease and to compare the activity of this enzyme with "normal" brain tissues from people ranging in age from 3 to 80 who died of non-neurological disease. The assay involves the use of the linoleoyl hydroperoxide as the substrate, with glutathione providing the reducing power, and coupling this to glutathione reductase and measuring the rate of disappearance of NADPH in a recording spectrophotometer. As Dr. Hochstein mentioned earlier, this should be the enzyme that is responsible for the abnormality. At least from what we know superficially about the disorder, you would expect, since peroxidized acyl moieties are accumulating and we know this enzyme is specific for that, glutathione peroxidase should be the defective enzyme. But when you measure the activity, the enzyme is not deficient. In fact, if you look at the activities we found for the controls, we get 483 units in normal brain, and for the Jansky-Bielschowsky brains we get 817 units, and as an extra pearl we did one progeria brain and got 1,093 units of enzyme activity.

Dr. Zeman: What part of the brain did you look at-- were those homologous parts of the brain?

Dr. O'Brien: Yes. They were cortical gray matter in all instances. Obviously, they are problems because the brains had been frozen. Mr. Ruddick did an experiment to indicate that if you look at the activity over a long time period in a normal control which has been frozen and thawed several times there is no significant diminution in activity. But my point then is this enzyme activity is present; now why doesn't that enzyme take the accumulated acyl hydroperoxide and get rid of it? The other question, too, is: if it's not the acyl hydroperoxide or linoleoyl hydroperoxide that's the problem, perhaps it's just hydrogen peroxide itself. Why doesn't the catalase that's present in these tissues in normal quantities take care of that, and why do these children then accumulate the substrate? The answer may be that we're looking at the wrong substrate. There may be a very specific acyl hydroperoxide that we have not defined that's part of the peroxidized lipoprotein varnish. It may be bound in some way so we can't determine exactly what it is, and that substrate may be very specific for this enzyme. The other enzymes that are present in normal quantities such as catalase and hydrogen peroxidase may not act upon that substrate. Therefore we have to really get down to the fine details of the molecular structure

285

of the accumulated product in relationship to the enzyme that
has been found deficient to understand this disorder. In
terms of therapy though, if we could somehow prevent that
unique hydroperoxide from accumulating, by preventing either
that accumulation by dietary means or some other means (knowing
that the disease has a very slow progression), we may be able
to suppress its accumulation by that route. Then the other
hydroperoxides that accumulate may be taken care of by catalase
and glutathione peroxidase. There is still an open good possibility that we could by preventive measures somehow deal
effectively with this disorder.

Dr. Zeman: The distributional features of this particular
disease seem to provide some clues as to what specific peroxide
we should be looking for. It must be a peroxide which utilizes
a substrate which has a particularly high concentration in
neuronal perikarya, and furthermore it must occur in particularly
high concentrations in the outer segments of the retinal rods
and cones. I think this is the type of approach Dr. O'Brien
has in mind, an approach which gets its clues from various
disciplines. It requires teamwork over a broad range of talent,
activity, and observation. How are you going to find this
particular substrate? Have you any ideas how this can be
done? Should we produce a variety of peroxides from various
types of tissue and have them react with the normal peroxidase
and with the deficient peroxidase, and then by analytical
procedures determine the difference in the reaction mixture?

Dr. O'Brien: One comment I'd make about the model you
drew with respect to distribution is that this may be a phenomenon which is related to the fact that these cells don't
divide. You do see trouble in dividing cells such as epithelial
cells and liver cells in small concentrations. It may be
that because the neuron isn't dividing that there is a particular
susceptibility for the stored substance. That's always been
something that I've thought in the back of my mind may account
for the particular predilection of this disease for the nervous
system.

To go on to your second question, obviously this enlightened
self-interest will dictate the way this problem is solved.
I think Dr. Armstrong indicated that he's starting to look
at isozymes. I think we need to sharpen the assay technique
to the point where you can really define the enzyme in the
test tube. Once you can do that, of course, that may make
it possible for you to do heterozygote detection and in utero
diagnosis. At least in those families in which you've got
tragedy, if you could diagnose this disease in utero, then
they could have another pregnancy and hopefully select only
those children that are unaffected by the disease. I would
put that as priority one, at least in terms of human need,
it's very important.

Dr. Zeman: It was my understanding, from what I have been able to read in the literature, that fetal tissue is not very active in peroxidases. Is that generally accepted?

Dr. Hochstein: Glutathione peroxidase is almost absent in fetal rat tissue, and then in the first week of life its activity increases enormously.

Dr. O'Brien: Well, I would suggest that we need to perfect an intrauterine diagnostic test for this disorder. With my experience with ganglioside storage disease, that has turned out to be one of the most promising and important things.

Dr. Rider: Well, that's prevention, of course, and that's a different aspect. I think I'd like to concentrate more on therapy.

Dr. O'Brien: There is no question in my mind that the therapy problem is going to be much more difficult to solve.

Dr. Rider: I'm sure that's true, but that's one reason we're all here.

Dr. Menkes: No, I agree with Dr. O'Brien. I think at this point we are on the verge of being able to prevent this disease, and I think our money should go in preventing this rather than treating. We have been successful in none of the CNS disorders, even though we have known the enzyme defect for a long time. Dr. O'Brien, how many years ago did you do this on Tay-Sachs? Six years, is it? You still have no treatment.

Dr. Dawson: Perhaps the late onset of this disease is going to be a problem in prenatal diagnosis unless you institute a massive screening program for heterozygotes. This may be justified if this disease turns out to be as common as recent work seems to indicate. You see, you have onset at about 11 or 12 years of age, by which time the family is usually complete.

Dr. O'Brien: Yes, although it's not as clearcut. You seem to have an ethnic predilection, with the Jansky-Bielschowsky patients being Anglo-Saxons and the Spielmeyer-Sjögren patients being of Scandinavian origin, but of course this doesn't seem to be as clear.

Dr. Rider: Obviously, therapy is very difficult--there is no question about it. I think I would still like a summary of the possible therapy. As you know, antioxidants and other treatments of this type may well ameliorate this disease.

Dr. O'Brien: Sure, both approaches ought to go on simul-

taneously. The therapeutic antioxidants constitute a shotgun
approach, because we really don't know what they do. We need
to isolate the enzyme in reasonably purified form, so that
the requisite kinetic studies can be done in order to elucidate
what the enzyme itself actually does. It is necessary to look
at it in terms of its substrate characteristics, the effective
inhibitors, its heat stability, the physical properties of
the enzyme in the normal. Having that, one can then begin
to start to make judgments with respect to whether particular
molecular compounds have important effects on that enzyme
in terms of activity, stimulation, or stabilization in the
normal case; these may then be extended to treatment of the
diseased patient.

     Dr. Menkes: What do we know about the substrate specificity
of glutathione peroxidase? Could you use linolenoyl hydroperoxide as one of the substrates? Does it react to that?

     Dr. Hochstein: Yes. I don't think there are important
differences with respect to the nature of the hydroperoxides.
The hydroperoxides used usually are the ones most easy to
prepare--and that's why they're used. Dr. O'Brien has looked
at a variety of hydroperoxides, and I don't think there are
important differences.

     Dr. Rider: I like to think of an analogous situation,
say, of L-dopa. It was postulated that dihydroxyphenylalanine
would be effective in Parkinsonism, and it didn't work. Once
the levo form was developed, it crossed the blood brain barrier
and was very helpful in these patients. I'm sure it doesn't
cure anybody, but it certainly prolongs the life of many of
these people with Parkinsonism. I think we just can't close
our eyes to something like that. Dr. Zeman mentioned the
possibility of joining the peroxidase, for example, to something
else which would cross the blood brain barrier.

     Dr. Hochstein: I'd like to make a suggestion with regard
to assays of enzymes like glutathione peroxidase. All of
us usually assay these enzymes under conditions in vitro at
high concentrations of substrate. I wonder if it wouldn't
be of value to do these kinds of assays under conditions where
substrate is limited perhaps so that you can see altered KM's.
Maybe activity of zero-order kinetics is fine, but when the
substrate is limited we might pick up things that we miss
at the present time.

     The other thing that occurs to me is that perhaps this
enzyme phenylenediamine peroxidase is not deficient--there
is activity there--and it may be that what we really should
be concerned with is the amount of enzyme present in relation
to the amount of hydrogen peroxide in the cell. Perhaps these
cells are producing too much peroxide for this amount of enzyme,

and it would be really of value to know the hydrogen peroxide level in these cells as compared with a normal cell.

Dr. Armstrong: Normal cells don't have any, at least that I can measure in that assay system.

Dr. Hochstein: No hydrogen peroxide? There are more sensitive techniques to measure peroxide: with aminotriazole or with scopolamine one can detect small amounts of peroxide.

Dr. Menkes: You're not just talking about hydrogen peroxide—you mean total peroxide, because I cannot see hydrogen peroxide accumulating with all the catalase around and other things.

Dr. Hochstein: As a matter of fact, hydrogen peroxide does accumulate in cells. If you look at liver, there is a steady-state level of hydrogen peroxide which is much higher than that in the red cell. Hydrogen peroxide is produced normally as a result of a variety of metabolic pathways: for example, when cells oxidize xanthine to uric acid, hydrogen peroxide is generated. It is always present in the cell. And all of it is not handled by catalase, because the catalase is isolated in the peroxisome under the subcellular compartmentalization of enzymes.

Dr. Menkes: Are there peroxisomes in the brain—in the neurons?

Dr. Zeman: De Duve claims[40] that there are no peroxisomes in the brain; and Müller, who works with De Duve, with whom I've had endless discussions, has never been able to provide evidence of peroxisomes in brain tissue in contrast to liver and kidney. But this, of course, is rat brain, and there are indeed species differences with respect to the oxidases. For example, Dr. Patel has not been able to find the PPD peroxidase in the dog, is that correct?

Dr. Patel: That's right, even in the mice.

Dr. Menkes: Is their catalase in the brain?

Dr. Zeman: Catalase is in the brain, and catalase shows a very specific distributional pattern which has received considerable attention. Glutathione peroxidase is in the brain and the distribution there also shows regional differences which span a range of one order of magnitude.

Dr. Rider: I still like the idea of using the model you have: you have affected children in which you can show decreased activity. Obviously, the defect is not absolute; it's not an all-or-none phenomenon; otherwise, they wouldn't have lived at all, and they've lived for many years. It seems

that you could very simply try to give large amounts of peroxidase and assay the white cells in these children again
in a week or two or a month. If there were to be a change
in white cells, it wouldn't necessarily follow that such a
regimen could effect changes in the brain, but at least you'd
be on the right track. If peroxidase does not cross the brain
barrier, it might be possible to join it to something that
does cross. If peroxidase didn't get in the white cell, that
probably would indicate that the approach wasn't going to
be fruitful.

Dr. Zeman: Even if we were to get it in the white cell,
the question is whether we could get it to that region or
structure where the damaging reaction takes place.

Dr. Austin: May I add here, just as a follow-up on what
Dr. Dawson was saying, that it may not be necessary to bring
the levels up to normal; it may only be necessary to bring
them up to a heterozygote's level. The point that there is
evidence of some enzyme activity to begin with is very hopeful;
it suggests that the enzyme protein in fact is there.

Dr. Rider: I'm sure we could get the patients and parents
willing to do something like this.

Dr. Hartroft: In your therapeutic approaches so far
you have only increased antioxidants; you have not decreased
the dietary levels of unsaturated fat. Is it conceivable
that, through whatever pathways you want to visualize, the
unsaturated fat is somehow increasing the requirement of activity
of this or other enzymes that may or may not be relatively
deficient? In your dogs, have you tried feeding them a completely semisynthetic diet without unsaturated fat?

Dr. Zeman: No.

Dr. Hartroft: It would have to be a semisynthetic diet
where you got rid of every bit of unsaturated fat. Use the
phenylketonuric approach, if you see the analogy, and try
it on your dogs. A diet completely free of unsaturated fat,
with all the fat in the form of saturated fat; and another
group, or dog, with all fat in the form of unsaturated fat
and no saturated; then a third dog, or group, free of fat
of all kinds, and then your normal control or regular control
or positive control, and compare their onset of symptoms.
Such an approach would be similar to handling of phenylketonuria
with a tryptophane-free diet.

Dr. Menkes: This is a simple thing, to us at least who
have used a phenylketonuric diet, but I think Dr. O'Brien
has just scotched this approach when he says that he has found

glutathione peroxidase, that this is normal; and when he says that glutathione peroxidase is active toward the fatty acid peroxides of the ω:3 and ω:6 series, then your essential fatty acid is not the problem, it's something else.

Dr. Hartroft: We do know, on the basis of a whole lot of evidence experimentally, that you cannot produce the pigment unless you have unsaturated fat as the starting material. Now you can't get rid of all the unsaturated fat in the body, but you can keep it to a minimum by dietary means, and this has been done in other situations. Is it possible that in raising the antioxidant levels in these patients and not at the same time removing as much as possible of the unsaturated fat a therapeutic opportunity is being missed?

Dr. Zeman: In these disorders of lipid peroxidation the electronmicroscopic evidence very clearly indicates that much of the polymerization and crosslinking of biological species does not occur with the unsaturated fatty acids in the cytoplasmic pool, but rather with subcellular organelles. That is, what becomes peroxidized are the unsaturated fatty acid moieties of the complex lipids in the subcellular membranes, notably the mitochondria and the endoplasmic reticulum.[58]

Dr. Hochstein: I know that one can readily alter the fatty acid composition of the membranes of red cells by diet, but how are such changes evoked in the brain?

Dr. Hartroft: Perhaps I could push my analogy with phenyl-ketonuria a little further. You cannot have a human being alive without all the essential amino acids, so in the thera-peutic approach to phenylketonuria one does not attempt to eliminate all tryptophane, only to reduce it to a minimum. This approach seems to work in a practical way with phenyl-ketonuria. I think it might be worthwhile to try the same approach in Batten's disease of reducing dietary unsaturated fat to the minimum of 1 or 2% of total calories, first in the dogs and later in humans if warranted.

Dr. Zeman: But if the nutritional intake of unsaturated fatty acid would be as important in bringing about the disease, wouldn't you expect to find the lesions in the liver rather than in the brain?

Dr. Hartroft: No, this would depend on the relative balance in the various tissues and their requirements, which I don't think at this stage we can predict or formulate.

Dr. Zeman: But let's go to the nutritional models of ceroid storage. If you look at yellow fat disease, for instance, the lesions are predominantly in the storage fats and in the liver, but not in the brain. If you look at cirrhosis in the choline-deficient liver the pigments are again in the liver and not in the brain. It seems to me that while I cannot directly refute this notion, that whatever evidence we do have seems to place the brain into the very last compartment in which any dietary changes could be brought to bear.

Dr. Hartroft: That's true, but on the other hand, by decreasing enzyme requirements in the body generally by reducing unsaturated dietary fat, possibly any enzymes present--even if only in small amounts--would then be more readily available to the newer tissue.

Dr. O'Brien: May I respond to your model? I think the model breaks down. In phenylketonuria you have a total deficiency of phenylalanine hydroxylase. In Batten's disease, as far as we know, we have an enzyme, the glutathione peroxidase, present in the tissue, that should take care of the polyunsaturated peroxides that accumulate, so the analogy is not complete. In one case you have zero enzyme for the substrate, and in the other we have at least evidence that the enzyme that takes care of these toxic products is present. There may be a subcellular distribution problem: we know that glutathione peroxidase is a cytosoluble enzyme, the lipopigments appear to be accumulating in lysosomes, and what Dr. Armstrong's enzyme may be is a lysosomal specific peroxidase and, therefore, hydroperoxides accumulate because the glutathione peroxidase doesn't get to the accumulated lipopigments and do its job because of the compartmentation problem. That is the case in Pompe's disease, where you see specific accumulation of glycogen in the lysosomes but not in the cytosol because the cytosol enzymes are able to break it down, so this may be the problem. I cannot see a relationship as simple as you draw it with total or marked restriction of polyunsaturated fatty acids. This is not to say it shouldn't be tried; I think it should be tried.

Dr. Zeman: Can I just make a remark here? I think, Dr. Hartroft, we would be happy to try the diet which is free of unsaturated fatty acids, and since you're a specialist in nutrition I would like to get your suggestion here.

It is true, Dr. O'Brien, that the pigments do accumulate in the lysosomes, but this does not necessarily mean that they are formed there. As a matter of fact, if you look at the electron micrographic evidence, the opposite is true; the pigments form in the cytoplasm and then secondarily are taken up by autophagic vacuoles, where the digestible moieties of the polymers are digested and the pigment becomes condensed.

Dr. O'Brien: I think the same thing is true of the gangliosidoses. There are membrane lipids that end up in the lysosome, and finally you can't cleave them because the enzyme in the lysosome is not there.

Dr. Zeman: That's right.

Dr. Rider: May I comment on that? Just because the yellow pigment accumulates doesn't necessarily mean anything; it can be the end product of a dead cell.

One other quick question: Have you tested your dogs to see if they lack this peroxidase?

Dr. Patel: We have tested a number of them, the results are rather inconsistent. However, the deficiency observed with p-phenylenediamine (PPD) is not as great as we would expect.

Dr. Rider: On the other hand, your dogs may not be the exact human model.

Dr. Hochstein: I'm really in sympathy, Dr. Rider, with your desire to push ahead with therapy simultaneously while we look at what's going on in cells, but I think the problem of direction of therapy cannot be resolved until we have further results. Dr. Armstrong has provided us with an important lead, but until we know something more of the nature of this enzyme, what it is, what it does, what is the nature of its substrates, we can't think any more constructively about therapy than a year ago.

Dr. Rider: I agree, I think that certainly is a first priority.

Dr. Hochstein: There's nothing I can see that can go on simultaneously until we know a little bit more about that enzyme and what it does.

Dr. Philippart: Such a diet free of unsaturated fatty acid, might create more confusion than anything else. There is an absolute requirement in mammals for unsaturated fatty acids in the diet--they are needed for building membranes and so on--you might create a new disease.

Dr. Hartroft: But you have the same two-edged sword in phenylketonuria. Uncontrolled therapy did more harm than good in some cases.

Dr. Philippart: But nobody has ever tried not to give any. There have been experiments in animals, mostly in the rat since the original observation of Burr and Burr.[59] Alterations of the skin, heart, liver, and kidney, growth, muscle tone, and cholesterol transport have been reported; there is increased fragility and permeability of cell membranes.[60]

293

The effect of essential fatty acid deficiency on the brain has not been extensively studied.[61] [62] Ataxia has been observed in the guinea pig.[63] There are few observations of human deficiency in the infant[64] or in the adult.[65] It might be more interesting to give an excess of unsaturated fatty acids.

Dr. Zeman: This has been done and it produced no changes in the overall picture. The dogs received an excess of unsaturated fatty acids; they had a fish diet.

Dr. Hartroft: You gave them an excess in the diet, but not the opposite--you did not create a deficiency. What diet do you give them routinely?

Dr. Zeman: We keep them on two different diets. They have a Purina main chow diet in our laboratory, but Dr. Koppang kept his dogs on a diet of horsemeat, which is relatively low in polyunsaturated fatty acids, in one situation, and on a diet of fish meal, which has about 10 times the concentration of unsaturated fatty acids, in another; there were no differences in the clinical course. There were differences in the clinical course if the animals were kept on antioxidants, and antioxidants significantly retard the age of manifestation of the disease. This is part of the rationale for using antioxidants in the treatment of the human disease.

Dr. Hartroft: These commercial chows have just barely enough essential fatty acid to prevent deficiency--which is about 2% of total calories--to minimize rancidity and thereby to extend shelf life. Dogs on any kind of a commercial pellet ration are receiving the lowest unsaturated fat diet compatible with normal growth and development.

Dr. Zeman: Dr. Armstrong, you have tried the antioxidant treatment; can you tell us about it?

Dr. Armstrong: I'll tell you about one case that we have: the young brother in case 1 (Fig. 28) who had the initial symptoms shortly after we measured his low peroxidase. He was put immediately upon Dr. Zeman's therapy of vitamin E, vitamin C, BHT (butylated hydroxytoluene), and DL-methionine. We had baseline peroxidase and baseline peroxide levels. The first time we reassayed this child, 60 days after initiating the treatment, the enzyme had not changed in terms of specific activity. However, the peroxide in this first analysis had decreased approximately 39%. He came in this week and we have drawn another white cell assay. When we return home after this conference we will measure again to determine whether the peroxide level has continued to drop. In any event, there was no change in the enzyme, but there was a 39% decrease in the level of peroxide, which we might attribute to the antioxidant therapy.

Dr. Rider: Could you explain what this treatment program was? I am generally familiar with it, but I want to know exactly what you gave this child.

Dr. Zeman: We gave him 2 g of vitamin E, 500 mg of vitamin C, 1000 mg of DL-methionine, and 200 mg of BHT or 100 mg of Santoquin as daily oral doses.

Dr. Hartroft: Isn't this the Tappel cocktail?

Dr. Zeman: Yes.

Dr. Armstrong: Clinically, before this child went on the antioxidant therapy, he had seizures, his electroretinogram was abnormal in both rods and cones, and he was beginning to have impairment of mental function: his I.Q. was not what it ought to be for age 3 years roughly. We have looked at those parameters again, too. His electroretinogram is now interpreted as normal; the rod system is normal, but the cone system is still abnormal. He has had no seizures in the 60 days that he has been on the therapy. The I.Q. testing is somewhat subjective, but the people who are testing think that he is improving in that area also; however, the parents have put a lot more into this child since the death of the other boy, so it's rather hard to evaluate that. Nevertheless, he hasn't had a single seizure since he went on the therapy. Now, granted, this is not quite 3 months yet.

I might emphasize that here is a patient who was probably diagnosed and put on treatment about as early as you could hope to find, so he's probably as minimally involved a patient as one could obtain. We have not tried this approach in any of the cases in which the disease is well advanced.

Dr. Austin: May I add something? He was not only caught early, but he also has a malignant form of the disease. His brother went downhill once he had the disease; it was very startling, very impressive. So one emerges with the feeling here that something has been going on.

Mr. Mark Ruddick: I'd like to mention another form of possible therapy and ask whether anybody's had any experience with it. I haven't been able to find any reference to it in the literature in relation to Batten's disease and the lipofuscinoses. There is a drug called centrophenoxine or Lucidril, which has been used in Europe. It's been shown to melt away lipofuscin in brains of aging animals quite dramatically; this has been confirmed on several occasions. I wonder in particular Dr. Zeman, if you've had an opportunity to try this drug on the dogs.

Dr. Rider: I can answer that with regard to a human.

We tried that on one patient both orally and by injection
over quite a few months, and it didn't seem to make any difference at all.

Dr. Zeman: I might add to that, that Dr. Isabel Rapin
at Albert Einstein has tried Lucidril as well and has not
observed any improvement. This seems to point out the fact
that we have suspected for a long time, that the pigment per
se is not necessarily causing the disease, but, rather, the
inactivation of biological species. I would certainly agree,
however, that once massive accumulation has occured, there
is a severe distortion of the geometry of the cell which impedes
diffusion and reaction paths on a very general level.

Dr. Menkes: What is that drug again?

Mr. Ruddick: It's called centrophenoxine or Lucidril;
it's a conjoiner of oxine or growth hormone; it's a very interesting subject.

Dr. Zeman: It's a phenoacetic acid derivative. The drug
was developed by Anphar Laboratories; it's marketed as Lucidril,
and it's used as an anabolic drug for the treatment of geriatric
problems.

Dr. Alan Percy: I think I could make some general comments.
I think until we reach the point where we're convinced that
we're dealing with one or more specific isoenzymes or protein
groups that we'll have difficulty in trying to interpret activities that we observe, which may represent multiple different
enzymologic reactions. So I think I would just like to echo
what Dr. O'Brien said, that we must stress the pursuance of
the observations that Dr. Armstrong has made to try to cone
down on the specific--if there are specific--isoenzymes that
are absent or deficient in their activity. I might step out
on a limb and be a little bit far out in terms of therapy;
if one really wants to entertain a dramatic mode of therapy,
that would be to add specific genetic material which would
compensate for the apparent deficiency of genetic material
in this group of diseases.[66]

Dr. Zeman: Do you have a virus which...

Dr. Percy: That's exactly the model which I think one
might be interested in pursuing, if one can be sure which
specific enzyme protein is deficient, and if one can find
a source which one can bind to a virus or some other carrier
of genetic material. I think as long as you have a reasonable
model--either that or the tissue culture system, if that might
turn out to be a useful system--those would be modes of eval-
uating...

Dr. Rider: Wouldn't it be hazardous to give a person

a virus that you hope to localize in the brain?

Dr. Zeman: No. Some people have been reasonably successful in treating with viruses.

Dr. Menkes: Can I add an anecdote here? I had a little girl who was coming down with some undiagnosable degenerative disease--seizures and everything--and we were considering brain biopsy. She got a very virulent case of chickenpox, and her disease was and has continued to be arrested since.

Dr. Zeman: This is not, however, unusual, because there are several interpretations for this. Of course, one would be that she did have a slow virus disease and the chickenpox infection induced interferon and arrested the situation. What is that amino aciduria which is treated with virus?

Dr. Philippart: Argininemia.[67]

Dr. Zeman: Argininemia.

Dr. O'Brien: It's a very bad example because it doesn't work.

Dr. Percy: In epidemiology or pediatric practice we have a history of 15 or so years of infecting the general population with SV-40 virus as a result of polio immunization, and at least to this point we have no evidence that there are adverse effects to that kind of an infection.

Dr. Zeman: Except for an occasional case of progressive multifocal leukoencephalopathy.

Dr. Rider: I'd like to throw out one wild thing, and that is when Chuck had surgery it was obvious that bleeding was prolonged and the prothrombin time was very low. He has been on vitamin K since then and his bleeding time is all right, but I never could understand why his prothrombin time was low because he was on a good diet at that time. I am asking whether there is any relationship between vitamin K and peroxidase.

Dr. Hochstein: Yes, I can say something. Vitamin K is one of those drugs which autoxidizes and actually produces hydrogen peroxide. In fact, in the newborn, vitamin K may be a hemolytic agent. It may be a potentially dangerous drug in terms of peroxide production. I remember when vitamin K or menadione was used in radiotherapy to enhance the hydrogen peroxide production, but this would be in the opposite direction.

Dr. Menkes: Wait a minute. If you're giving a lot of antioxidants, wouldn't you expect the level of vitamin K to be low?

Dr. Hochstein: The problem is that nobody really knows what the role of vitamin K is in prothrombin synthesis, whether it's the reduced form or the oxidized form. It may be that it's the oxidized form in vitamin K quinone that's important and, therefore, with any antioxidants you'd be preventing the formation of that, too. It might be interesting to do an experiment with antioxidants and look at clotting time.

Dr. Rider: I'll have to check back, but I think he was on vitamin E at that time, but I don't think he was on BHT.

Dr. Dawson: It's a little late in the day to present any data, but perhaps a few general comments about possible brain lipid abnormalities in this disease might be in order, since we seem to have decided that essentially the brain is the most affected organ. Is there anything specific about brain lipids which might be more susceptible to peroxidation? One can demonstrate apparent lipid storage in the neurons by, say, light microscopy histology, and this is very easy to do. On looking at neutral lipids one finds an increased level of esterified cholesterol which is presumably a secondary phenomenon related to the demyelination and the macrophage invasion that has taken place. One thing we have found is a marked diminution in the level of the trisialoganglioside (GT_1a), which is a specific brain glycolipid. In our hands this is almost diagnostic.[37][68] We have obtained brain biopsies and found this abnormal pattern, and then predicted accurately that the pathologist would find curvilinear bodies. It's difficult to think of an explanation for this apparent loss of trisialoganglioside (GT_1a), which we believe has something to do with neuronal function; it may be a neuronal component. Its synthesis may be under the control of prostaglandins which could conceivably be affected by unsaturated fatty acid abnormalities, since prostaglandins are derived from unsaturated fatty acids, such as arachidonic and arachidonate. It seems to be fairly specific for this disease, although it may be a secondary effect. I think that perhaps considering things like this may give us some sort of clue as to the pathogenesis of what's taking place in the brain. The other thing we have noticed, particularly in the more severe forms, is very, very low levels of ethanolamine plasmalogen. Ethanolamine plasmalogen seems to be the first phospholipid to go. Phosphatidyl serine has also been low in some of our terminal cases, but not quite so low in the biopsies. Even in the two biopsy samples that we have examined, the plasmalogen content seems to be very low. I would like to ask if anyone else has noticed this sort of finding. It could be an artifact due to our techniques, but we have large numbers of pathological controls. Again, plasmalogens are very highly concentrated in the brain, much more so than in other tissues (with the exception of erythrocytes), and it is conceivable that this could again be some pointer to why this disease has a special predeliction for the brain.

Dr. Austin: May I ask Dr. Dawson if included among your controls were other equally severe poliodystrophies, in which there is this same outstanding neuronal loss in the cortex.

Dr. Dawson: Probably nothing quite as dramatic as some of these Bielschowsky-Jansky's. For instance, in one case at autopsy it was almost impossible to find anything resembling an intact neuron. We've examined a whole range of lipid storage diseases for other reasons, and brains in similar states of demyelination. I think loss of ethanolamine plasmalogen has been reported in various dystrophies; in multiple sclerosis plaques particularly they are notoriously low. This could well be a nonspecific finding related to just the generally bad shape of the brain, but it might be something worth considering since the plasmalogens do have an extra double bond that isn't found in other phospholipids.

Dr. Hochstein: Perhaps I could add to that. We've found that in the red cells during the course of peroxidation one of the first phospholipids to be lost is phosphatidal ethanolamine.

Dr. Zeman: I can add that in the dogs with the neuronal ceroid-lipofuscinosis there is a marked diminution of phosphatidyl ethanolamine. With respect to the trisialogangliosides, I just wonder whether the following explanation could be considered. The distribution of this particular ganglioside is heavily slanted toward the periphery of the cell, especially the synaptic parts--the synaptic acceptor sites--and it is that part of the nerve cell which the histologists never see but in these diseases is most severely damaged, whereas the perikaryon which we look at in our histological preparation seems to be relatively well preserved. However, its content in trisialoganglioside, as per unit surface area, is small. In other words, what your data indicate is the tremendous retraction in surface area of the nerve cells in this disease. I might add to that, that this is associated with a staggering decrease in the concentration of γ-aminobutyric acid, which is also localized in the synaptosomes.[58] These findings could go hand in hand and, as you suggested, would indicate secondary phenomena of the disease. The phosphatidyl ethanolamine situation might be more specific in the respect that this compound is particularly easy prey to peroxidative mechanisms.

Dr. Hartroft: Has anybody measured cerebral prostaglandins in these cases?

Dr. Zeman: No, we've talked about that, though.

Dr. Philippart: Regarding the trialoganglioside I remember one case of Kufs disease in which we found indeed a rather low level, but there was a very striking high quantity of

the GD_1b the slower moving disialoganglioside. However, we
had a problem there because this is one of the species which
increases with age. Since we don't have many controls in
the 50-year old age group, I don't know the significance of
this finding. On the other hand, in Tay-Sachs disease, for
example, trisialoganglioside levels are very low too.

Dr. Dawson: I don't recall the exact quantitative figures.
Usually you have to put so much of the Tay-Sachs ganglioside
there.

Dr. Philippart: Yes, but we have calculated the absolute
amount and expressed it as a function of the dry weight or
fresh weight to confirm that it was actually decreased. Regarding the ethanolamines, we have occasionally found decreased
plasmalogen in the lipofuscinoses. However, studying red
cell lipids, which are probably one of the richest sources
of ethanolamine plasmalogen, we did not find anything abnormal
in families with different types of Batten's disease.[69] But
you may look in your cases and see; it would be interesting.

Dr. Dawson: You do find the ceramide trihexosides and
also globoside, which I think Suzuki and others have reported
in Tay-Sachs brain.[37 70 71] Again this seems to be a function
of the general disarray of the neurons in this disease, but
I think these secondary phenomena are interesting, since they
might give some reason for the neuron specific nature of this
disease.

Dr. Austin: I was wondering if Dr. Patel was going to
say something more about the vitamin B_{12} situation.

Dr. Patel: We don't have our own observation as to its
effect on the peroxidase per se, but there are reports in
the literature which indicate there is a four- to fivefold
increase in the peroxidase activity, measured in the submaxillary
gland and thyroid gland, both iodinating as well as when the
peroxidase activity was measured with guaiacol as hydrogen
donor, which of course would indicate that there is true peroxidase activation.

Dr. Zeman: How about diaminobenzidine?

Dr. Patel: No, they did not use diaminobenzidine.

Dr. Zeman: This would be crucial, I suppose.

Dr. Patel: Yes, it would be very crucial, of course,
but another thing is with experimentation with vitamin E,
which suppresses the peroxidase activity with all three hydrogen
donors we have measured, which includes dianisidine, p-phenylenediamine, and guaiacol, but suppression comes after about 10

300

days. In other words, there is transient activation or transient increase in activity in the first 10 days when you put normal individuals on vitamin E treatment. However, as you prolong the treatment--we have continued about 2 months--there is depression, close to 15-20% of the control (that is, previtamin treatment) activity. This may be due to the reduction in the peroxides in the system; this is speculation on my part.

Dr. Rider: If it didn't reduce the peroxide, then you'd have a detrimental effect if you were going to reduce the peroxidase.

Dr. Patel: That's exactly right.

Dr. Austin: What is the mechanism postulated by which the vitamin B_{12} increases the peroxidase?

Dr. Patel: I think it was de novo synthesis . This might be a very good thing to look at.

Dr. Austin: Whose studies were these?

Dr. Patel: They're from experimenters in the Department of Physiology at the Indian Institute of Experimental Medicine in Calcutta;[72] they have collaborated here also with Dr. Barker in the University of California at Berkeley. This should be an interesting study, I would think.

Dr. Zeman: What was the concentration of vitamin B_{12}?

Dr. Patel: It was physiological. They gave about 44 µg/kg body weight. They received vitamin B_{12} intravenously, which really is very promising.

Dr. Zeman: Over what period of time did those studies extend?

Dr. Patel: I think several weeks. I don't know the time exactly, but it's in terms of weeks.

Dr. Zeman: Of course, with many enzyme inducers we do see this effect, that the efficacy becomes less with time, and there is habituation. This is particularly true for alcohol oxidase, alcohol dehydrogenase, as shown by Krebs, and for a variety of other enzymes which are concerned with the metabolism of cytotoxic drugs.

Dr. Rider: I'd like to ask Dr. Armstrong and Dr. Austin what are you going to do next, in the sense of what are you going to pursue now?

Dr. Austin: I think the important thing to do at this

301

stage, Dr. Rider, is to have a period of incubation. Let
these ideas swirl around a bit and collide in new patterns.
At the end of that time I think one stands a chance of having
something come out of it that makes rational sense. I think
it's important to sort of let things simmer and float around
a little bit.

Dr. Zeman: I think we should ask Dr. Armstrong whether
he would welcome specimens from various patients and confirmed
heterozygotes. If yes, in which form should these be shipped
to him.

Dr. Armstrong: I'd like to have some referred to me
but at a later date; I'm loaded with work right at the moment,
but I would like to do some of those and see if we can transport
such specimens and still get valuable answers from the assay.
We've had some materials shipped to us and they appear to
be all right.

Dr. Zeman: How are they shipped, as a pellet or as a
suspension?

Dr. Armstrong: We've been shipping them as the final
purified pellet and then freezing it as the pellet, and then
shipping it down to our laboratory where we can just freeze
and thaw five more times, spin it down and get the supernatant,
then assay it.

Dr. Zeman: Would this require a known number of cells
per unit volume?

Dr. Armstrong: Yes. I ask that you count the number
of cells in there to begin with so I can adjust the assay;
also, send along a CBC.

Dr. Zeman: There is one more question. Is this enzyme
activity the same in lymphocytes and in polymorphonuclear
cells?

Dr. Armstrong: There is apparently no activity in lymphocytes; there is a small amount in monocytes, and there is
activity in eosinophils but it's a different kind of peroxidase;
the basophils have some, too.

Dr. Rider: This is in the polys?

Dr. Armstrong: Yes, this is all in the neutrophils.

Dr. Menkes: Is this enzyme from fibroblast cultures?

Dr. Armstrong: We looked at only one fibroblast culture;
it was a whole roller bottle on a cystinuric patient I think,

and we didn't get any activity even when using the entire bottle, but I don't know how many passages it had been through or anything else. I think that this needs to be looked at again, but it was the only one shot we had at it.

Dr. Zeman: Have you looked at amniotic cells and fetal tissue?

Dr. Armstrong: No. Amniotic fluid per se; if you just aspirate out some amniotic fluid and assay it, it has very good peroxidase, but we have not done the cells.

Dr. Zeman: Well, then, if you have good peroxidase in the amniotic fluid, maybe we don't need the cells.

Dr. Armstrong: That's right.

Dr. Zeman: How do you express the activity, as a function of protein concentration?

Dr. Armstrong: Yes, in specific activity.

Dr. Zeman: And how does it compare to the polymorphs?

Dr. Armstrong: It's a little lower; there's a lot of protein in the amniotic fluid, but in terms of raw activity it will give you optical densities in the range of 0.5-0.7, so it has a lot of activity.

Dr. Zeman: In other words, this would be a very simple procedure for the prenatal diagnosis on the fluid.

Dr. Armstrong: That's right. We don't do anything. We take 0.5 cc of amniotic fluid and just add it to the incubation mixture and go; there is no preparation or anything.

Dr. Zeman: Then you can start measuring at zero time. Have you seen a homozygous affected yet in the amniotic fluid?

Dr. Armstrong: No.

Dr. Zeman: I want to begin this summary by thanking the participants for having come to San Francisco, and for their important and certainly striking contributions. We have discussed here a relatively narrow aspect in the pathogenesis of neuronal ceroid-lipofuscinosis, namely, the causative aspects of the pathogenesis, and have expanded then on the conclusions which can be drawn from the work of Dr. Armstrong and his associates. The assumption that an important part in the pathogenesis of neuronal ceroid-lipofuscinosis is associated with an increased rate of peroxidative events has been materially strengthened by Dr. Armstrong's observations

of a deficiency of a peroxidase which, for want of anything
better, we have decided to call p-phenylenediamine (PPD) peroxidase, the natural substrate of which is not yet known.
This would then permit a number of conclusions and would explain
the obvious hereditary nature of these conditions as an expression of a gene for polypeptide deficiency whereby the
system of peroxidases would be deficient in one or perhaps
more of its isoenzymes or components. This observation itself
dictates the further approach we have to take in order to
elucidate the chemical pathogenesis of this disorder with
respect to the specific activity of this enzyme, on which
we can only speculate at the present time.

Here I feel that the suggestion made by Dr. O'Brien,
namely, that we have to expect to find a very specific peroxide
or hydroperoxide which this particular isozyme detoxifies,
is a most important consideration and is fully backed up by
the fact corroborated in his laboratory and in ours. Namely,
the seemingly more important and more generally active peroxidase
systems--such as catalase on the one hand, and glutathione
peroxidase on the other hand--are not only entirely normal
in the tissues of these patients and in their blood, but are
even increased--at least in men, and this increase may be
considered to be the result of an enzymatic derepression by
substrate accumulation. So what we are looking for now is
the specific biological substrate of Dr. Armstrong's peroxidase,
and we will have to leave it up to our biochemically oriented
enzymologists to devise the procedures and techniques to go
about this.

Hand in hand with this development, a number of therapeutic
possibilities have been discussed: enzyme replenishment or
substitution or, in view of the partial deficiency of this
enzyme, enzyme induction. The latter, a priori, would appear
to be the most promising, and there is ample evidence from
analogous situations that this may work. The other side of
the coin would be, as pointed out by Dr. Dawson, the reduction
in the concentration of the natural substrate for the deficient
enzyme; but inasmuch as we do not know the substrate, there
is nothing specific we can do. Therefore, the "shotgun" approach
at the present time still seems to have some conceptual support.

Probably the most fascinating thoughts which spring from
this remarkable discovery, and which Dr. Hochstein has been
pointing out so succinctly, are the possible implications
for the problem of physiological peroxidation and certain
phenomena of aging and involution. In this respect it is
perhaps fitting to take a somewhat broader view of the entire
problem. It was pointed out by Dr. Hochstein that it is a
remarkable feature that organisms have developed which depend
on unsaturated fatty acids on the one hand, and on oxygen

on the other, and yet these two compounds together are almost incompatible with each other. The wisdom of this evolutionary process is not quite apparent to my feeble mind at the present time, but I'm sure that it will give rise to some learned discussions and reflections. I think we have made considerable progress, and I ask your indulgence that I look back some 5 years ago when we started these discussions when we were faced with a great problem, but we really could not ask pertinent and intelligent questions because we did not have he necessary data. We have come a long way, and I still remember when Dr. Hartroft first tried to point out the problem. He made a sweeping gesture to the wall and said, "Here is your problem on the wall--it's paint." What you are faced with here is the problem as to how paint is generated in cells and how paint is removed from cells. Well, we have come a long way and now we know how paint is being produced in cells, and how paint is being produced in the cells of patients with neuronal ceroid-lipofuscinoses. It has boiled down to what appears to be a relatively simple defect of an enzyme.

We do not know whether it is a deficiency of a protein or whether it is a defectively constructed protein.

These are questions which will eventually be resolved and will at the same time open up entirely new vistas with respect to the biological activity of various peroxidases.

The observations of Dr. Armstrong have now made not only a dent but a big crack in the concept of myeloperoxidases as we find it in the literature, and I'm personally grateful to all of you for having been re-educated in this respect and been helped to overcome many prejudices.

I think we can now look forward to a period of solidification of ideas and concepts into a more directional approach, which should lead to faster progress than was hitherto possible because we now have available a testable hypothesis.

REFERENCES

1. Tappel, A. L. Lipid peroxidation and fluorescent mole-
    cular damage to membranes. In: Pathological Aspects of
    Cell Membranes, B. F. Trump and A. Arstila, Eds., Vol.1,
    Academic Press, New York, in press.

2. Zeman, W. Presidential Address: Studies in the neuronal
    ceroid-lipofuscinoses. J. Neuropathol. exp. Neurol., 33,
    1-12 (1974).

3. Armstrong, D., S. Dimmit, L. Grider, D. E. VanWormer, and
    J. H. Austin. Leukocytic peroxidase deficiency of homo-
    zygotes and heterozygotes with Batten's disease. Trans.
    Amer. Soc. Neurochem., 4, 89 (1973).

4. Hartroft, W. S., and E. A. Porta. Ceroid. Amer. J. Med.
    Sci., 250, 324-345 (1965).

5. Hagberg, B., P. Sourander, and L. Svennerholm. Late
    infantile progressive encephalopathy with distrubed poly-
    unsaturated fat metabolism. Acta Paediat. Scand., 57,
    495-499 (1968).

6. Svennerholm, L. Personal communication.

7. Hochstein, P., and L. Ernster. Microsomal peroxidation
    of lipids and its possible role in cellular injury.
    Ciba Foundation Symposium on Cellular Injury, 123-
    134 (1964).

8. Gonatas, N. K., R. D. Terry, R. Winkler, S. R. Korey,
    C. J. Gomez, and A. Stein. A case of juvenile
    lipidosis: the significance of electron microscopic
    and biochemical observations of a cerebral biopsy.
    J. Neuropathol. exp. Neurol., 22, 557-580 (1963).

9. Hartroft, W. S. Personal communication.

10. Cohen, G., and P. Hochstein. Glutathione Peroxidase:
    The major pathway of peroxide destruction in erythro-
    cytes. Biochem., 2, 1420-1428 (1963).

11. Stossel, T. P. Phagocytosis. N. Engl. J. Med., 290,
    774-780 (1974).

12. Pritchard, E. T., and H. Singh. Lipid peroxidation in tissues of vitamin E deficient rats. Biochem. Biophys. Res. Commun., 2, 184-188 (1960).

13. Hartroft, W. S. In vitro and in vivo production of a ceroidlike substance from erythrocytes and certain lipids. Science, 113, 673-676 (1951).

14. Casselman, W. G. B. The in vitro preparation and histochemical properties J. Exptl. Med., 94, 549-562 (1951).

15. Casselman, W. G. B. Factors influencing the formation of ceroid in the livers of choline-deficient rats. I. Dietary fats. Biochim. Biophys. Acta, 11, 445-446 (1953).

16. Casselman, W. G. B. Factors influencing the formation of ceroid in the livers of choline-deficient rats. II. Dietary antioxidants. Biochim. Biophys. Acta, 11, 446-447 (1953).

17. Porta, E. A., and W. S. Hartroft. In: Pigments in Pathology, M. Wolman, Ed., Academic Press, New York, 1969, 123-154.

18. Suzuki, Y., and H. Suzuki. Partial deficiency of hexosaminidase component A in juvenile GM_2-gangliosidosis. Neurol., 20, 848-851 (1970).

19. Okada, S., M. L. Veath, and J. S. O'Brien. Juvenile GM_2 gangliosidosis: partial deficiency of hexosaminidase A. J. Pediat., 77, 1063-1065 (1970).

20. Philippart, M. [14]C incorporation into brain explants from lipofuscinosis and sulfatidosis. In: Proceedings 3rd International Meeting of the International Society for Neurochemistry, Budapest 1971, J. Domonkos et al., Eds., Akademia Kiado, Budapest, 1971, p. 343.

21. Paoletti, R., and C. Galli. Effects of essential fatty acid deficiency on the central nervous system in the growing rat. In: Lipids, Malnutrition, and the Developing Brain, K. Elliott and J. Knight, Eds., Elsevier, New York, 1972, 121-132.

22. Svennerholm, L., C. Alling, A. Bruce, I. Karlsson, and O. Sapia. Effects on offspring of maternal malnutrition in the rat. In: Lipids, Malnutrition, and the Developing Brain, K. Elliott and J. Knight, Eds., Elsevier, New York, 1972, 141-152.

23. Hartroft, W. S., and J. H. Ridout. Pathogenesis of the cirrhosis produced by choline deficiency. Escape of lipid from fatty hepatic cysts into the biliary and vascular systems. Amer. J. Pathol., 27, 951-989 (1951).

24. Hartroft, W. S., In: Liver Injury, Hoffbauer, Ed., 1950, 109-150.

25. Hartroft, W. S., and E. A. Porta. Unpublished data, 1960.

26. Kristensson, K., S. Rayner, and P. Sourander. Visceral involvement in juvenile amaurotic idiocy. Acta Neuropathol., 4, 421-424 (1965).

27. Porta, E. A., and W. S. Hartroft. Early deposition of ceroid in Kupffer cells of mice fed hepatic necrogenic diets. Can. Med. Assoc. J., 88, 1167-1169 (1963).

28. Hagberg, B., P. Sourander, and L. Svennerholm. Late infantile progressive encephalopathy with disturbed polyunsaturated fat metabolism. Acta Paediat. Scand., 57, 495-499 (1968).

29. Yavin, E., and J. H. Menkes. The culture of dissociated cells from rat cerebral cortex. J. Cell Biol., 57, 232-237 (1973).

30. Menkes, J. H., D. R. Harris, and N. Stein. Biochemical studies on brain explants and fibroblast cultures in Batten's disease. In: Sphingolipids, Sphingolipidoses, and Allied Disorders, B. W. Volk and S. M. Aronson, Eds., Plenum Press, New York, 1972, 549-560.

31. Yavin, E., and J. H. Menkes. Polyenoic acid metabolism in cultured dissociated brain cells. J. Lipid. Res., 15, 152-157 (1974).

32. Yavin, E., and J. H. Menkes. Effect of temperature on fatty acid metabolism in dissociated cell cultures of developing brain. Pediat. Res., 8, 263-269 (1974).

33. Tappel, A. L., B. Fletcher and D. Deamer. Effect of antioxidants on lipid peroxidation fluorescent products and aging parameters in the mouse. J. of Gerontology, 28, 415-424 (1973).

34. Bailey, J. M., and L. M. Dunbar. Essential fatty acid requirements of cells in tissue culture: a review. Exptl. Molec. Pathol., 18, 142-161 (1973).

35. Armstrong, D., S. Dimmit, and D. W. VanWormer. Studies in Batten's disease. 1. Peroxidase deficiency in granulocytes. Arch. Neurol., $\underline{30}$, 144-152 (1974).

36. Baudhuin, P., H. Beaufay, and C. de Duve. Combined biochemical and morphological study of particulate fractions from rat liver. Analysis of preparations enriched in lysosomes or in particles containing urate oxidase, amino acid oxidase, and catalase. J. Cell Biol., $\underline{26}$, 219-243 (1965).

37. Lenn, J. J. and G. Dawson. On the significance of curvilinear bodies in late infantile lipidosis. Amer. J. Ment. Defic., $\underline{77}$, 597-606 (1973).

38. Patel, V. Unpublished data.

39. Müller, M. Biochemical cytology of trichomonal flagellates. J. Cell. Biol. $\underline{57}$, 453-474 (1973).

40. De Duve, C., and P. Baudhuin. Peroxisomes (microbodies and related particles). Physiol. Rev., $\underline{46}$, 323-357 (1966).

41. Hruban, Z., and M. Rechcigl, Jr. Microbodies and Related Particles, Academic Press, New York, 1969.

42. Zeman, W. Historical development of the nosological concept of amaurotic familial idoiocy. In: Handbook of Clinical Neurology, Vol. 10, P. J. Vinken and G. W. Bruyn, Eds., North-Holland, Amsterdam, 1970, 212-232.

43. Batten, F. E. Family cerebral degeneration with macular change (so-called juvenile form of family amaurotic idiocy). Quart. J. Med., $\underline{7}$, 444-454 (1914).

44. Siakotos, A. N., H. H. Goebel, V. Patel, I. Watanabe, and W. Zeman. The morphogenesis and biochemical characterization of ceroid isolated from cases of neuronal ceroid-lipofuscinosis. In: Sphingolipids, Sphingolipidoses, and Allied Disorders, B. W. Volk and S. M. Aronson, Eds., Plenum Press, New York, 1972, 53-61.

45. Zeman, W. Proceedings of the 2nd Conference on the Clinical Delineation of Birth Defects. In: Part IV, Nervous System, Vol. VII, Williams and Wilkins, Baltimore, 1971, 23-30.

46. Boehme, D. H., J. C. Cottrell, S. C. Leonberg, and W. Zeman.

A dominant form of neuronal ceroid-lipofuscinosis. Brain, <u>94</u>, 745-760 (1971).

47. Jansky, J. Sur un cas jusqu'à présente non décrit de l'idiotie amaurotique familiare compliquée par une hypoplasie du cervelet. Sborna. lék. <u>13</u>, 165-196 (1908).

48. Bielschowsky, M. Über spät-infantile familiäre amaurotische idiotie mit kleinhirn-symptomen. Dtsch. Z. Nervenheilk. <u>50</u>, 7-29 (1913).

49. Sjögren, T. Die juvenile amaurotische idiotie. Klinische und erblichkeitsmedizinische untersuchungen. Hereditas (Lund) <u>14</u>, 197-426 (1931).

50. Karnovsky, M. Personal communication.

51. Dawson, G., R. Matalon, and Y. T. Li. Correction of the enzymic defect in cultured fibroblasts from patients with Fabry's disease: treatment with purified α-galactosidase from Ficin. Pediat. Res., <u>7</u>, 684-690 (1973).

52. Philippart, M. Fabry disease: kidney transplantation as an enzyme replacement technique. Birth Defects, <u>9</u>, 81-87 (1973).

53. Clarke, J. T. R., R. D. Guttmann, L. S. Wolfe, J. G. Beaudoin, and D. D. Morehouse. Enzyme replacement therapy by renal allotransplantation in Fabry's disease. N. Engl. J. Med., <u>287</u>, 1215-1218 (1973).

54. Desnick, R. J., K. Y. Allen, R. L. Simmons, J. E. Woods, C. F. Anderson, J. S. Najarian, and W. Krivit. Treatment of Fabry's disease: correction of the enzymatic deficiency by renal transplantation. J. Lab. Clin. Med., <u>78</u>, 989-990 (1971).

55. DiFerrante, N., B. L. Nichols, P. V. Donnelly, G. Neri, R. Hrgovcic, and R. K. Berglund. Induced degradation of glycosaminoglycans in Hurler's and Hunter's syndromes by plasma infusion. Proc. Nat. Acad. Sci. U.S., <u>68</u>, 303-307 (1971).

56. Erickson, R. P., R. Sandman, W. v. B. Robertson, and C. J. Epstein. Inefficacy of fresh frozen plasma therapy of mucopolysaccharidosis. II. Pediatrics, <u>50</u>, 693-701 (1972).

57. Little, C., R. Olmescu, K. G. Reid, and P. J. O'Brien. Properties and regulation of glutathione peroxidase. J. Biol. Chem., <u>245</u>, 3632-3636 (1970).

58. Zeman, W. The neuronal ceroid-lipofuscinoses. Batten-Vogt syndrome: a model for human aging? Adv. Geront. Res., 3, 147-170 (1971).

59. Burr, G. O., and M. M. Burr. A new deficiency disease produced by the rigid exclusion of fat from the diet. J. Biol. Chem., 82, 345-367 (1929).

60. Holman, R. T. Essential fatty acid deficiency. Progress in the Chemistry of Fats and Other Lipids, Vol. 9, 1968, 279-348.

61. Anonymous. Rat brain fatty acids in essential fatty acid deficiency. Nutrit. Revs., 30, 18-21 (1972).

62. White, H. B., M. D. Turner, and R. C. Miller. In: Society for Neuroscience, 3rd Annual Meeting, San Diego, 1973, 426.

63. Crawford, M. A., C. A. Lloyd, and L. V. Springett. Dietary alterations in polyunsaturated fatty acids in guinea-pig brain, liver and muscle. Biochem. J., 122, 11P (1971).

64. Paulsrud, J. R., L. Pensler, C. F. Whitten, S. Stewart, and R. T. Holman. Essential fatty acid deficiency in infants induced by fat-free intravenous feeding. Amer. J. Clin. Nutrit., 25, 897-904 (1972).

65. Collins, F. D., A. J. Sinclair, J. P. Royle, D. A. Coats, A. T. Maynard, and R. F. Leonard. Plasma lipids in human linoleic acid deficiency. Nutrit. Metabol., 13, 150-167 (1971).

66. Merril, C. R., M. R. Geier, and J. C. Petricciani. Bacterial virus gene expression in human cells. Nature, 233, 398-400 (1971).

67. Rogers, S., A. Lowenthal, H. G. Terheggen, and J. P. Columbo. Induction of arginase activity with the Shope papilloma virus in tissue culture cells from an argininemic patient. J. Exptl. Med., 137, 1091-1096 (1973).

68. Dawson, G., and N. J. Lenn. Lipid abnormalities in four cases of late infantile cerebroretinal degeneration with multilamellar cytosomes. Trans. Amer. Soc. Neurochem., 2, 66c (1971).

69. Philippart, M. Unpublished data.

70. Suzuki, K., and G. C. Chen. Brain ceramide hexosides

in Tay-Sachs disease and generalized gangliosidosis
(GM_1-gangliosidosis). J. Lipid Res., **8**, 105-113 (1967).

71. Dawson, G. Glycosphingolipid levels in an unusual neuro-
visceral storage disease characterized by lactosyl-
ceramide galactosyl hydrolase deficiency: lactosylcera-
midosis. J. Lipid Res., **13**, 207-219 (1972).

72. Banerjee, R. K., and A. G. Datta. Effect of cobalt and
vitamin B   on the peroxidase and iodinating activity
of mouse thyroid and submaxillary gland: in vitro
stimulation of vitamin B   coenzyme on the iodination
of tyrosine. Endocrinology, **88**, 1456-1464 (1971).

PARTICIPANTS
SIXTH ROUND TABLE CONFERENCE ON BATTEN'S DISEASE
SAN FRANCISCO, CALIFORNIA
February 22-23, 1975

Donald Armstrong, Ph.D.
Department of Neurology
University of Colorado
Denver, Colorado

Glyn Dawson, Ph.D.
Department of Pediatrics
University of Chicago
Chicago, Illinois

Irwin Fridovich, Ph.D.
Department of Biochemistry
Duke University Medical Center
Durham, North Carolina

W. Stanley Hartroft, M.D., Ph.D.
Department of Pathology
University of Hawaii
Honolulu, Hawaii

Paul Hochstein, Ph.D.
Department of Pharmacology
University of Southern California School
  of Medicine
Los Angeles, California

William G. Hoekstra, Ph.D.
Department of Biochemistry
University of Wisconsin
Madison, Wisconsin

John H. Menkes, M.D.
Department of Pediatrics
University of California
Los Angeles, California

Jaime Miquel, Ph.D.
Experimental Pathology Branch
NASA, Ames Research Center
Moffett Field, California

313

Lester Packer, Ph.D.
Department of Physiology
University of California
Berkeley, California

Vimal Patel, Ph.D.
Department of Pathology
Indiana University School of Medicine
Indianapolis, Indiana

Michel Philippart, M.D.
Department of Pediatrics
University of California
Los Angeles, California

Anver Rahimtula, Ph.D.
Department of Biochemistry
Memorial University of Newfoundland
St. Johns, Newfoundland, Canada

J. Alfred Rider, M.D., Ph.D.
Children's Brain Diseases Foundation
Franklin Hospital
San Francisco, California

George Rouser, Ph.D.
Section of Lipid Research
City of Hope Medical Center
Duarte, California

Gregory R. Schonbaum, Ph.D.
Department of Biochemistry
St. Jude Children's Research Hospital
Memphis, Tennessee

Frank Yatsu, M.D.
Department of Neurology
University of California
San Francisco, California

Wolfgang Zeman, M.D.
Department of Pathology
University of Indiana School of Medicine
Indianapolis, Indiana

SIXTH ROUND TABLE CONFERENCE ON BATTEN'S DISEASE

Dr. Zeman: At the occasion of the last conference, all of us were quite elated about the findings of Dr. Armstrong, namely that in Batten's disease, there is a reproducible deficiency of a peroxidase which for want of anything better we have termed p-phenylenediamine-mediated peroxidase. This enzyme was measured in leukocytes of patients and adequate controls and was found to be severely depressed in activity to approximately 8-12% of normal controls. At that time it seemed that this might be a genetically controlled enzyme deficiency and that whatever residual enzyme was present was not sufficiently active to prevent the peroxidation or to detoxify a specific peroxide. So it appeared that the biochemical pathology of this group of diseases, which we rather generously call Batten's disease, would be fully satisfied, namely that there is a continuous high rate of peroxidation, not only of the specific peroxide but also, by way of a chain reaction, of other cellular components, in particular, subcellular organellar membrane systems. Such a process would lead to the continuous accumulation of lipid polymers, of cross-linked proteins and of acidic polymerized lipid substances which then eventually become incorporated into tertiary lysosomes and distort the geometry of the cells. At that time it was already known that the enzyme defect did not exactly behave as the textbooks tell us, that is to say when we tested ascertained heterozygotes such as biological mothers of patients, they would not in all instances show dosage compensation for the activity of this particular enzyme. More disturbingly, it was found that the enzyme was also deficient in various forms of Batten's disease which for very good reasons we believe may be genetically heterogeneous. On account of these observations which have been subsequently extended to include the same enzyme defect in a highly inbred strain of English Setters and also in a dominantly inherited adult form of Batten's disease, it was obvious that further studies must be undertaken in order to clarify the nature of the deficiency of PPD- or p-phenylenediamine-mediated peroxidase. What was proposed was that perhaps one or two isozymes of this particular peroxidase system may be deficient or actually absent. The possibility was raised as to whether a modifier gene was required in order to explain the onset of the disease at widely differing ages, ranging from infancy to late adulthood. Therefore we have come together here in order to further discuss

315

the implications of these various findings with the hope to
develop testable hypotheses and to forge ahead with our quest
for a complete elucidation of the chemical and genetic pathogenesis of this group of diseases. What we hope to achieve
today and tomorrow is essentially to reconcile current available
information with current concepts of the mechanisms by which
a genetically controlled defect expresses itself in the parameters that we have established for this particular group
of diseases.

Last time, Dr. Armstrong not only reported his very
fascinating data to us, but he also indicated certain prospective
studies which may enable us to come somewhat closer to grips
with the conceptualization of this particular enzyme defect.
There are in particular two studies which I have in mind:
a further refinement and perhaps sophistication of the isozyme
determinations and a series of hybridization experiments utilizing deficient enzyme preparations from patients who clearly
suffer from different forms of Batten's disease, such as for
instance the dominantly inherited form and a recessively inherited type.

Dr. Armstrong: Our data obtained since last year's meeting has indicated that the usual soluble peroxidase enzyme
that we have measured in the past is deficient and continues
to decline as the disease progresses. At the same time, we
have noted that an insoluble peroxidase fraction subsequently
increases, as the disease progresses, so that it appears at
this point there is some sort of shift from the normal soluble
peroxidase fraction to some bound or insoluble enzyme fraction.
In addition to that, we have some preliminary data now on
the isoenzyme separation of leukocyte peroxidase in a soluble
fraction, and I would like to ask my collaborator Dr. Reigh
to comment on our findings.

Dr. Reigh: If a deficiency of peroxidase exists as such,
we were interested in the mechanism responsible for it and
wondered whether it could be attributed to some isozyme deficiency. Accordingly we began to try to separate leukocyte
isoperoxidases and the slides summarize some of the findings
for white cells. The bands shown for white cells were obtained
from white cells prepared from blood bank blood. These cells
demonstrated as many as 6 isozymes and this inconsistency
is typical for blood bank type preparations. White cells
from Batten's patients seem to show all the isozymes present
as in the normal controls, but it appears that in each case
the isozymes are diminished. It takes a lot of white cells
to do these separations, about 45,000,000 cells, a problem
which has prevented our performing more extensive and a larger
number of experiments.

Dr. Zeman: Dr. Reigh, could you perhaps interpret the

316

slide for us because I don't think everybody is familiar with microelectrophoresis. First of all, is that in agar gel?

Dr. Reigh: This is polyacrylamide.

Dr. Zeman: Polyacrylamide. And then, how many different bands can you distinguish in your control preparations, in comparison to the preparation from the Batten's patient?

Dr. Reigh: Well, there are at least four bands in the control. With the initial staining you see that there are two bands present in the top group, and there are also two bands in the lower area. In the Batten's patient there also appear to be four bands, two toward the top and then you see two at the bottom. The Rf values do not exactly correspond with those of the normal controls. However, it is very possible that this is an artifact due to the curving effect of the migratory front. At this time we believe that these bands are probably the same, but in the Batten's patient you have a decreased amount of each isozyme. No particular isozyme is missing.

Dr. Zeman: In other words, the original notion of yours, Dr. Armstrong, that there might be some isozymes missing is not substantiated by the more recent studies.

Dr. Armstrong: We looked at those initial ones last year. They were done on cellulose acetate, and we didn't have enough cells on them, I don't think. We have been able to put more cells on now, so that the bands we didn't see last year are really there.

Dr. Hoekstra: I'd like to ask whether you have looked at the effects of reducing agents, particularly sulfhydryl compounds such as mercaptoethanol and cysteine--whether this causes any change in these isozymes?

Dr. Reigh: Well, mercaptoethanol and cysteine tend to be inhibitors of peroxidases and they would inhibit the staining, but I haven't looked at that.

Dr. Rouser: Now, it seems to be that central to your thesis, the slide actually shows different, that the bands don't match. Now, your interpretation was that had you applied the normal control in the well where you have your Batten's preparation now, it would have given the same result.

Dr. Reigh: What do you mean? Why the bands didn't exactly correspond?

Dr. Rouser: Yes.

317

Dr. Reigh: Sometimes the migrating front is curved, so that the outside preparations seem to run slower.

Dr. Rouser: Alright, so you have put them in different positions, and they do match up.

Dr. Reigh: I haven't done that because like I say you have to get 45 million cells from a kid, and he doesn't go along with it. Next time I get enough cells to run I'll put it in the center well so that you won't get that effect.

Dr. Rouser: Well, I think you really should do that because that is very central to the thesis here, because it may still be possible that you have different isoenzymes, and that would go along with your original idea.

Dr. Armstrong: The sensitivity in the assay is a problem that we face.

Dr. Hochstein: If I understood Dr. Armstrong correctly, what we are now talking about is not a deficiency of peroxidase but rather an altered distribution of the peroxidase from soluble to particular fractions of the cell, and in that case isn't it rather important to look at the particular isozymes before one makes any conclusions about what's deficient?

Dr. Reigh: At least in the soluble fraction we see a deficiency revealed by the gels. Solubilizing the enzyme in the membrane fraction is a big problem. You can assay it simply by taking the pellet and putting it into an assay system and measuring the activity obtained from the membrane-bound fraction, but solubilizing the enzyme for electrophoresis is very difficult. EDTA does not work. Sodium dodecyl sulfate, sodium deoxycholate--any of these solubilizing agents aren't particularly good for freeing the enzyme. It stays bound to the membranes even under sonication--you get a large amount left stuck to membranes.

Dr. Rouser: Have you tried potassium chloride--you know, ionic, just straight ionic dissociation (SIS).

Dr. Reigh: No, I haven't done that. I have considered it.

Dr. Rouser: Well, if you utilize SIS, etc., you're breaking apart the so-called intrinsic protein and not necessarily removing the extrinsic, which your enzyme might very well be. Therefore, high or low salt would be the way to do, but I'd like to add one other thing that I think is of outstanding importance here. You see, one thing you have to decide on when you show this change in your patient, you really should know what the change with age is in the normal population.

The question being then, is this one of those programmed enzymes that normally goes down with age?

Dr. Armstrong: The normal curve, I said, represented patients from a couple of years of age up to 50 or 60.

Dr. Rouser: You can't group them in any way according to age.

Dr. Armstrong: No, there's overlap.

Dr. Rouser: That's the problem: the normal range is so broad, but if in fact you do plot activity as a function of age and accept this broad range, you will see that there is a change with age, just the lowest part of the high end may match the low end, but still you can show change with age.

Dr. Zeman: It appears that the concept of the peroxidase deficiency has been subject to a major change of direction and I think it cannot be taken lightly in view of Dr. Armstrong's report and certainly of what Dr. Hochstein has just pointed out, namely that total enzyme activity may not change at all, but what changes is the physicochemical behavior of the enzyme and under those circumstances I believe we should now hear from Dr. Schonbaum, relative to his concern about the validity of this particular assay.

Dr. Schonbaum: Enlarging on some of the remarks that have been made before, let me ask a simple question. I understand that the deficiency is apparent only in the p-phenylene-diamine assay but not with dianisidine or guaiacol.

Dr. Reigh: No, recently I've used guaiacol and demonstrated the deficiency also, in one case. I just started using guaiacol.

Dr. Schonbaum: Well, that would seem to be a rather crucial point because my remarks before were simply addressed in reference to the so-called specificity of peroxidases and I believe there would not be any difference in phenaromatic amines, particularly if you take something like 3'3'-diamino-benzidine or p-phenylenediamine. Now, of course, if there is a parallelism between the deficiency as measured via one assay and another one, this situation is entirely different. The crucial question is that: is there or is there not dif-ferentiation in apparent activities by using different sub-strates. In this respect also, I would like to address perhaps a question to Dr. Zeman, because I believe that in the setters, there was again a difference between so-called typical substrates of peroxidase and p-phenylenediamine. The explanation which would be very plausible is the total peroxidase remains constant, but the insoluble fraction is different in normal and diseased individuals. This does not seem to hold, if differentiation between substrates is not obtained. Dr. Patel, you have had considerable experience with various hydrogen donors.

Dr. Patel: Well. to date, we tested three different hydrogen donor substrates which include guaiacol, diaminobenzidine, and p-phenylenediamine. As we indicated in our report, we haven't really observed the deficiency with guaiacol in the soluble enzyme fraction. That is, we haven't looked at the insoluble, which was just described by Dr. Armstrong, so at this point I could only say that the deficiency in the English Setters can be demonstrated with p-phenylenediamine, only, whatever that means, I could not really explain.

Dr. Dawson: Initially it looked quite striking. With o-dianisidine, the activity in human patients was completely normal, in fact greater than normal. With p-phenylenediamine there was quite a marked deficiency. Unfortunately, we haven't pursued this with other patients, but now I am sort of intrigued by Dr. Armstrong; if I get you right, you assay the 10,000g pellet from these patients and they have completely normal activity.

Dr. Armstrong: They had a greater than normal activity. I reported the percentages. The normal individual has 87% soluble and a 13% insoluble activity and it is 25% and 75% for the Batten's patients, or something like that.

Dr. Hochstein: I wonder if someone could comment on the relationship between the peroxidase that is being described and the well known myeloperoxidase of white cells. There are individuals known who are deficient in myeloperoxidase and these individuals have a very severe disease characterized by inability to destroy bacteria. They have chronic infections. That enzyme is assayable by guaiacol and a variety of hydrogen donors. This enzyme, whose distribution is changed--I am not even going to talk about deficient enzyme anymore--is this related in some way to myeloperoxidase, is there some information at all? Do these children for example, have problems with infections? Do the English Setters have problems with infections?

Dr. Zeman: I can only answer Dr. Hochstein with respect to the incidence of infection. We have not observed a higher frequency of infections in human patients nor in the dogs and I am not aware of any literature reports which would indicate, either directly or indirectly, that there is a deficient myeloperoxidase in patients with Batten's disease or in the dogs with a similar condition. Does anyone have any remarks as to the myeloperoxidase situation?

Dr. Philippart: Well, I think the observation that the soluble activity decreases during the course of the disease, is a very interesting one. It suggests that the enzyme may actually be trapped like lipids in the pigments that accumulate which might be the first site to look at for these enzymes. I wonder if there is any suitable histochemical technique to search for peroxidase, perhaps with p-phenylenediamine or whatever substrate it takes, especially in the regions with accumulation of pigment.

Dr. Zeman: I have no data which would answer your question. Does anyone have any observations along those lines?

Dr. Rouser: I just want to make an obvious suggestion. Certainly what Dr. Philippart says is one of the things you should do, that is, find out if this phenomenon is some kind of a storage thing. In other words, it could be that in the course of the disease, with all this cross-linking that we assume to be going on, that the soluble enzyme which must really do its thing in the soluble phase, is becoming attached more and more to membranes, where, being removed from its true site of action, it is just less efficient, although in vitro, the activity might be measured as normal.

Dr. Zeman: Would you expect that if an enzyme becomes cross-linked by malonaldehyde or other carbonyls, that it would lose its activity?

Dr. Rouser: No, there are quite a number of enzymes that do not, particularly if it is done with glutaraldehyde and certain other aldehydes. This is one of the things that Sjöstrand has been studying.

Dr. Hoekstra: This brings up the point I was going to make, which has perhaps already been discussed. Rather than being the cause of the disease, couldn't the decreased PPD-peroxidase activity be the result of the disease and might not the insoluble form be partially oxidized, disulfide-bridged, perhaps to cell particulates or aggregated, but still carrying enzymatic activity?

Dr. Hochstein: Sure. Along those lines, if I understood your slides correctly, Dr. Armstrong, you said the thyroid peroxidase was also diminished in activity, so that perhaps the soluble enzyme becomes fixed. The patients who have this disease, are they hypothyroid?

Dr. Zeman: No, they are not hypothyroid; however it is true that the thyroid, together with brain and testes, shows the highest degree of accumulation of autofluorescent lipopigments or cross-linked polymers.

Dr. Rouser: In line with the suggestion that this might be just a part of a major picture, not necessarily the cause, it seems to me that by determining other soluble enzymes you could gain some valuable information on that point. Because if it is a rather nonspecific linkage effect, perhaps other soluble enzymes could be subject to a similar process.

Dr. Zeman: I think this is certainly logical reasoning. Now, as I understand it, glutathione peroxidase is a soluble enzyme and we have reports from several independent laboratories that glutathione peroxidase is not reduced in this particular disease, neither in tissue such as brain, nor in leukocytes. Likewise, so-called true peroxidase and catalase are normal, and perhaps sometimes increased in these patients. This was reported by Dr. O'Brien. Dr. Patel found it in the dogs, and if I am not mistaken, Dr. Armstrong looked at these systems too.

Dr. Philippart: I have looked at acid hydrolyases but these enzymes don't have many sulfhydryl bridges, so they wouldn't very likely be involved, but it might be very interesting just to try to use a normal leukocyte extract and let it set with increasing amounts of peroxide for an increasing amount of time and see if this is one way to make it insoluble.

Dr. Zeman: This is a good suggestion.

Dr. Armstrong: Pursuing this line of thinking in a rather non-specific way, and referring to the proceedings of the previous conference, where it was suggested that a change in carbohydrate metabolism might easily do the job, I just would point out that perhaps some glycolytic enzymes are being attached to membranes thus losing their normal sequence, in which they behave properly.

Dr. Hoekstra: Could I make one more point on this assay. I am not an expert on peroxidase assays, but as I studied some of the material sent, I went back to the older literature of Chance on assaying peroxidase, horseradish peroxidase, etc. and I found that the rate that you measure depends on the rate of combination or reaction of the peroxide with the enzyme in some cases, the so-called K1, and in other cases it depends on the final reaction of the enzyme complex with the hydrogen donor, the so-called K4. You can measure K1 or K4 with the same substrate, hydrogen peroxide plus specific hydrogen donors, by changing the relative concentrations, and absolute concentrations of the hydrogen donor and the hydrogen peroxide. Now if, as a result of peroxidation or increased oxidants in the cell, you would partially denature or damage the myeloperoxidase such that you might change the reaction rate between peroxide and the enzyme, you may pick up an entirely different result, depending on the rate of reaction with a particular hydrogen donor. Now what I am asking is: has anybody got a good kinetic study with both guaiacol and p-phenylenediamine, varying the hydrogen donor concentration over a very wide range, to know whether there is a specific difference here or is it just a matter of the concentration of the substrates used?

Dr. Zeman: Dr. Armstrong, would you like to address yourself to that question?

Dr. Armstrong: I thought you could answer that.

Dr. Zeman: Then I will ask Dr. Patel, he has done something along those lines.

Dr. Patel: We have changed hydrogen peroxide concentrations, keeping constant the p-phenylenediamine. As you can see, in the diseased animal, the inhibitory effect of peroxide is marked. The percentage inhibition of peroxidase activity is much more prominent in the diseased than in controls. I must admit that this was not intended to be a kinetic but just a comparative study, so I really couldn't comment on whether this was due to compound II or compound I.

Dr. Hoekstra: I believe that as you increase the hydrogen peroxide concentration you would tend to more nearly measure the K1.

Dr. Patel: That is probably true.

Dr. Hoekstra: I think it would be necessary to vary both the concentrations of the peroxide and of the hydrogen donor over a wide range.

Dr. Patel: We have done that to find out the optimum activity, keeping constant the leukocyte peroxidase concentration in extracts from normal individuals, just to find out how much p-phenylenediamine would give the maximum optical density change.

Dr. Hoekstra: Do you have any data on the concentration of the hydrogen donor you have examined?

Dr. Patel: I don't, but it is obvious that if you dissolve the maximum amount in your medium, you get maximum optical density change. You really have to compromise on the solubility of p-phenylenediamine in order to get the optical density change you really want. The procedure Lück has described, we want to stick to, because of its diagnostic value, so we kept everything constant in a comparative sense.

Dr. Schonbaum: Following Dr. Hoekstra's remark, perhaps
I can enlarge a little bit on it. The rate limiting step
in most peroxidase reactions, particularly those measured
by Chance, was the reduction of compound II by the donor and,
at least for plant peroxidases, the rate constants are generally
in the order of about 10^5, that means about 10 times lower
than reduction of compound I to compound II. That simply
means that, providing the donor concentration is high enough,
let's take for example something like millimolar concentration,
and assuming a rate constant in the order of about 10^5, you
have a pseudofirst order constant of around $10^{-2} sec^{-1}$.
Now, since the combination of enzyme with the peroxide very
rarely would exceed $10^7 M^{-1} sec^{-1}$ and using 10^{-3} molar hydrogen
peroxide, it would give you a pseudofirst order of about 10^4
sec^{-1}. That means, I should have remarked before, that you
will not be measuring the rate of combination of enzyme with
the peroxide, but rather its reduction. Well I don't know
what the rate constants are for myeloperoxidase or any other
type of peroxidase you have here, and therefore the kinetic
discussion is very difficult to put in concrete terms without
having those studies. I would imagine that variations of
the donors would be an important parameter in those studies--
variations in concentration. It still brings me to the original
question. I still cannot readily reconcile in my own mind,
that if there was a limitation of this sort, then we must
necessarily find parallel difference in normal and abnormal
cells, using different substrates. I am a little confused
now. If I follow Dr. Reigh correctly, there are such differences. If I follow Dr. Dawson there are no differences.
Couldn't we settle this question first, whether such a difference
exists, or doesn't exist?

Dr. Zeman: Dr. Reigh, would you please make a definitive
statement giving absolute specific activities relative to
different substrates for the soluble enzyme.

Dr. Reigh: I won't argue the point with you. It is
apparent to me that if a reduced activity can be shown with
p-phenylenediamine it can be shown with any other hydrogen
donor. I think that the problem lies with different techniques
for isolating the white cells, different techniques of breaking
the white cells, and the release of enzyme. As Dr. Armstrong
has talked about the bound fraction; if you use some very
rigorous technique for breaking white cells, you may dump
out all the peroxidase. I made one determination with guaiacol
and I did show that there was also a deficiency...a parallel
deficiency...using p-phenylenediamine for this one particular
patient. But that is the only one I have done so far, but
as far as I am concerned, you should be able to demonstrate
it with all of them and I am going to look at the whole range,
under the conditions that we isolate the white cells and under
the conditions that we release the soluble enzyme.

Dr. Zeman: Dr. Reigh, you did not make a definitive statement. May I ask you again, what were the specific activities you measured with guaiacol in the patient, as compared to controls and what were the specific activities as measured with p-phenylenediamine?

Dr. Reigh: I don't carry the numbers around with me. It was about on the order of 50%, enough to show that there was a definite difference kinetically.

Dr. Zeman: When we speak of enzyme defects in genetically controlled diseases, the·specific activity we measure in the homozygous affected is usually in the range of a few percent up to perhaps 10 or 15 percent. A 50 percent reduction on the other hand, we associate, at least in our minds, with a heterozygous state. I seem to recall that Dr. Armstrong reported specific activities in p-phenylenediamine-mediated peroxidase in homozygous affecteds in the range of 8-12% of normal controls and my question is: was the reduction which you measured with guaiacol of the same range as you got in the same patient with p-phenylenediamine, and was it also in the range of the affecteds as previously reported by Dr. Armstrong and his associates?

Dr. Reigh: This was considered to be a heterozygous carrier and in this case, I had about 55% of control activity with p-phenylenediamine, and with guaiacol.

Dr. Zeman: Thank you.

Dr. Schonbaum: Another question, perhaps just a point of clarification. In your kinetic assays in carriers, at around 20 to around 40 seconds perhaps, there is a very rapid decrease in apparent activity. If I am correct, such a pronounced decrease in activity is not observed in normal cells nor with enzymes extracted from normal cells. Have you any information on the level of residual peroxide at the time of this apparent decrease in activity?

Dr. Armstrong: We haven't calculated that data yet. I am going to look at them at each point in time on that curve. Right now there are just the 100-second values, so I don't know.

Dr. Schonbaum: You haven't tried by any chance to use alkyl peroxide like methylhydrogen peroxide instead of hydrogen peroxide in your assays?

Dr. Armstrong: No.

Dr. Zeman: Before we return to the general discussion,

I would like to ask Dr. Armstrong to report to us whether
he has performed any mixing experiments of enzyme preparations
from patients with different clinical diseases, belonging
to the Batten group. These experiments had been suggested
on the basis of the so-called Neufeld principle or Neufeld
experiment where Dr. Neufeld has shown that cells kept in
tissue culture from two very closely related conditions, namely
Hunter's disease and Hurler's disease, are capable in co-cultivation to correct for the enzymatic defect. Under the assumption
that this defect in PPD-mediated peroxidase activity may be
different in the different clinical forms, Dr. Armstrong said
he was prepared to do such experiments.

Dr. Armstrong: I'm not sure I understand, Dr. Zeman,
you mean the stuff we showed last year?

Dr. Zeman: No. You reported last year mixing experiments
which indicated that there was at least no inhibitor involved
in your observations and by the same token we wondered whether
you would mix, for instance, an enzyme preparation from a
patient with the so-called Jansky-Bielschowsky type and a
preparation from a patient with the Spielmeyer-Sjögren type,
whether the enzyme activities would come out as the arithmetic
mean or whether there were any corrective factors involved
in your system.

Dr. Armstrong: No, since last year we have not done
any further mixing experiments. The initial ones were a control
with a late infantile or a control with a juvenile. We have
not tried any further mixing experiments.

Dr. Zeman: Thank you. Then I will call on Dr. Fridovich,
who has analyzed Dr. Armstrong's data and has hopefully come
to some very enlightening conclusions.

Dr. Fridovich: I'm surprised Dr. Armstrong didn't comment on it since we spoke of it just before the meeting.
If you look at figure 40 on page 276 this presents the mixing
experiments. There is in fact clear evidence for an activation
of the enzyme in the diseased sample by something which is
present in the normal sample, because the same total number
of cells are used in preparing the extract of the normal and
the homozygote and the same total number are present when
they're mixed; that is to say, half as much of the normal
and half as much of the homozygote. When these two preparations
are mixed together, what one would ordinarily expect is the
arithmetic mean of the sum. In fact, what is shown, however,
is the sum of activities of the unmixed preparations, with
twice the number of leukocytes. So I take this as clear evidence
for an activation or an activating factor. Of course, I got
kind of excited when I saw that because it made me think about

a paper I had published in 1963. This had to do with the horse-radish peroxidase and the observavation was, that the activity optimum occurred at pH 5.8 with p-phenylenediamine or o-di-anisidine; if one raised the pH significantly above that, there was sharp loss of activity. This loss of activity could be prevented by adding nitrogenous ligands. The net effect then is that the activity of the horseradish peroxidase toward certain substrates--p-phenylenediamine and o-dianisidine--but not towards other substrates such as guaiacol, can be remarkably activated by adding certain nitrogenous ligands which act therefore as allosteric effectors, positive allosteric effectors and what I'm suggesting only as a possibility, of course, I may be dead wrong, is that there is not a defect in the level of the enzyme, but a defect in the level of the activator, the activator being present in the normal and absent from the diseased homozygote and that activator might work something like the activators worked that were described in this paper. The possibility is easy to test.

Dr. Hochstein: Isn't this data kind of consistent with the idea that there's an inhibitor present which is diluted two-fold and therefore permits the inhibited enzyme now to be activated, or is that what you were saying? You say acti-vator. Are you talking about an activator or an inhibitor?

Dr. Fridovich: I suppose there are two ways to look at it. One could have the absence of an inhibitor or the presence of an activator, either way, but I don't think that a two-fold dilution of an inhibitor would give you the full activity which is really seen in that experiment, but the absence of an activator which is present in the enzyme prepara-tion of normals, that could do it.

Dr. Rider: Dr. Fridovich, do you think that this could possibly have some practical value, as you know, we're all concerned with these children with Batten's disease and trying to figure out ways of treatment which might theoretically be of benefit to them and we have been feeding children per-oxidase and we have been giving them foods high in peroxidase, for example, and I see here your ligands, you used ammonia, pyridine, imidazole and hydrazine. I don't know whether any of those could be ingested, or whether on theoretical grounds similar compounds could be used as donors and might influence the peroxidase reaction.

Dr. Fridovich: I think, of course, the first thing would be to demonstrate that there is in fact the absence of an activator. I don't know--let's assume that there is. The next step, of course, would be to find out what the natural activator is and this could be done by isolation. Of the compounds I tested, I would suspect probably that the most innocuous would be imidazole which probably would be fairly well tolerated and not have side effects and so if it is the absence of an activator, something like imidazole could well be used to replace the missing natural activator, whatever it is.

Dr. Rider: This, of course, is extremely intriguing because as I've seen Dr. Armstrong's data, I'm impressed with the fact that the mother or father of these children have a low peroxidase level, yet they have no manifestations of the disease. So obviously they have something that's protecting them or activating this low level of peroxidase. Then they have a child, who has the same level as the mother or father and yet he has the disease so he is missing something which the mother had or the father had that protected them from the disease and this would fit right in, I think, with your idea there.

Dr. Fridovich: I'm not sure, that's the way I understand the data that I've heard and that is to say that if the level of activity which is normally present represents an excess, that is to say, there's a beefing factor, a safety factor, then one could well do with half that much and not see symptoms whereas a tenth that much would be over the line, so to speak, and I thought the heterozygotes had half the normal level and homozygotes less than 10 percent.

Dr. Rider: No that's not true. Some of the mothers or fathers are as low if not lower than the children.

Dr. Fridovich: I didn't realize that.

Dr. Rider: Am I not right, Dr. Armstrong?

Dr. Armstrong: That's true and I think Dr. Dawson has found that too.

Dr. Rouser: I would like to add, the substances as you note here, one of them being ammonia, I think might be considered more of a physiological substrate since there is a fair amount around and this can be made in huge quantities as you see by things like glutaminase and so on.

Dr. Fridovich: Yeah, but the trouble with free ammonia is that, in fact, the level of free ammonia in normal liver for example is essentially zero, almost unmeasurable simply because it's removed very quickly in the synthesis of urea, for example.

Dr. Rouser: But what I'm saying is: it might be the generating system and not the absolute amount. In other words,

if you have something there that works with ammonia and you're
making ammonia, some of it goes to the peroxidase.

Dr. Fridovich: I guess the important thing would be
to first establish that that is the case.

Dr. Packer: This question is asked out of complete ignorance. See the strategy is to feed the peroxidase or foods
containing high levels of peroxidase to patients. Now the
enzyme being a protein, of course will not cross the gut.
So the only effect I could see is that it would use up substrates
which you hope would cross the gut. I think that would be
the wrong way to do it, but maybe I don't understand it.

Dr. Armstrong: The horseradish peroxidase, at least,
does in fact cross the gut very nicely. There are some reports
in the literature, using rats or mice, it is species-specific,
we've shown it in our patient also at least in terms of increasing his circulating leukocyte peroxidase activity.

Dr. Packer: Is it certain that that is due to the move-
ment of the enzyme into the animals' circulation or rather
some induction phenomenon that the feeding of this enzyme
might have had on the levels of enzymes?

Dr. Rouser: You only move it one step, if you say it
can cross the gut. As it goes through the other compartments,
it might be using up a lot of these substrates, say in the
blood and so on, before it actually got into the intracellular
compartment.

Dr. Armstrong: It's quite possible. In any event, one
child has been treated with horseradish peroxidase over about
a year and a half. We started giving him a very small amount
of horseradish dissolved in his milk which he took three times
a day, and have increased it over this period of time from
1 mg per day of the Sigma Type II horseradish peroxidase to
56 mg. What we have plotted here is enzyme activity at 20
seconds of incubation. The initial baseline activity was
in fact deficient. He then went on the vitamin E antioxidant
therapy and his enzyme jumped up a little bit. Although he
was maintained on antioxidant therapy, the enzyme activity
fell and about a year later was down at terribly low levels.
We then put him on horseradish and as we increased the dose,
his activity has continually risen and is now way up into
the normal range, if not the very high normal range. All
this means is that the enzyme has gotten across the gut and
was phagocytized by the neutrophils. We could prove that
by running isoenzymes patterns on it and see if they match
horseradish rather than natural leukocyte, but we haven't
done that yet. I think of very great importance is that as

we did each one of these assays, we always do the peroxide
assay at the same time, and this boy initially had a very
high peroxide level. After 5 months of peroxidase administration
he had no demonstrable peroxide, which means that the horseradish
peroxidase has gotten into the white cells.

Dr. Rider: Dr. Armstrong, with respect to those two
points where the enzyme activity rose rapidly, did you increase
the dose at both places and if so what was the amount of increase.

Dr. Armstrong: Before the first rise, he was on about
30 mg a day. Then he went to 56 mg and was kept there but
the activity is still going up without increasing the dose
of enzyme.

Dr. Rider: But if you hadn't changed the dose, enzyme
activity might still have gone up. What was the clinical
response?

Dr. Armstrong: He was severely clinically involved.
As his enzyme levels dropped, he became very ill and stayed
that way until around June or August of that year and he clinically started to look a little better. He has not continued
to improve. The only thing that I can tell you and the only
frame of reference we have as to whether this treatment is
doing any good or not, is that his older brother died of this
disease at about 4 years and about 4 or 5 months. As Dr.
Zeman has pointed out, if there are more than one patient
in the family they usually get sick at the same time, have
a very similar course and usually die very close to each other.
This young boy is still ambulatory and he's pushing 5. His
clinical course is still going down, but it may be going down
at a slower rate than it would have had we not given peroxidase.
There's no way to equate that.

Dr. Dawson: Is there any evidence that peroxidase gets
across the blood-brain barrier? Do you know?

Dr. Armstrong: There are some recent reports now by
Westergard and Rappaport that it does go across some cerebal
arterioles with a certain diameter, it does not get across
capillaries--the tight junctions are too tight for that, but
even if it gets across, I don't know that there's evidence
that it would get from the extracellular space into the neuron
itself, but it will get across the blood-brain barrier as
of the reports I read in 1974.

Dr. Philippart: Did you feed peroxidase to normal controls, specifically the parents to see if you can boost the
leukocyte peroxidase activity?

330

Dr. Armstrong: No, the decision was made on those low enzyme values, also, that the patient was clinically in trouble and we just started giving it to him.

Dr. Hoekstra: Were there any side effects?

Dr. Armstrong: None at all and we had checked for the antibody and there isn't any. That is, he has not produced any antibodies against the horseradish during the course of his treatment, and he has never been febrile.

Dr. Zeman: We have also been treating patients with dietary peroxidase supplementation, but with a disease of this type which is chronically progressive, it is very difficult to really make sure that the effects you may observe are due to the treatment or in spite of the treatment and it is not possible, at least we have not been able, to set up double-blind controlled experiments. So I would like not to stick my neck out and make any observations with respect to the efficacy, but what we are planning to do, is at least to test the efficacy of dietary horseradish peroxidase on the rate of lipid peroxidation by monitoring the ethane evolution in the lung and thus, at least get an indication whether it reaches the lung. These experiments have all been protocolled, but have not been performed.

Dr. Hoekstra: Evolution of what?

Dr. Zeman: Ethane. Evolution of ethane is a direct measure, I think on a stoichiometric basis, of peroxidation. I think we should go back at least for a moment and ask Dr. Armstrong about his reaction to Dr. Fridovich's suggestion that he may be dealing with the presence of an activator in normal and its absence or at least relative lack in the Batten's patients. After all, he did the measurements and he made the observations and I think we would like to hear his comments on that. Do you think this is a reasonable suggestion, Dr. Armstrong?

Dr. Armstrong: Yes, as Dr. Fridovich and I discussed earlier, I was so intent on looking for an inhibitory effect there, I guess I simply missed looking at this possible stimulation. It may well be that there's something there to look into.

Dr. Rouser: I'd like to make what seems to me to be a fairly obvious suggestion, namely, that those who are most interested in the therapeutic approach make two lists, one list being those things that cross the blood brain barrier and could therefore be of use and the other list is any of those substances that might possibly have anything to do with

331

the activation of the enzyme that perhaps is involved. That, to me, seems to be the direction for those interested in therapeutic work.

Dr. Dawson: I suppose one of the more interesting aspects of this enzyme, I think Dr. Armstrong has some data, is its actual subcellular location. I don't think the evidence is completely clear about the location of the storage material. Are the bodies which contain the curvilinear bodies really lysosomes or are they some sort of membranous organ other than lysosomes. I guess most of us are used to working with lysosomal storage diseases and Batten's disease appears quite different. I think you alluded to this sort of thing with your discussion of factors produced by cultured cells which can then cross-correct the other cells, the business with Hunter's disease and Hurler's disease. Do you believe that lysosomes are involved? I think the evidence is that peroxidase is not lysosomal although electromicroscopically it might be.

Dr. Zeman: I believe we are all more or less agreed on the following: the acidic lipid polymers which form a large part of the autofluorescent pigments that accumulate in nerve cells in particular, but also in other tissues, form in the cytosol without participation of lysosomes. Now as these cross-polymers accumulate within the cytoplasm, and we very frequently see them attached to subcellular membrane structures, such as endoplasmic reticulum and mitochondria, they become successively incorporated into autophagic vacuoles. This occurs presumably on the basis of programmed focal lysis. As these autophagic vacuoles fuse with primary lysosomes, part of the, what we have called, pre-pigment is digested and presumably the non-catalyzable cross-polymerized material is retained. This process of "garbage removal" results in a selective accumulation of the cross-polymers in tertiary lysosomes. Now, we do have evidence that these tertiary lysosomes with the pigments inside do show all the enzyme activities that we find in other tertiary lysomes. They contain various acidic lysosomal hydrolases in relatively normal proportions. There are very high specific activities of acid phosphatase, hexosaminidases and comparatively low activities for mannosidase and fucosidase. I believe that the evidence does not point to the fact that cross-polymerization occurs within the autophagic vacuole or in the tertiary lysosomes. There might be some further rearrangement on a molecular basis, but the original cross-polymerization happens in the cytosol.

Dr. Dawson: It is presumed that peroxidase will be taken up by pinocytosis and end up in a secondary lysosome or heterophagic vacuole. Although the enzyme might be taken up in the cell, it might be compartmentalized in the wrong compartment.

Dr. Zeman: I realize the rationale of your argument.
I think we might even go further and say, and this has been
brought out by Dr. Hartroft, that there might be a factor
already present in the plasma which initiates peroxidation
of unsaturated fats after it has been taken up by the cell.
Now, I would think that if free radicals are involved in this
process they could easily attack the smooth endoplasmic reticulum
which forms the membranes around the secondary or tertiary
lysosomes and may even get into cytosol. What this discussion
really leads us to is that we have reverted back to factors
of secondary and perhaps tertiary rank in the pathogenesis
of the disease and it seems that we have gotten farther away
from a consideration of the expression of the genetic defect
in terms of a biochemical lesion.

Dr. Packer: I don't know if this is worth considering
or not, but a whole new technology has been developed in recent
years.   It has had spectacular success in immobilizing and
stabilizing individual enzymes.   For example, such an approach
has been used in some cancer chemotherapy where stabilized
and immobilized asparaginase has been encapsulated and injected
into animals.   Likewise, people are considering developing
artificial kidneys with stabilized and immobilized urease,
and so on.   This is a whole new way of tackling problems.
Now, it occurs to me that perhaps some research would be worth
embarking on, where peroxidases and catalases, enzymes that
are important perhaps in this disease, could be stabilized
and immobilized and encapsulated and their effects in experimental animals evaluated.   That is a forerunner to trying to mani-
pulate, if you like, the capacity of an animal to handle free
radicals.

Dr. Philippart: I'd like to comment specifically on
the lysosomal involvement in a disease like Batten's. Although
much emphasis over the last few years has been given to genetic
inherited deficiencies, it is clear that there is a large
number of diseases of the lysosomal system which involve entirely
different mechanisms. So, we need specific enzyme, but we
also need proper substrate. That is to say, anything which
would denature the substrate--and Batten's may be a very good
example of this--could result in a substrate which can no
longer be digested. If we want to prevent the progress of
Batten's disease, the only hopefully beneficial action, would
be to prevent the formation of the peroxide, whatever it may
be. This is the way we have to stop the mechanism. Once you
have denatured lipids inside lysosomes, you have a basically
lipofuscin-like material which will never be digested by any
method, even in vitro. There are diseases which develop secondary to different types of chemicals which interfere with a
normal lysosomal function. Among these, chloroquine is one
of the best studied examples. These components, however,

all interfere with the digestion inside the lysosome. The chemical reaction of denaturation produces permanent changes. If we want to prevent the lysosomal indigestion we have to prevent the primary denaturation. The idea to inject the peroxidase and hope that it will help to digest the denatured material will lead us nowhere because no enzyme can break down these denatured lipofuscin materials.

Dr. Zeman: I follow your argument. I do agree with everything you have said. However, our working hypothesis in the past has been that the presumed high rate of peroxidation does lead to the formation and accumulation of products which in themselves are toxic to the cell and I believe it is fairly well established that the formation of peroxy radicals and similar products of peroxidation is entirely a biological mechanism. Normally, these substances are readily detoxified by a number of enzyme systems. So what we have pursued then, is precisely what you say, namely the prevention of peroxidation. The question which you raised, namely is there any extrinsic factor involved which produces these undigestible polymers, that is different from the mechanism of peroxidation, has not been explored. The reason for this omission is that Dr. Tappel's data, in particular, looked so convincing, i.e., the formation of peroxidized lipid polymers from the interaction of hydroperoxy fatty acids, interacting with not only simple biochemical species but whole subcellular organelles, such as endoplasmic reticulum, ribosomes and mitochondria.

Dr. Hochstein: Do I understand that you're saying the working hypothesis is that there's an accumulation of peroxidizable, or peroxidized lipids and products that cause cell damage and that this accumulation takes place because there's an excess of hydrogen peroxide in the tissues of patients with Batten's disease? Is that the fundamental concept?

Dr. Zeman: No, that is not precisely what I have tried to say. What I am saying is this: in this group of diseases we have evidence of two apparently conjugated phenomena, namely the accumulation of autofluorescent lipopigments and a commensurate loss of cytoplasm and its organelles. This is in contrast to the age-dependent accumulation of lipofuscin in aged individuals where we also have an accumulation of lipopigment but no demonstrable reduction in the volume of the cytoplasm of the affected cell. Now, then, what we have assumed is the following, that peroxidation in these patients with this group of diseases proceeds at a rate which is equal or perhaps greater than the synthetic rate of the cell to replace the cross-linked or otherwise inactivated biological species. In other words, peroxidation under those conditions cross-links, inactivates or otherwise alters biological constituents, including subcellular organelles, which are lost

to the cell as functional elements. These polymers form the
backbone of the pigments and the cell is not able by its synthetic
ability to overcome the continuous loss of biological constituents. Whether this process is initiated by hydrogen peroxide,
whether it is due to unsaturated fatty acid hydroperoxides
or whether it is due to any other initiator, we do not know.
What we do know, however, is that in measuring the amount
of accumulated peroxidized biological material we use the
specific fluorescence of a Schiff-base amino-imino-propene
which is a condensation product of malonaldehyde with, perhaps
phosphatidyl ethanolamine, or perhaps with the amino group of
lysine.

Dr. Hochstein: If I can take a simple-minded look at
what I hear now, it seems to me that I know about peroxidation,
that either, there are two processes involved in the accumulation of peroxidized products, either initiation and the effectiveness of initiators in inducing peroxidation and the
effectiveness of chain-breakers in stopping peroxidation or
antioxidants. If I understand the clinical situation, these
patients in fact do not respond to vitamin E, which is a highly
lipid soluble antioxidant--does it penetrate into the brain,
does anybody know?

Dr. Zeman: Well, it must go into the brain tissue, there
is no question about it, because it's part of lipoprotein
membranes, you see.

Dr. Hochstein: Well, in the one other instance that
I know about where patients have been shown to be sensitive
to oxidant damage, and this is the anemia associated with
prematurity, these infants do respond to vitamin E, and the
red cell membrane does not peroxidize when these babies are
treated with vitamin E. So there is no question in my mind
that vitamin E does penetrate into body compartments, and
yet if it is not effective in these patients, the patients
with Batten's disease, somebody is trying to say something
to us. I mean, in other words, antioxidation is not the problem,
it seems to me.

Dr. Packer: Maybe the vitamin E doesn't get exchanged
into the brain and a mechanism needs to be sought to facilitate
the exchange of hydrophobic molecules like vitamin E into
the brain.

Dr. Rouser: In general, the brain can be considered
to be permeable to lipid soluble material.

Dr. Packer: Well, maybe in this particular disease what
we have to do is get increased levels, higher levels. Maybe
more efficient means of exchanging the vitamin E than just
feeding it in their diet.

Dr. Rouser: Yes, I would certainly buy that plus the cross-linking idea. That certainly could decrease the transport of lipid soluble substances across the brain.

Dr. Zeman: Dr. Hochstein, I think there might be a misunderstanding. I did not say, nor did anyone else, that vitamin E is not effective in this disease. What we can say with definity is that it is not curative but we do have the distinct impression that relatively high doses of vitamin E will delay the manifestation of the disease, at least in dogs. High doses of vitamin E together with other antioxidants seem to slow down the progression of the disease in men. Now, the question really is how high a dose of vitamin E should be given. There is little doubt from the clinical observations of Dr. Armstrong, that antioxidants will reduce whatever amount of peroxides he finds in leukocytes.

Dr. Hochstein: I am confused about terminology now. I'm not following you, Dr. Zeman. I have a problem with the concept of a peroxidase as an enzyme which functions in the detoxification of hydrogen peroxide. Peroxidases are usually involved in specific functions within the cell, like thyroid peroxidase, or the myeloperoxidase of the white cells involved in iodination reactions. There are enzymes that are involved in hydrogen peroxide detoxification, and these are glutathione peroxidases, and probably to a lesser extent catalase, although this one can argue about, but it doesn't seem to be that a deficiency of this enzyme, the leukocyte peroxidase that's been described, really reflects a lowering of the amount-- or can reflect a lowering of the amount of hydrogen peroxide in cells; I don't think it follows. I think what would be of interest is the natural substrate for this enzyme and what effect does that natural substrate have as an antioxidant or a pro-oxidant. Do you see what's bothering me? I don't understand the terminology we're using, I don't understand how peroxidases result in a decreased level of hydrogen peroxide in cells. It doesn't make sense to me. Does it?

Dr. Fridovich: Well, just from the point of view that peroxidases, all peroxidases consume peroxide, and if there were a sufficient level of the hydrogen donor then this would certainly result in the net consumption of hydrogen peroxide. Now, whether or not the specific peroxidase that we're talking about here, the one that uses p-phenylenediamine, is a significant factor in the scavenging of peroxide, that I could not say, but you have data yourself in the erythrocyte which show that glutathione peroxidase certainly functions in this way in the red cell and that catalase does to a lesser extent.

Dr. Hochstein: Well, that's true in the white cell, also.

Dr. Fridovich: Then why shouldn't that be true also in the brain?

Dr. Hochstein: I am asking what are the functions of these peroxidases, the leukocyte peroxidase, what does it do? I don't think it plays a major role in hydrogen peroxide detoxification.

Dr. Fridovich: Why do you say that?

Dr. Hochstein: I say that because one can account for the consumption of hydrogen peroxide formed in a leukocyte and granulocyte in terms of oxidized glutathione. There is no evidence for other endogenous substrates for peroxidases in leukocytes, and I don't know what the substrate for the PPD-mediated peroxidase is and therefore I don't know what we're asking of this enzyme. Am I not being clear?

Dr. Fridovich: Not entirely. Try me again. What I understand you to say is that in a particular kind of cell, for example in the erythrocyte you can account for all the peroxide consumption in terms of reduced glutathione converted to oxidized glutathione, but are you prepared to say that in the brain it is glutathione peroxidase which is the major scavenger for peroxide or might it not be another kind of peroxidase with a different specificity predominance.

Dr. Hochstein: Alright, I have to accept that there might be something else. So we're saying then that the white cell peroxidase deficiency or altered distribution reflects something that's going on in the brain also. Is that the idea?

Dr. Zeman: That is, at least as I understand it, the working hypothesis and this brings me back to a question which I wanted to raise before when Dr. Armstrong presented his measurment of the activity of this peroxidase in various parts of the brain tissue. Were these units expressed as percentage of the control? Can you tell us what the specific activities were in relationship to the leukocytes.

Dr. Armstrong: In the brain, they are much lower. These are very low activities, and I am simply making a comparison with some control tissues. Until we can measure isoenzyme patterns or inhibitors or things like this, we ought not to say that these peroxidases are really peroxidases. In the p-phenylenediamine system they will give some color changes and there is much less color produced by the tissue from a Batten's patient than there is from a control patient.

Dr. Zeman: In order to come back to Dr. Hochstein's

conceptual difficulties, we have assumed and I believe this
has been stated so by Dr. Hochstein and Dr. Fridovich as well,
that peroxidation reactions in life systems can be initiated
and once the initiation has taken place the process for all
we know may continue on a simple thermodynamic principle without
any enzymatic activity, and that for instance a hydroperoxy
radical may enter into a chain reaction affecting several
molecules and that the peroxidation of a vitamin E molecule
represents a chain-breaking mechanism which prevents further
peroxidation. So we discussed the possibility that this enzyme
may have a very high specificity for its natural substrate
which we do not know and that the natural substrate--a peroxide
or hydroperoxide--may indeed be the initiator for a chain
reaction.

Dr. Rahimtula: I would like to comment about the lipid
peroxidases. I give you an analogy with the liver cells.
The amount of lipid peroxidation, at least that initiated
by iron, depends upon the addition of extrinsic iron, if not,
the peroxidation will attenuate itself. It can be shown that
the iron that is added, binds to apoferritin and is removed
from circulation and therefore you don't have any further
peroxidation. I am wondering if something similar occurs
in the brain of patients with the disease, perhaps an absence
or alteration of an apoenzyme which can bind to the iron or
something else, and thus sustain continued peroxidation.
It is also not true that once a chain reaction has started,
it can keep on going, because you do have antioxidants and
so on, and I think these would terminate the reaction unless
a continuous source of radicals is present. So I don't think
it is so simple as that. And the other thing is, although
you say that glutathione peroxidase which detoxifies peroxides
is normal, what about glutathione levels. In hepatocytes,
once you oxidize glutathione, it can leave the cell more readily.
Maybe that is another problem

Dr. Fridovich: I would agree with you that one needs
a continuing source of radicals to initiate the peroxidation
and I would like to suggest that there is a continuing source
of radicals, and that is that during the reduction of oxygen
and during metabolism, certain fractions of the oxygen are
reduced univalently to form superoxide and these radicals
are fairly reactive themselves. Even more, they can react
with hydrogen peroxide to give hydroxyl radicals. These could
certainly act as an initiator of lipid peroxidation. As defenses
against this very damaging occurrence, one would require enzymes to scavenge the superoxide and, of course, there are
superoxide dismutases, and one would require enzymes to scavenge peroxide, and there we would have catalases and the
whole host of different peroxidases. So the reaction of superoxide and hydrogen peroxide to hydroxyl would be made very

unlikely by keeping the two reactants at low concentration. Nevertheless, there is in any case a continuing source of radicals during normal aerobic metabolism.

Dr. Schonbaum: I would like to ask a couple of questions. I agree solidly that you can have a source of free radicals arising from a variety of reactions. But it would seem that in a cell with a normal component of glutathione, the dissipation of such radicals would presumably proceed most effectively through the sulfhydryl group oxidation rather than say with a lipid peroxidation. In this context, perhaps somebody could tell us what is the level of reduced glutathione in the diseased cells or in the cells which are deficient in peroxidase.

Dr. Zeman: Dr. Patel, you have determined glutathione peroxidase in brain tissue, did you do that by adding glutathione or did you just add the acylperoxides.

Dr. Patel: Well, I really didn't determine the reduced glutathione content. We determined activity, that is in vitro activity of glutathione peroxidase which was normal, and Dr. Zeman pointed out there are a number of laboratories who have also shown that. As far as I know, nobody has determined the reduced glutathione content in the patient.

Dr. Zeman: That's not quite true, but I'm not sure how valid this data may be. About 8 years ago I had some specimens of brain tissues from patient's with Batten's disease examined by column chromatography for amino acids, in which process glutathione concentration was also determined. I can only say that I do not recall that there was any significant deficiency in glutathione in comparison to controls and to brain tissues affected by other diseases. The only thing I do recall is that in all instances we did find a very significant reduction in the concentration of gamma aminobuteric acid, but this is a different story, and I believe I do have the explanation for this finding. As far as glutathione is concerned, I don't recall any degree of lowered concentration. Now the problem with all these determinations is that there are rather marked chemical changes occurring in frozen tissues as a function of time, especially if they are frozen at temperatures higher than -78° C. Our tissues were, and that is one of the reasons we have never reported this data.

Dr. Miquel: I just would like to comment on a couple of points that I think are rather important. The first is about the effectiveness of the antioxidants, which incidentally is difficult to prove. We have spent a few years working on the effects of antioxidants on the longevity of drosophila. These insects become loaded with pigment, as they get old and Siakotos showed this to be ceroid rather than lipofuscin.

I think drosophila is a rather elegant model for diseases
with ceroid accumulation on which we have tried about twenty
different polar and non-polar antioxidants. The best results
that we have obtained so far is a 22% increase in the life
span of fruit flies treated with tocopherol and thiazolidine
carboxylic acid, which is a sulfhydryl derivative of cysteine.
We assume that we are slowing down the aging processes by
about 20%. An effect of a comparable magnitude in Batten's
disease would be difficult to prove. Nevertheless these drugs
should be tried. Dr. Zeman mentioned that in normal aging,
lipofuscin accumulates in neurons with no loss of organelles
in contrast to Batten's disease where the lipopigment storage
is accompanied by loss of organelles. However, several recent
papers from England indicate a similar inverse relationship
between the contents of lipofuscin and RNA in individual cells
of normal human brains. So I think that it has been proven
now that wherever you find lipofuscin, the nerve cell is losing
organelles at the same time, not just in the areas where the
lipofuscin accumulates but even in areas of cytoplasm that
seem to be well preserved. If you quantitate RNA, you see
loss even in these other areas. We have data on aged mouse
brains which confirm this inverse relationship between the
amounts of lipofuscin and RNA, so I really think that Batten's
disease and normal brain aging may be even more closely related
than we thought before. The last point is about the site
of lipid peroxidation. Is it extra- or intralysosomal? We
are getting rather interesting results with centrophenoxine.
This drug is supposed to remove age pigment. Obviously, lipofuscin is extremely hard to digest, so I cannot believe that
centrophenoxine is extracting the lipofuscin from the lysosomes.
What may occur is that peroxidation occurs outside the lysosomes
but keeps on going inside. Centrophenoxine may then slow
down intralysosomal peroxidation.

Dr. Zeman: Thank you, Dr. Miquel. We have gotten a
little bit away from the peroxidase situation. I think that
Dr. Hoekstra is going to put us back on the right track.

Dr. Hoekstra: I'm not sure that I'll put it back on
the track. I have two comments to make: 1) from our studies
in animals, the amount of glutathione peroxidase in brain
is low and others have reported this as well, in fact, so
low that some investigators question whether it exists at
all except in the blood that happens to be in the brain.
We're convinced that there is more than just what is in the
blood and that it's low. I don't know the glutathione concentration in brain, but concentration of glutathione is just
as important as that of the enzyme because you can't saturate
glutathione peroxidase with glutathione. The breakdown is
proportional to the glutathione concentration so it is just
as important and could be of significance. The other point--

340

maybe this is a good time to mention another possible model. The way I see it, there are three primary possibilities: 1) overabundance of radicals, oxidants, what have you. 2) lack of protective systems and 3) an inherent alteration in the lipid membrane. I'm sure this last one has received some attention and the implication is that probably there isn't any big change. But the model that this brings to my mind is some work being done by Dr. Kenneth Munkres at our University with Neurospora and he has various mutants of Neurospora that show early death, very much earlier than the normal. One of these is inositol-less. It can't make inositin. So the assumption is that there is something wrong with the phospholipids. A second one is leucine-less, it can't make leucine. This doesn't make quite as much sense but as Munkres thinks the inability to make leucine might have something to do with alterations of the proteins of the memrane. For the third one, the mutational defect is unknown. They call it a normal death. It dies very early. In all of these cases, they find evidence of lipid peroxidation, increased fluorescent pigments, etc. In all cases, they can prolong the life of the mutants with antioxidants, including vitamin E, as well as synthetic lipid antioxidants and they have some evidence they can do the same thing, providing extra selenium, by as much as 200%. But despite the presence of antioxidant you finally reach the point where those cells will die and they die in the presence of antioxidant, showing evidence of extensive lipid peroxidation. He's done a very interesting thing recently and this is unpublished but I talked to him and he said I could mention it, that is, he has fed these molds, Neurospora, amino acid analogs of phenylalanine and methionine and the old idea is that these would foul up the protein synthesis. But he finds that they will shorten lifespan of the normal wild type Neurospora but that that shortened lifespan can then be prolonged with antioxidants and, again, it's his concept that these amino acid alterations are of particular significance in the structure of the membrane, in some way changing the sensitivity of the lipid to oxidation.

Dr. Zeman: These observations are in good agreement with the studies of Barber who has found that certain changes in the tertiary protein structures in lipid protein micelles will facilitate peroxidation of the hydrophobic moieties of the complex lipids just by conformational changes in the apparently protective protein moiety of the micelle. This seems to be an explanation for the observation on the Neurospora fed amino acid analogs. So this would make sense in view of the work and findings of Barber.

Dr. Fridovich: I wonder if Dr. Hoekstra can tell us how the survival of the Neurospora is measured? What conditions are imposed to keep them from dividing and growing, if you know?

Dr. Hoekstra: As I say, this isn't my work, this is Dr. Munkres and I've cooperated with him on some aspects but I'm not an expert in the field. However, I gather that what he does is he simply inoculates the Neurospora into what he calls a race tube which is a narrow caliber tube that he can extend out for meters and meters clear across the room, if he wished, and the normal wild type will just keep growing and probably grow clear around the block through one of these small capillaries, whereas the early-death mutants grow only a certain distance and then they die and when they start to die it's a sort of an exponential thing and they die faster and faster with time, and they just quit.

Dr. Rouser: With regard to the work on yeasts generally: They have a very high content of phosphatidyl inositol. Many fungi do, as a matter of fact. Now, secondly, those inositol-less organisms--what has been reported that I recall is that they keep going and keep diluting out their phosphatidyl inositol until they just don't have any more. They gradually lose organelles, etc. This would make sense with regard to what is being found now with the specificity for various lipid types for activation of enzymes. This is a rapidly enlarging field. Many people, I think, have in the past considered lipid as something that was just a part of the membrane and that was it. However, the picture that's emerging now is totally different, that all the enzymes that are intrinsic proteins, actually have a very definite lipid requirement. Now, phosphatidyl inositol has been implicated in one most interesting requirement in animals. It has been reported that adenocyclase would not respond to a whole series of hormones, if phosphatidyl inositol is not there. Another set of enzymes will not respond to hormones unless phosphatidyl serine is there. The general picture is that certain enzymes will depend entirely on phosphatidyl choline, the classic example being β-hydroxybuteric dehydrogenase. There are enzymes that seem to bind specifically only to sphingomyelin and so on. Now then, the implication of this is very broad for disease and this is a concept that I would like to introduce because I think it's an important one--that if this is true that there are only, you see, seven different types of phospholipids, counting all of the minor components as one unit, then that means that there must be a variety of enzymes all dependent on the same lipid and if this lipid is abnormal then you can expect many enzymes to be affected and so we might be going all the way around and saying that we do, in fact, have some kind of a lipid defect which feeds back into many enzymes and would therefore be rather hard to unravel.

Dr. Philippart: Regarding lipid abnormalities in such diseases, there is only one well-documented example. It was a case first reported by Hagberg and Svennerholm about 10

342

years ago, a child who died from a disease similar to Batten's disease and in which they found a striking deficiency of poly-unsaturated fatty acids. Recently about 30 such cases have been reported in Sweden and Finland. Little new data are available on the brain but clinically it seems to present a somewhat different form. Ultrastructually this disease is different too, because the pigment is mostly granular, not curvilinear in structure. We don't know if this is related at all to the peroxidase deficiency described in Batten's disease. I think that Dr. Dawson may also make some comment on some abnormalities on polyunsaturated fatty acids in the blood of some patients who may be more prone to pigmentary degeneration, retinal pigment being very rich in polyunsaturated fatty acids and so very susceptible to any peroxide type damage. On the other hand, lipid studies in Batten's disease have been very disappointing, that is to say, they are normal. If you have good fresh material or biopsy material you just can't find any lipid abnormalities there, distribution is normal, levels are normal and the fatty acid distribution is essentially normal, as well.

Dr. Zeman: The particular case that Dr. Philippart cited may really be pivotal with respect to the glutathione. There is one relation which is reasonably well established and that is that lack of glutathione in brain tissue prevents myelin formation. Vice versa during early life, glutathione concentra-tion, that is, free glutathione in brain tissue is very high during the process of myelination which is at its maximum rate shortly before birth up to about the age of 18 months. Now in the case which Dr. Philippart made reference to we found two things which may go along with a glutathione def-iciency, namely, a complete or almost complete lack of myelin on the one hand and an enormous accumulation of lipopigments, the result of lipid peroxidation, on the other. Now in the other types of Batten's disease, myelin is more or less normal. This would indicate that glutathione levels at the time the disease process becomes active, there would, at least by im-plication, be no major deficiency of glutathione.

Dr. Packer: I ask for a point of information. A group of patients have been discovered in Japan to have a catalase deficiency. Have any studies been done of the proclivity of such people to develop Batten's disease? That might be interesting.

Dr. Philippart: As far as I know, it is just a curiosity. They are quite susceptible to infection but it is a pretty mild disease and I don't know of any neurological complication described in such patients.

Dr. Hochstein: There are families who are acatalasic

343

known not only in Japan but also in Switzerland and Israel.
There are, I've forgotten how many now, but there are quite
a few in the world who are acatalasic. The Swiss and the
Israeli families do not have these problems with gum infections.
They appear to be perfectly normal, healthy individuals and
we presume they are so because they have glutathione peroxidase
present which handles the peroxides at least in their red
cells. I think catalase is an enzyme looking for a function
and we don't know what it is yet.

Dr. Packer: Well, I know that generally it is very difficult to saturate catalase with a substrate; generally even
low levels of catalase might be sufficient to handle the damage
that might be inflicted by hydrogen peroxide except perhaps
in ionizing radiation.

Dr. Fridovich: The comment I wanted to make is that,
first of all, with respect to other species, ducks for example
normally have 1/500th the level of catalase that, say, mammals
have and they suffer no apparent problems from this lack.
The other thing with respect to the Km of catalase for peroxide,
it's over one molar, so what you say about the inability to
saturate is true but what this really means is that at very
low ambient steady state levels of peroxide the efficiency
of catalase as an enzyme is low, whereas peroxidases which
may have a low Km for peroxide could be operating much more
rapidly.

Dr. Schonbaum: I wouldn't want to start a discussion
here on catalase versus glutathione peroxidase. These are
conflicting views that I don't think are reconcilable in any
way. Nonetheless, the very low level of catalase in avian
erythrocytes, has not, and should not be taken to mean necessarily that catalase in other tissues is equally low or ineffective. For instance, glutathione peroxidase is much higher
in avian erythrocytes and forms compensatory mechanisms.
Number two, which perhaps ought to be considered is that through
direct studies, spectrometric studies in perfused liver, you
can actually identify formation of catalase peroxide derivatives,
showing that it is playing a role, it is functional and whether
it functions in the oxidation of alcohols or other substrates
is a moot point at this stage but, nonetheless it is functional.
Number three which I shall like to bring out is so-called
"absolute acatalasemia" which I think is probably a misconception
because there are various forms of acatalasemia. In some
individuals there is structually defective catalase which
when assayed through an ordinary classical method is very
rapidly inactivated. In fact, it is fully viable but more
fragile and therefore it appears as if there were some deficiency
when you use it under high peroxide conditions. In other
words, the acatalasemia has proved that catalase is an enzymological

appendix, if you will. I think it would be a little too premature to conclude that from the genetic point of view nonetheless, there is an interesting question and that is that
both glutathione peroxidase and catalase have the primary
step approximately the same rate constant, around 10^7. Therefore
catalase and glutathione peroxidase should compete almost
equally effectively for peroxides in the primary step, that
is, formation of enzyme peroxide derivative. In the presence
of excess glutathione, no doubt glutathione peroxidase can
function more effectively. However, under oxidative assault,
for instance in antimalarial treatment where glutathione levels
drop very rapidly, the catalase then expresses its function
to a greater extent. So it depends very much what is the
rate of peroxide generation, what is the level of glutathione
peroxidase, what is the level of glutathione reductase and,
of course, NADH and NADPH. It is a complex system and therefore
to conclude that either glutathione peroxidase or catalase
are not effective in a given system, would be totally erroneous.

    Dr. Zeman: What you are suggesting is that we haven't
done our homework. We have looked at bits and pieces and
have been overambitious in drawing unwarranted conclusions.
The right way to do this is to look at the whole system of
enzymes and cofactors and activators and so forth, in order
to develop a more meaningful and more accurate picture of
the situation.

    Dr. Hochstein: I really don't think that we should en-
gage in an argument about catalase and glutathione peroxidase
but I must disagree with what Dr. Schonbaum said, that, in
the case of the antimalarial drugs which are peroxide-generating
compounds, that glutathione gets oxidized and is not available
as a substrate for glutathione peroxidase, because it can't
be regenerated by the sensitized cells, sensitized to peroxide,
despite the presence of catalase, despite the presence of
Compound I, the peroxide catalase complex, because it is
not the first rate constant that is relevant--it is the second
one. Well, obviously this argument could go on, Dr. Zeman,
but I think the biological evidence in terms of cell damage
done suggests strongly that when the glutathione levels in
a cell fall then the catalase doesn't stand up as a protective
agent.

    Dr. Schonbaum: I am sure Dr. Fridovich would mention
here that in very severe oxidative assaults you would have
also superoxide radical formation which neither catalase nor
glutathione peroxidase break down. So the question of control
of peroxide metabolism is far more complex than just simply
assigning it to one or other group of enzymes. The fact is
that catalase did suffice to stage evolution, perhaps it is
just simply not perfectly effective in all phases of peroxide

decomposition. It is widely distributed, not just simply in
red cells, not in the liver or kidney only, but in a variety
of other tissues. I think that the most comprehensive study
by George on the distribution of catalase and superoxide dismutase in a variety of tissues bears on this point and I would
feel very strongly that any data on the presence of peroxides
in diseased cells would be difficult to reconcile with the
presence of catalase in those cells at the same time and I
am talking about hydrogen peroxide. If you have other peroxides,
alkyl, azo, etc., catalase will work in a primary reaction
step in forming Compound I, but only providing that such peroxides are of low molecular weight--either lower aliphatic
peracids or lower alkylperoxides. On the other hand, glutathione
peroxidase in a primary step appears to be far less discrim-
inatory. It will work with very large peroxides and therefore
its presence is absolutely essential for the dissipation of
such derivatives. Catalase in those systems will be completely
ineffective. It would not decompose linoleic acid hydroperoxide or things like that very effectively.

Dr. Philippart: Well, I think that one important consideration is not only to have enzyme in the cells but their site.
As far as I know, catalase is essentially a peroxisomal enzyme
and I don't know if there is much found in the soluble cytoplasm,
for example.

Dr. Schonbaum: Yes, they are found. In some species,
you find catalase predominantly in peroxisomes. In others,
you find actually far higher amounts of catalase in cytoplasmic
compartments. In fact, there is a great deal of discussion
going on now as to whether it arises through the breakdown
of peroxisomes or whether there are two separate pools, which
are biosynthesized separately. Masters does believe that
there are two separate pools. Of course, we do know that the
subunits of catalase are synthesized in the cytoplasm,
are transported into peroxisomes where the heme is interpolated
into the apoprotein followed by the polymerization of the
subunits into the tetramers. The possibility that a considerable
number of subunits is diverted into the cytoplasm is not totally
unlikely as Masters would have it. So there are different
pools of catalase, not only peroxisomal but also very high
cytoplasmic in some cases.

Dr. Packer: What is known about the levels of these
enzymes we've been talking about in autopsy specimens of patients
who have had Batten's disease, compared with similar autopsy
specimens from healthy individuals? I presume it would be
difficult to get information on the steady state level of
metabolites, but it certainly should be possible to get some
information on the total levels of enzymes, perhaps not their
latency, which is important. Secondly, what is the composition

of the cytochrome components, the main system that delivers free radicals.

Dr. Zeman: Dr. Patel, would you answer that question please.

Dr. Patel: I suppose you missed the first part of the talk--it was extensively discussed that the dog model we have has normal glutathione peroxidase, this is in leukocytes.

Dr. Packer: I'm talking about brain tissue.

Dr. Patel: Brain also has normal glutathione peroxidase and catalase. However, we could not demonstrate p-phenylene-diamine-mediated peroxidase, and with guiacol there is no deficiency. In other words, the peroxidase enzymes we mentioned, that is glutathione peroxidase, "true" peroxidase, and catalase are within normal range.

Dr. Packer: How about the enzyme that delivers the free radicals, like the cytochrome components?

Dr. Patel: I think Dr. Tappel has looked at it, and I believe they are within normal range too--I'm not too sure about that.

Dr. Zeman: Since we mentioned what we have looked at, I might add that we also looked at brains from human patients for activity of glutathione peroxidase and catalase, and found this to be normal, in fact catalase activity in brain tissue is so high that it is very easy to demonstrate considerable differences in specific activity from one part of the brain tissue to another. What we have not done, and this is the question which has been raised repeatedly, is to measure con-centrations of reduced and oxidized glutathione in the same specimens. Neither have we been able to get reproducible data on the p-phenylenediamine-mediated peroxidase in tissues, because the activity proved to be very low.

Dr. Packer: I'd like to suggest we pay more attention to this part of the problem, it is really very important. For example it's recently begun to emerge that the iron-sulfur components, non-heme iron components, of the electron trans-port chain are probably the most important factors in the generation of free radical-mediated damage in those membranes, probably this spreads to other membranes. There is also a very close correlation between the levels of these non-heme iron-sulfur components and vitamin E, which is also interesting. For example, in vitamin E deficiency, the non-heme iron-sulfur components practically drop to zero. It is very dramatic and very important I think, and so studies like that would be perhaps diagnostic.

Dr. Philippart: Another important piece of information that we would like to have is where do peroxides accumulate, what is the level in different tissues, in the body fluids, in the subcellular organelles?

Dr. Fridovich: A number of years ago when I first heard of Batten's disease I contacted you, Dr. Zeman, you sent me some samples which I assayed for superoxide dismutase and I found that there were no differences between the homozygote and the normal but I have forgotten which tissues you sent me--do you remember?

Dr. Zeman: There were 2 types of tissue we sent you. We did send you cultured brain cells from newborn homozygous affected dogs. On those you reported 0.5 activity. We also sent you leukocytes and brain tissues from dogs and from patients and the striking results were that on the specimens from affected homozygotes you invariably reported very low activities, anywhere from 0.5 to 2.5, whereas in the controls, you found high activities; however there were some controls which had very low activity but they definitely did not have the disease. That was the situation.

Dr. Fridovich: It sounds as though the results are confusing and it may possibly be worthwhile doing it again on the basis of blind assays, which was the situation then, so I never knew what I was assaying.

Dr. Rider: We're getting near the close of today's session, and I will try to bring us back on the clinical track since I am primarily a clinician. I think there is pretty good evidence for low peroxidase level in the white cells of the subjects with Batten's disease, and also of the parents, but occasionally only of either the father or the mother. Now, assuming this is true, then we have to think about what protects the parent with this low enzyme level--why don't they have manifestations of the disease. The other thing that's bothering me now, is that Dr. Armstrong has shown that he could raise the level of peroxidase in the white cells, and yet there was no dramatic reversal of the clinical course. Maybe the disease has been slowed down but this is difficult to tell. Let me say again, there's got to be something different between the child with Batten's disease and his father or mother with a similarly low level of enzyme and even if you increase the enzyme activity to normal you still haven't converted the patient to a normal person, so there must be additional factors related to peroxidase. So let's think in terms of what factors these might be, and what possibilities exist to make the peroxidase more efficient or permeate the cell membrane more easily.

Dr. Fridovich: Perhaps you are asking for too much,
that is to say, if the damage represents an irreversible accumulation of the material which is not metabolized, you may prevent its further accumulation but you may not hope for a
reversal, unless perhaps this drug centrophenoxine which has
been reported by Nandy and others can actually clear the cell
from accumulated lipofuscin. Perhaps it might work in con-
junction with administered peroxidase.

Dr. Rider: But you should be able to stop the disease
in its tracks--maybe you don't improve the coordination or
function or vision, but it shouldn't continue to deteriorate
if you've really gotten at the basic cause of it.

Dr. Fridovich: But that was what was reported--that
is to say, that the progression was slowed down.

Dr. Rider: Well, but there shouldn't be any progression
if you've solved it, you see? Just like if you have a diabetic
under good control, there shouldn't be any progression of
the degenerative features any more than in any other person.

Dr. Fridovich: Has centrophenoxine been tried?

Dr. Rider: Well, I used it on my own son, Charles, for
awhile by injection, and we saw absolutely no benefit from
that. I think we must consider these other factors, activators,
co-enzymes, things that potentiate. Would you agree with
that, Wolf?

Dr. Zeman: Yes, I agree with the fact that the pigments
are, at best, the indicators of something going basically
wrong in the cell, but the pigments themselves are probably
quite inert and do not produce any severe dysfunction of the
cell unless they reach very large proportions.

I think we should close now for today. you have all
heard the evidence which has become increasingly confusing,
and somewhat muddled. Tomorrow we'll meet here at 9 o'clock
and hope to come to grips with the problem of the peroxidases
to the extent that we can resolve what types of studies may
further the understanding of these conditions in the light
of what has been discussed today.

Dr. Zeman: The discussions which we held yesterday cast
considerable doubt on the concept that the p-phenylenediamine-
mediated peroxidase abnormality which has been found by Dr.
Armstrong and confirmed by other laboratories, represents
indeed the expression of the genetic defect in this group
of diseases. I should mention that the hereditary nature
of all forms of neuronal ceroid-lipofuscinoses is well established,

so that it is by no means far-fetched to assume an underlying enzyme defect. However, we all feel that the peroxidase data are not as clearcut as we wish them to be, especially if compared with enzyme defects which have been found in other recessively inherited diseases, for example the lysosomal disrders. Under the circumstances, I feel that before we try to either resuscitate the concept or put in on a new basis, we should exploit the fact that we do have experts on the chemistry and physical chemistry of peroxidases, and shall now enter into a discussion as to peroxidase chemistry which would be fairly comprehensive. I'm calling on Dr. Schonbaum to give us his views.

Dr. Schonbaum: Before entering into a discussion of peroxidases, I wonder whether we might clarify some aspects of peroxide assays in the system described by Dr. Armstrong. It is my understanding that the abnormal leukocytes contain some peroxides as gauged by formation of some color derivative upon addition of p-phenylenediamine to the system without supplementing it with exogenous peroxide. My question, specifically, would be this: How much peroxide is present in that system; have any titrations been made of the amount of the peroxide? The second question will be: Suppose you add catalase to the system prior to the addition of p-phenylenediamine; is there still formation of color derivatives observed? Have any studies been done on oxidation, let's say, of added cytochrome C to your assay mixture? Perhaps in this context also, I might ask yet a fourth question, that is, is there any consumption of oxygen taking place in your homogenate before addition of hydrogen peroxide or p-phenylenediamine?

Dr. Armstrong: We have considered all of those questions, too, Dr. Schonbaum, and we have no data on many of those yet. Since last year we have been working on a specific assay just for hydrogen peroxide, and the assay is now ready and usable, and so we will be putting this into operation very shortly, so we have no information as to the concentration of the peroxide at this time in the white cell.

Dr. Schonbaum: You don't know whether this is hydrogen peroxide or any other type of peroxide?

Dr. Armstrong: Not at this point.

Dr. Schonbaum: I do believe that several relatively simple analytical procedures would lend themselves to a very rapid determination as to the nature of the peroxide, and to the quantitative evaluation of its effects. For example, I think that the cytochrome C system offers a very sensitive way of measuring a variety of peroxides other than hydrogen peroxide; it does not preclude, of course, hydrogen peroxide.

Pretreatment with catalase would eliminate hydrogen peroxide
and give you some measure of other peroxides. The effect
of reducing agents before addition of p-phenylenediamine to
the system would also suggest perhaps as to what type of peroxide
it might be; some peroxides, for example, are very readily
reduced by agents like borohydrite, others are very resistant.
And of course it is a difficult, rather ambitious way of doing
it through the polarography examinations, where different
peroxides have different redox potentials, and therefore one
can separate them. But that may be very difficult to do in
a particular system.

Since we have no information on the type or the properties
of those peroxides, perhaps I will now briefly review some
of the properties of peroxidases.

Dr. Rider: Can you give us some examples of other kinds
of peroxides?

Dr. Schonbaum: One type of peroxide which we mentioned
already several times here, for instance are alkyl peroxides,
linoleic acid peroxides. You could have some azo-peroxides,
particularly if the system undergoes rapid auto-oxidation
with formation of aldehydes, you might have traces of peracids
in the system. A very common type of peroxide which is found
in a variety of biological systems are disubstituted peroxides:
ROOR; an example of a peroxide of this type comes from Samuelson's
work on prostaglandin peroxide intermediates. There are also
peroxides which can be conceived as arising in the course
of biological redox reactions. It is quite possible that
the peroxide which is present in Dr. Armstrong's system is
hydrogen peroxide. But, this being the case, it will be very
easily eliminated by the addition of a trace amount of catalase.
You need something in the order of 10^{-9} or 10^{-8} molar to eliminate peroxide in a matter of seconds. On the other hand,
it is not entirely clear to me whether the continuous generation
of peroxide takes place, and this was the reason for asking
whether oxygen consumption occurs on isolation of your homogenate. If oxygen consumption does take place other than
through the normal metabolic pathways, which would have to
be differentiated, the way which one can estimate formation
of peroxide is in the presence and absence of catalase. The
rate of oxygen uptake in the presence of catalase would be
somewhat slower than in its absence, because catalase would
decompose the peroxide, regenerating back some oxygen. So
the problem of determining whether peroxide generation does
take place and how fast, is not an insoluble one, but should
be quite amenable to rigorous experimental study.

Dr. Zeman: Dr. Schonbaum, could the presence of increased
amounts of methemoglobin in these patients indicate the pre-

sence of peroxides? We have measured methemoglobin in patients'
and dogs' blood, and find it to be around 5% in all affecteds,
as compared to about 1-2.2% in our normal controls.

Dr. Schonbaum: That certainly will be one of the possible
interpretations. I would imagine that Dr. Fridovich might
agree that formation of superoxides would also be consistent
with increased formation of methemoglobin. There are a variety
of other ways in which methemoglobin can be formed, for example,
in the presence of nitrite which would pass through that system,
that's one of the well delineated systems in which rapid increase
of methemoglobin occurs. What is definitely indicated is
a defective control of the redox systems which maintain hemoglobin in its reduced state; in other words, you do have to
have a reducing system which readily reduces methemoglobin
back to the ferrous state. In other words, there's a balance
between the oxidative and the reductive pathways. So if one
is defective you might see increased amount of methemoglobin
or apparently we can say there is increased oxidative pathway
whereby the reductive pathway which is normal cannot maintain
that hemoglobin in its reduced state.

Dr. Rider: Dr. Schonbaum, one other quick question.
I missed what you said would inhibit peroxide. You said only
tiny amounts like 10^{-8}, but of what?

Dr. Schonbaum: It does not inhibit, it actually mediates
the decomposition of hydrogen peroxide. The catalase which
I have alluded to is an excellent system for decomposition
of hydrogen peroxide, without necessitating a secondary reducing
agent. Now, the case of glutathione peroxidase, which is
an equally effective mediator of hydrogen peroxide decomposition,
generally of peroxide decomposition, the reaction occurs in
two steps. First, interaction of peroxide with glutathione
peroxidase, presumably oxidizing the enzyme; the second state
is the reduction of the oxidized glutathione peroxidase by
reduced glutathione, with regeneration of the active enzyme
and conversion of reduced glutathione to the oxidized form.
In the case of catalase, hydrogen peroxide serves both as
an electron donor and electron acceptor. In the first stage
of the reaction, hydrogen peroxide interacts with catalase
forming a derivative discovered by Britton Chance 25 years
ago, which is commonly referred to as Compound I. In the
second stage of the reaction, Compound I is reduced by hydrogen
peroxide with liberation of oxygen. Thereby you have a very
efficient cycle of hydrogen peroxide elimination. Since the
reactions are very rapid, in fact, they are not entirely,
but always diffusion-controlled, you need only trace amount
of the enzyme for the very effective decomposition of hydrogen
peroxide.

Dr. Zeman: Dr. Schonbaum, would you like to show your material?

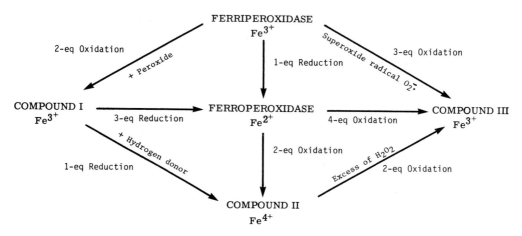

Figure 41. Schematic representation of peroxidase action.

Dr. Schonbaum: To summarize briefly some of the catalytic properties of peroxidases, I invite you to consider some of the data on Fig 41. As far as we know, most peroxidases, in contrast to hemeproteins such as myoglobin, hemoglobin, exist in a ferric oxidation state, designated as ferric per-oxidase, and in this form they engage in a very facile reaction with a variety of peroxides, not only hydrogen peroxide, but also with alkyl peroxides like methyl, ethyl, propyl, butyl, amyl, and equally with peracids, peracetic, perpropionic, any of the higher, and also with aromatic peracids like per-benzoic, forming a derivative first observed by Professor Theorell and kinetically defined by Britton Chance. The de-rivative is known as Compound I. It is not an enzyme peroxide complex; it is an oxidized form of an enzyme in which the redox components are distributed between the methyl ion and the porphyrin microcycle of the prostethic group, which in peroxidases, at least of plant origin, is invariably iron-protoporphyrin 9. I'd like to emphasize this point because the peroxidases with which I believe you are mostly concerned, of the myeloperoxidase type, contain a prostethic group whose chemical nature has not been identified definitely. It is a porphyrin, but unlike protoporphyrin 9, the substituents at the peripheries of the pyrrol rings appear to be different. Compound I can enter into one electron redox reaction forming a spectroscopically distinct derivative which we call Compound II, and in which the redox equivalents appear to be mostly centered at the methyl ion. It is this Compound II which is in most peroxidase reactions the rate limiting intermediate in the course of enzyme mediated reactions. The conversion of ferric peroxidase to Compound I and thereby to Compound II occurs in a stoichiometric relationship, one peroxide molecule giving you one Compound I, which in the presence of a single reducing equivalent can give you Compound II. However, in the presence of excessive peroxides, particularly--not particularly but exclusively--the presence of hydrogen peroxide, another derivative appears, designated as Compound III. It is only observed under conditions of large hydrogen peroxide excess. I mean something in the order of 1000:1 ratio of peroxide to enzyme, that means at least millimolar since most of the reactions of peroxidases are done with micromolar levels of the enzyme, therefore we need approximately millimolar hydrogen peroxide to form Compound III. Compound III is variously designated as oxyperoxidase or peroxidase in an even higher oxidation state than Compound I. I think that Compound III needs perhaps some greater attention than it has received to date, because unlike the difficulty which attends its formation through the hydrogen peroxide pathway, it is very readily generated in the presence of superoxide radical. As you notice, formation of Compound III from ferric peroxidase can be achieved in the presence of dihydroxymaleic acid, oxygen, and trace metal ions, generally manganese. The reaction appeared puzzling for many years, and some decade ago Yamasaki had suggested that the effective oxidant in this system could be superoxide radical, at that time considered a little bit of a curiosity, and I am told by Dr. Fridovich, there were some doubts as to the correctness of this interpretation. His proposal appears to be far more justifiable now, and is believed to be correct. In other words, you could form Compound III through the interaction of ferric peroxidase with superoxide radical. I bring this point to attention for the single reason that p-phenylenediamine is one of the few substrates that reacts fairly readily with Compound III, unlike most other donors. Of course, p-phenylenediamine will also react quite happily with Compound I, and Compound II.

I will now try to develop the evidence which, in my opinion, indicates that p-phenylenediamine is a poor choice for measuring peroxidase activity. The first step in the oxidation of this molecule produces a radical, which subsequently loses an electron. Now what is the fate of this radical? It can, of course, interact with itself, giving you conjugated derivatives. They would be readily oxidizable in the presence of oxygen with the loss of protons and you'll get an azo derivative. Such an azo derivative can be subject to further oxidation

and conjugate your derivatives in various ways. What is not
very clear to me at that stage, is which product is actually
observed in the course of the p-phenylenediamine reaction,
because there is by no means a single derivative at any point.

In other words the radicals produced in the oxidation
of p-phenylenediamine and other unsaturated aromatic amines
and phenols can give rise to a host of conjugated derivatives
with different spectroscopic properties. Under changing experimental conditions a shift from one type of derivative
to another type can readily occur. We can have the whole
gamut of derivatives of this type as emphasized by B. C. Saunders
in the course of his painstaking work in trying to identify
varieties of dyes which might be formed. As an aside, perhaps
I should mention that a great deal of this type of work had
originated some 60 to 70 years ago, following the observation
that peroxidases mediate oxidation of a variety of aromatic
amines and phenols with the formation of colored derivatives.
The dye industry was extremely interested in colors in those
days which provided the impetus for this work. Most of the
assays which we use today, date back to these times.

When we come to consider what is going on in the assay
system and how we could interfere readily with the transformation of one derivative into another, thereby giving somewhat different spectroscopic features...for example, I am
not sure whether the spectra of the derivative formed in
the normal cell extract and defective one are identical or
not. For instance, when you follow the spectrum at 480 nm,
does it mean that you've got simply one type of a derivative
which absorbs much of the energy at 480 nm and another part
at 520 nm, or is there a possibility that derivatives of
different types are formed and give this absorption? Of
course, one of the oxidation products I think which has been
specifically mentioned here was an imine, an analogue of
benzoquinone, and as we know an imine of this type will also
conjugate with the reduced molecule, it will also undergo
hydrolysis to give you quinones. In short, the reaction
is complex.

In the case of o-dianisidine the number of products
is known, it is somewhat smaller, I believe, but it is also a complex
reaction. If we have to limit ourselves to the aromatic
amines for our assay purposes I would like to suggest for
your consideration perhaps a somewhat different amine which
is a substituted derivative, four methyl groups in the ring,
2,3,5,6-tetramethyl-p-phenylenediamine. The virtue of this
compound as I see it would be to eliminate some of the potential
substitutions in the ring, leaving perhaps only the conjugated

chromophore to be considered. Even more attractive might
be to consider oxidation of some dyes, like crystal violet.
The leuko-crystal violet upon oxidation gives you a crystal
violet, a compound which is very readily assayed around 600
nm, which is characterized by very high extinction coefficient
on the order of about 75,000 which, in fact, could be even
suitable for the determination of peroxide. The merit of
a system of this sort is that it does not undergo polymerization
and therefore the reaction is limited to a single oxidation
step. These are some remarks which I would like to leave
you with as to the chemistry of peroxidase and some of its
substrates and perhaps provide some basis for the reservations
which I expressed today regarding p-phenylenediamine.

Dr. Zeman: Thank you Dr. Schonbaum. If I understand
correctly what you are saying, the way to look at the peroxidase
activity is by using hydrogen donors which by virtue of a
single derivative give you a more correct and truer picture
of the kinetics.

Dr. Schonbaum: Might give you...we don't know.

Dr. Zeman: Hopefully so, yes. Thank you. Does anyone
have any comments? Yes, Dr. Rahintula.

Dr. Rahintula: If I understand correctly, the problem
seems to be excess of lipid peroxidation in your disease
and in view of that I'd like to ask Dr. Armstrong and Dr.
Patel if it might not be more relevant to assay using linoleic
acid hydroperoxide than hydrogen peroxide.

Dr. Zeman: I believe we have touched upon this particular
problem and both Dr. Hoekstra and Dr. Fridovich uncovered
some flaw in the data which has been obtained hitherto by
determining acylperoxidase, such as glutathione peroxidase
with linoleic peroxide. The problem which has been completely
neglected in these studies, which incidentally turned out
to show normal enzyme values, is that no consideration has
been given to the concentration of glutathione in the tissues.
The in vitro systems which have been used, and let me repeat,
which have shown normal glutathione oxidase-reductase activity,
are artificial systems and do not, or may not reflect the
situation at the level of the tissue. So, I believe that
we may have to scratch all this data and start from the beginning by first determining glutathione concentration and
availability in the tissues in which we determine the peroxidase
activity.

Dr. Fridovich: I would like to return to something
that was presented by Dr. Armstrong yesterday because I'm
just wondering about the possible explanation and that was

the statement that in the case of a diseased cell there was
a decrease in the soluble PPD-peroxidase but an increase
in insoluble activity. I'm just wondering whether in the
latter case you were certain that a control had been done
in which peroxide was omitted. I'll tell you what I'm thinking
about is an old reaction which used to be called a Nadi reaction. What it is really based upon is p-phenylenediamine
will very readily reduce cytochrome C and, of course, if
there is a little cytochrome oxidase as there would be in
an insoluble, membranous preparation, cytochrome C could
be reoxidized again by cytochrome oxidase and then reduced
again by the p-phenylenediamine and so one could have a p-
phenylenediamine oxidase activity due to the combined presence
of the cytochrome and the cytochrome oxidase. Could you
comment on that?

Dr. Reigh: I think you have to allow for any possibility
with all the oxidating processes that could occur in a pellet.
I'm not sure exactly how you would control this. You could
try to dialyze away peroxide that might be present but then
you also dialyze some of the components which might be necessary for the cytochrome system so you'd eliminate their
activities also. I'm not sure exactly how you could attack
the problem.

Dr. Fridovich: Just following a comment made by Dr.
Schonbaum a very short time previously, and that would be
that the addition of a small amount of catalase would, of
course, take care of any endogenous peroxide and if you then
had activity, you could be certain it was due to something
like the Nadi reaction.

Dr. Reigh: Right. Well, the question I had for Dr.
Schonbaum before is that in these preparations we have normal
catalase activity, but we assume we have peroxide available;
I wonder if there is a possibility that because of the high
Km for catalase that you still have what might be a relatively low concentration of peroxide due to the equilibrium
involved but it would be sufficient to demonstrate peroxidase
activity due to the lower Km of peroxidase.

Dr. Fridovich: Well, I'm trying to focus on the pellet
activity because that very much beclouds the issue of whether
or not there is really a decrease in the level of an enzyme
and I'm trying if possible to find a basis for eliminating
that. The fact that you have normal catalase applies only
to the supernatant fraction because catalase is a soluble
enzyme, but it doesn't apply to your washed pellet, so you
would still have to do the experiment of adding exogenous
catalase.

Dr. Reigh: Yes, I realize you will, but I'm still a
little bit concerned whether it will eliminate all of the
peroxide present.

Dr. Schonbaum: Just a couple of very brief minutiae.
There is no equilibrium between catalase and hydrogen peroxide.
The Km is at first pretty well an operational term rather
than defined in a typical Michaelis-Menten sense.   As I mentioned before, the reaction with hydrogen peroxide is diffusion-
conrolled.   Therefore once the peroxide gets to the catalase
active sites, as far as we can gauge, it never gets out.
The way in which you work, you can have a small stationary
amount of hydrogen peroxide in the presence of catalase if
it is continuously generated.   If you do have a large concentration of competing substrate with hydrogen peroxide,
for instance, some alcohols, formate, formaldehyde,very effectively will compete with hydrogen peroxide for the second
stage of the reaction.   For this reason I have mentioned
a variety of tests for peroxides, first hydrogen peroxide,
alkylperoxides, azoperoxides which would differentiate between
some of those oxidants, but as I have remarked yesterday,
and I am in thorough agreement with Dr. Fridovich on this,
that another pathway of handling p-phenylenediamine oxidation
would be through direct entry into the cytochrome chain.
As we well know, the phenylenediamine derivatives have been
used extensively as an entry into cytochrome C system for
study of site 3 in oxidative phosphorylation.   So there is
a very distinct possibility that you do have oxidation occurring
in this manner which raises an intriguing question, why is
it specific or peculiar to your diseased cells?

Dr. Zeman: In other words, Dr. Schonbaum and Dr. Fridovich, what you are now raising is the possibility that the
p-phenylenediamine reaction, as has been practiced by several
of us, may not even be indicative of enzyme activity, but
of an oxidation-reduction mechanism involving cytochrome
C and cytochrome oxidase.   In order to sort this out, we
would have to perform the experiments which you have suggested;
that is, first to get rid of hydrogen peroxide by the addition
of traces of catalase and then by perhaps poisoning the cytochrome oxidase system or something of this type.

Dr. Schonbaum: Yes, I'll agree with that.   I think
p-phenylenediamine is just a very powerful and relatively
nonspecific reductant.   I should add that some of the compounds
which I have mentioned fall pretty much in the same category
and therefore would not be necessarily sufficiently discrimina-
tory to eliminate some of the questions which we have raised
today.

Dr. Fridovich: The point to be emphasized is that this

problem of this artifact applies specifically to the activity in the insoluble rather than to the activity in the soluble, because cytochrome oxidase is not a soluble enzyme unless one uses detergents to bring it into solution. So it seems to me that the original observation that there is a decrease in the peroxidase activity in the soluble fraction should be held on to as something valid and real, which we now need to find out whether it's due to lack of an activator or it's truly due to a defect in the enzyme or not. I think that is still an important point for investigation.

Dr. Reigh: Yes, one comment is that when we take the pellet fraction we add phenylenediamine first, we observe no color formation until the peroxide is added. I think the suggestion of the best way to do it would be to poison the cytochrome oxidase system to make sure that it does not function after addition of the peroxide. But we do not get just activity from adding the phenylenediamine, the peroxide must be added before we get activity, but to confirm this peroxidase, I think poisoning the cytochrome C oxidase system would be the ideal way.

Dr. Zeman: Dr. Schonbaum, just one brief question. Can you give us a quick reference to the crystal violet substrate for peroxidase activity?

Dr. Schonbaum: Crystal violet had been used for estimating hydrogen peroxide in the presence of peroxidases but not as an assay system some years ago and I can't offhand recall the reference which I'll be glad to send you. However, Bob White working in my laboratory had been intrigued by this reduction and he has some data on the conditions, optimal conditions for the assay. There appear to be some differences in the effectiveness of crystal violet in different peroxidase systems and perhaps it might be relevant in this context because lactoperoxidase appears to be a relatively poor mediator of crystal violet oxidation whereas horseradish peroxidase is a very excellent one. I have no way of guessing what would happen with myeloperoxidase.

Dr. Fridovich: I just wanted to comment that this general type of assay in which one uses a leukodye has been used extensively with different dyes and so, for example, leukomalachite green has been used and it has the same advantages that the leukocrystal violet has. Dihydrofluorescein has been used, in which case the product is fluorescent and one gains several orders of magnitude in sensitivity. Leuco-2,6-dichlorophenol indophenol has been used, so this is really representative of a whole class of assays, any one of which is much more sensitive and to be preferred to these assays in which the oxidation product as described by Dr. Schonbaum can polymerize and give a variety of products which become finally insoluble.

Dr. Schonbaum: Yes, I'm very glad you brought this point up which I haven't made very clear.

Dr. Dawson: Do you have any comments about the pH optimum of some of these peroxidases? That might be an interesting point.

Dr. Schonbaum: Well, I believe already Dr. Hoekstra has made some remarks which bear on that issue and that is that under a variety of conditions you can shift your rate limiting step from the formation of Compound I to the reduction of Compound I or II. Secondly, when you start working with aromatic amines you run into secondary problems and that is that most of the aromatic amines are weak bases with pKs in the region of around 4 to 5 and that means that you have to start taking into account the ionization properties of your substrate, the ionization properties of your products, the susceptibility to secondary reactions. To give you a very simple answer, a variety of phenols appear to be relatively pH independent over a wide range, let's say from about 4 to 8 or thereabouts. As Dr. Fridovich had brought yesterday in the reaction of o-dianisidine the pH optimum which is observed around 6 or 5.8 is no longer seen in the assay that is carried out in the presence of some additives such as ammonia, imidazole, or what have you. So you have to specify the conditions very precisely before giving you sort of a clear cut answer of what is going to be the pH optimum for a given reaction. I understand that from the operational point of view you choose one particular pH and you just simply compare it, assuming that all the other parameters stay constant then everything is OK. But I think in the paper by Dr. Patel and Dr. Zeman the reaction had been examined with p-phenylene-diamine between pH 4 and 8 or thereabouts with very small difference in the rates of oxidation except around 7.5 when the point was strikingly sharp.

Dr. Fridovich: That was seen only with the normal sample. That is to say, there wasn't a sharp peak with the abnormal sample and another thing which worried me, of course, was that that peak was defined by single point. I didn't have a point going up the hill and another one coming down and that always makes one wonder about the validity of that single point, so that should be looked at again.

Dr. Schonbaum: Well, perhaps I can amplify on the question of pH-dependence. Let's say you take a substrate like 2,4,6, trimethylaniline. It's an intriguing substrate because unlike very many other peroxide donors, it does give you a single derivative. It has some nice spectroscopic properties and has been very thoroughly studied by Saunders and Holmes. The pH optimum in that reaction, unlike in many other peroxidase reactions is around 4.5 and whether that reflects to some extent the coupling step or whether the disproportionation of radicals formed in the course of this reaction, is less effective at pH 4.5 is very difficult to say. We do not have the thorough kinetic description of this process. Like in most peroxidase reactions, once you get yourselves in free radical chemistry with a variety of products, the kinetics are hardly measurable.

Dr. Dawson: Certainly the product at pH 6 with p-phenylenediamine is quite different from the one formed at pH 7.3. The color at pH 6 is sort of dark blue, whereas at 7.3 it's more of a reddish brown type of chromogen and we've had reasonable success in demonstrating deficiency in Batten's disease at 6.0.

Dr. Schonbaum: Let me ask you this question. The product formed at 7.3, when you lower pH to 6, what sort of spectroscopic properties has it got?

Dr. Dawson: We haven't really checked that.

Dr. Schonbaum: Do you have products which alter their spectroscopic properties with pH or have you just simply changed the reaction pathways as I have indicated before?

Dr. Dawson: Well, it's just sort of one of the worrying aspects of the reaction.

Dr. Fridovich: What Dr. Schonbaum has suggested to you is your product may act like lithmus or phenolphthalein and in itself be an indicator and so change its color with pH and the thing for you to do then is, to form it at one pH and then see if its color changes when you go to the other pH.

Dr. Dawson: Yes, I think it probably will.

Dr. Armstrong: I would like to comment on Dr. Fridovich's statement about pH optimum. Ours is likewise a single point at 7.3 in the normal, however, we looked at several children with Batten's over the pH of 3.5 to about 10 also, and while their activity is low and it's hard to find a peak, nevertheless, the highest optical density also occurred at 7.3. When we did all the siblings and parents in those two families... they also peaked at 7.3, even though it was a single point, everybody consistently peaked at 7.3.

Dr. Zeman: I think that Dr. Fridovich's remarks as
to the pH dependency of the color and optical density of
the reaction product cannot be taken very lightly.   Indeed
both Dr. Dawson and Dr. Patel did observe these color changes.
It seems to me that it is one more reason to use other substrates and in vitro systems that have been suggested.   Perhaps
Dr. Fridovich could now discuss the possibilities of implicating
superoxide dismutase in this group of disorders.

Dr. Fridovich: If you have the patience to listen for
a few minutes, I'll just give a little background on superoxide
dismutase because it may not be entirely familiar to everybody
here.   I think I should start with oxygen.   Oxygen in the
ground state is a biradical.   It has two unpaired electrons
and the result of this is that it is very much less reactive
than it would otherwise be towards pairs of electrons.   If
you try to reduce oxygen, ground state oxygen, by inserting
a pair of electrons, you run into what is generally called
a spin restriction.   This is best explained in terms of quantum
mechanics, but it finally has to do with the fact that you
would, without inverting one electronic spin, be in the position
of trying to put two parallel spinning electrons in the same
orbit which is forbidden.   As a result of this spin restriction,
it is actually easier for oxygen to be reduced by steps which
are univalent and involve therefore one electron transfer
at a time.   Now if this is the case, and if we start with
molecular oxygen, and we have to consider adding four electrons
to go to two molecules of water, we have to consider intermediates, and these intermediates include the superoxide
radical which is reduced from oxygen by one electron, hydrogen
peroxide, which is a 2 electron reduction product and hydroxyl
radical which is the 3 electron reduction product.   Now it
has been known of course for a long time that hydrogen peroxide
was a frequently met intermediate of oxygen reduction and
the thing that is now apparent, that has been known for not
that long, the last decade only, is that the superoxide radical
is also a fairly common intermediate of oxygen reduction.
Just as we have catalases and peroxidases of various kinds
to function as defenses against the accumulation of hydrogen
peroxide by scavenging it, we have superoxide dismutases
which function in a similar way towards superoxide and scavenge
it.

The superoxide dismutases are of several different kinds.
They all carry out the same reaction, which is an oxidation-
reduction reaction between two superoxide radicals in which
an electron is transferred from one through the enzyme to
the other so that the product of the dismutase reaction are
oxygen and hydrogen peroxide. The catalases and peroxidases
have to take it from there and get rid of the hydrogen peroxide.

Now, I started to say that there are several different kinds of these enzymes and the distribution is as follows: In the cytosol of all eukaryotic cells there is a superoxide dismutase which contains copper and zinc and is blue-green in color and has a molecular weight of 32,000. It is made up of two subunits. In fact it is identical with the proteins known for a long time as hemocuprein, cerebrocuprein, hepato-cuprein, erythrocuprein. These were proteins isolated on the basis of copper content without known function. They are identical with the cytosol superoxide dismutase. Now that is in eukaryotes. In bacteria, there are two different kinds of superoxide dismutase which are similar to each other. These contain two different metals. One contains iron as the prosthetic group and the other contains manganese, but otherwise the proteins are similar, that is to say in terms of molecular weight, the subunit composition, even amino acid sequence. Now let's consider E.coli as an example. It has both of these superoxide dismutases, the manganese containing one and the iron containing one and you might inquire whether they may not be in different places in the E.coli. In fact they are. The manganese-containing one is in the matrix of the cell, and the iron-containing one is in the periplasmic space. In fact there is good data to show that the function is divided between these two enzymes. The one that is in the matrix, the interior of the E.coli, protects the cell against superoxide which is made internally as a consequence of its own restoration... its own reduction of oxygen. The periplasmic enzyme, that is the iron enzyme, functions to protect the cell against superoxide which comes at it from the outside, that is superoxide generated in the medium as the result of a variety of autooxidation processes.

So far I have spoken of 3 kinds of superoxide dismutases and I will throw in the 4th as there is actually a lot of interest in it. If one looks at mitochondria of any eukaryon, mammalian, plants, yeast, or whatever, one finds there a manganese-containing superoxide dismutase which is remarkably similar to the one found in the matrix of the bacteria. The reason I say there is a great deal of interest in this enzyme is related to the theory that mitochondria might have originated as symbions: prokaryons that entered into an en-dosymbiosis with a protoeukaryote. The fact that the mito-chondria have a superoxide dismutase very much like the bacterial one, of course, supports this notion and the similarity has now been investigated down to the level of amino acid sequence. There is in fact 80% absolute sequence homology between the bacterial types and the mitochondrial types of superoxide dismutase, but no homology between the mitochondrial and cytosolic enzymes, which is very nice to report.

I don't know what more I should say about this, except

that it has been our hope for a long time that one might
be able to observe with a higher animal, something that we
were able to do on purpose with bacteria and that is, we
have been able to generate mutants with defects of the superoxide dismutase. The expectation was that these mutants
would then have a decreased tolerance for oxygen. This has
been done and observed and of course there is good evidence
that the enzymes are absolutely essential for survival by
respiring cells. We had hoped that perhaps something like
this would be found as a naturally occurring mutant in a
higher animal. So far there isn't any evidence for this.
Perhaps because the defect, certainly the full defect in
the enzyme, would be absolutely lethal and the homozygote
would never survive past the one-cell state, but it may be
that some such disease, as the Batten's disease we are discussing, might depend upon a partial defect in the superoxide
dismutase or a partial defect seen only in one tissue such
as in brain. This is an old idea, we have partly investigated
it, but I think it is worth more serious efforts to find
out if the level of the enzyme is perhaps abnormal in the
tissues of the homozygous dogs.

Dr. Zeman: Thank you Dr. Fridovich. Perhaps we can
clarify one question which arises from the observation that
the pigments which we believe are due to peroxidation of
unsaturated fatty acids do occur already in utero. We have
been able to demonstrate this at least in dogs. So the question
is: What can you tell us about the age-dependent activity
of this set of enzymes and would there be evidence of superoxide
dismutase activity in embryonic or fetal tissue, which would
explain our morphological findings?

Dr. Fridovich: With respect to whether or not the enzymes
would be present in embryonic or fetal tissues, I think I
can answer absolutely that it would have to be. Among the
things that have been done, is to survey a wide range of
organisms and the superoxide dismutases are present in absolutely all respiring organisms. This includes various
types of bacteria, fungi, plants, fish, birds, insects, and
so on. The only organisms in fact which have ever been found
not to contain the enzyme are organisms which are sensitive
obligate anaerobes. I am quite certain that both the egg
and the sperm would have superoxide dismutase and the fertilized
egg would have superoxide dismutase in it.

If I may, I would like to make a comment with respect
to the lipid peroxidation. We can show that if one takes
an unsaturated fatty acid, let us say, linolenic acid, and
exposes it to any system which is making the free radical
superoxide, we have most often used xanthine oxidase which
is an enzymatic reaction known to make this radical, if one

364

does that, it is possible to show that peroxidation of the unsaturated fatty acid occurs, that the first product of this is the conjugated diene-hydroperoxide that we can see on thin layer chromatography or follow at 235 nm. Superoxide dismutase, if added to such an in vitro reaction system, inhibits the formation of the hydroperoxide of the fatty acid, therefore inhibits the peroxidation, but so also does catalase.

This brings me back again to what I was saying yesterday, that perhaps the worst thing about both superoxide radical and hydrogen peroxide is that they may react together to generate hydroxyl radical, which then by hydrogen abstraction could initiate lipid peroxidation. Therefore we should look upon superoxide dismutase as one barrel of a double-barrel defense against oxygen toxicity. I guess what I am really trying to say is that I could as easily explain excess lipid peroxidation in terms of a deficit of superoxide dismutase as I could in terms of a deficit of a peroxidase, either could do.

Dr. Zeman: I think the concept of a double-barreled mechanism preventing the destructive effect of peroxidation on cellular components is rather enticing with respect to the explanation of the pathogenesis of these diseases. There is abundant evidence that lipid peroxidation is not as lethal to the normal cell as it could be, if there were no protection whatsoever. So really what we are talking about is an insufficient partial protection which, integrated over time, produces a progressive lesion, which in itself shows only a superficial correlation with the manifestation of the disease. In other words, we have evidence, at least in the dogs, but also in man, that products of lipid peroxidation occur already during the fetal period and continue to accumulate to rather massive proportions, but it is another 15 months after birth in the dogs, and several years in human patients, until the disease becomes manifest clinically, and at that time, the damage of course has already been done.

Dr. Fridovich: I wonder whether this kind of chronic experiment has ever been undertaken in dogs, and that would be to see if it would be possible to exacerbate the symptoms and the rate of development of symptoms, by keeping the dogs at an elevated partial pressure of oxygen, say in an atmosphere containing 60 or 80% of oxygen, rather than air which is only 20%. Or of course one could go in the other direction and wonder whether a decrease in PO_2 would ameliorate the development of symptoms.

Dr. Zeman: Neither of those experiments have been done. We have considered them, but these are rather difficult experiments to perform.

Dr. Hoekstra: I'd like to ask Dr. Fridovich about the hydroxyl radical. If this is potentially the most damaging species, or the one most likely to abstract the hydrogen and initiate lipid peroxidation, what factors would affect the amount of it, relative to the amount of hydrogen peroxide and oxygen? Also is it feasible to measure the amount of hydroxyl radical in preparations from control and diseased subjects?

Dr. Fridovich: There is one great problem with the hydroxy radical, and that is that it reacts rapidly with everything. Leon Dorfman has gotten together a tabulation of at least 150 different compounds with measured rate constants for reaction with the hydroxy radical and I have looked that list over from one end to the other and I don't think that there is anything on it that reacts with less of a rate constant than 10^4 and 10^5 M^{-1}sec^{-1}, most reactions are going faster, like 10^9 or 10^{10} M^{-1}sec^{-1}, so that if hydroxyl radicals form, about the best hope you have for measuring it, is to put in a fairly high concentration of something that can scavenge it, which would then give a known product. We very frequently for example, use benzoate in this way. Benzoate reacts at about 6.6×10^9 with OH· so that if I had a process like the production of ethylene, which I suspect is dependent on OH·, if one can inhibit that by adding benzoate, then one has gained some confidence that perhaps it was really OH· which was involved. But a note of caution is required here, because it being so reactive, it could easily be overlooked if there was lots of the substrate that was doing the scavenging.

Dr. Patel: I was going to comment on the previous question asked, namely keeping the animal under high and low partial oxygen pressure. This has been done with normal rats, and you can see oxidative damage when you keep the rats in high oxygen. This can be prevented by feeding with antioxidants such as vitamin E. The reverse is true for keeping them at lower oxygen pressure which extends life expectancy.

Dr. Zeman: This is for normal animals but the problem we are faced with is that we should perform this experiment in a genetically controlled disease in which we have reasonably good evidence for peroxidation being one of the major pathogenic mechanisms and one way of finding out precisely whether there is peroxidation by oxygen toxicity is to perform the experiments which have been suggested by Dr. Fridovich.

Dr. Philippart: I have a question for Dr. Fridovich. Is the effect of copper deficiency on superoxide dismutase known?

Dr. Fridovich: Well, you mean has it been looked at.

Dr. Philippart: Yes.

Dr. Fridovich: Dr. Cartwright in Salt Lake City, has been studying copper deficient swine for quite a long time and at one point I did contact him to get samples and the results were as follows: When the copper deficiency was moderately severe, such that the ceruloplasmin level was O, the superoxide dismutase level was still normal. When the copper deficiency became more severe, cytochrome oxidase began to decrease and the superoxide dismutase level was still normal. Finally, when the animals were very sick, close to death, superoxide dismutase level fell to about 1/2 or 1/3. This was as low as we ever saw it go, probably because the animals couldn't survive with a greater decrease than that.

So that is one part of it. The other half is that I mentioned that there is also zinc in the cytosol enzyme and there is an investigator at the VA Hospital in Baltimore who studies zinc-deficient rats. He sent the samples for that material, and again, only when the animals were almost moribund did we start to see a decrease in the superoxide dismutase of the cytosol.

Dr. Rahimtula: Dr. Patel mentioned that a decrease in partial pressure of oxygen would prevent lipid peroxidation. The Km for oxygen is only about 5 micromolar for lipid peroxidation and I am wondering if just decreasing the pressure slightly would bring such a big change.

Dr. Fridovich: I think the important point here is not the Km for oxygen for lipid peroxidation in an in vitro system, but rather the Km for oxygen for those reactions that are making the radicals that initiate lipid peroxidation in an enzymatic system. And so for example, with several enzymes that we've looked at, xanthine oxidase, aldehyde oxidase and dihydro-orotic dehydrogenase, although the Km for oxygen in the normal oxidase pathway--oxygen to hydrogen peroxide--is rather low, about 10^{-5} molar, the percentage of the total electron flux to the enzyme, which is making superoxide, continues to increase with increased partial oxygen pressure up to higher than 1.5 atm. So I think that based on the way these enzymes act in vitro, the expectation would certainly be that the respiring cell would make more and more of the superoxide, the higher the partial pressure of oxygen.

Dr. Rahimtula: I would like to ask you another question. You just mentioned sometime back that superoxide would react with hydrogen peroxide and produce the hydroxyl radical. I presume you are referring to the Haber-Weiss reaction. Has his reaction ever been demonstrated and its product identified as hydroxyl radical?

Dr. Fridovich: Let me give you the data that is on hand. Suppose we took a xanthine oxidase system which we know is making both superoxide and peroxide. If to this I add methionol, I can observe the production of ethylene... right... so that the actual thing being measured is the rate of production of ethylene by gas chromatographic assay. Put in superoxide dismutase, it inhibits ethylene production, therefore hydrogen peroxide is required for ethylene production. Now both the Haber-Weiss reaction and the superoxide and the hydrogen peroxide reaction are giving me the material which is truly the attacking species that makes the methionol into ethylene. How do I test that? Well, I say let me take some things which I know to scavenge hydroxyl, but react neither with superoxide nor with hydrogen peroxide and see if they inhibit ethylene production. And so ethanol, mannitol, benzoate were tested, all of which have this property of scavenging hydroxyl radicals and they do inhibit ethylene production. Now that is the kind of evidence that I have. I have it for several other reactions besides ethylene production. But that is the evidence. Now whether you find it satisfactory or not, I can't tell. I find it rather difficult to explain any other way.

Dr. Schonbaum: In raising a hypothesis of hydroxyl radical participation, Dr. Fridovich has also presented the extensive data particularly those of Dorfman on the extraordinary activity of hydroxyl radicals, as we know the homolytic scission energy of H-O bonds is in the range of 110 Kcal. The hydroxyl radical is one of the most powerful oxidants which we have. But under those circumstances, one would expect that the lesions would express themselves in a variety of other ways. In this context perhaps, in the diseased system, is there evidence for any other type of deficiency or any other enzyme abnormality except those which you have referred to as peroxidase or lipid peroxidation? Is there anything else with any other enzyme assayed for or are they all normal? Are they the only systems which would show abnormalities, simply lipid peroxidation or peroxidation without any other abnormality?

Dr. Zeman: Quite a few enzymes have been looked at in this particular disease. On the assumption that the initiator of the peroxidative reaction may be ferrous iron, we have looked at the vitamin E dependent enzymes in hemesynthesis, such as δ-aminolevulinic acid synthetase and dehydratase and indirectly, ferrochelatase. At one time it appeared that these enzymes might be deficient in patients with Batten's disease, but strangely enough, the patients do not show the hemolytic anemia which you would associate with a deficiency of these hemesynthesizing enzymes.

Further more, quite a few hydrolases have been examined and found normal. From a survey of enzyme activities emerged the fact that the isolated pigments, namely the cross-linked polymers have very high activities of cyclic 2'3'-AMP hydrolase, which is a marker enzyme for myelin. So your question, which I believe tries to aim at the inactivation of enzymes by the process of homolytic scission and formation of dialdehydes and of other carbonyls and inactivation by cross-linkage, is not demonstrable, at least not in the system that we have looked at.

Dr. Schonbaum: Well the question was simply based on the proposition that the hydroxyl radicals being nonspecific, produce damage which is perhaps more general than the one which we have been told about.

Dr. Fridovich: I would just like to comment on this. I certainly agree with the notion expressed by Dr. Schonbaum that since hydroxyl is reactive towards so many things, it should do many things, but I would like to raise two points and one is that if one were imposing a low level of continuous damage across the board in many different enzymes, that enzyme which would suffer the greatest decrease in its steady state activity would be that one whose turnover rate was slowest, that is to say the one whose rate of resynthesis was therefore slowest so that perhaps what one should do would be look at half-lives of a number of enzymes. This would mean to look at the list and pick an enzyme whose half-life is the longest and see if that is diminished somewhat. That is the first point.

The second point is quite different and has to do with the fact that probably the distance that a hydroxyl radical could diffuse before it reacted with something in a cell would be rather small, simply because of the great abundance of things that it could react with and its great reactivity and so this point has to do with where the localization...where the hydroxyl radical is generated. For example, if you have a membrane with a lipid hydroperoxide then it would certainly react at the membrane rather than out in the cytosol.

Dr. Zeman: I am afraid that we do not have the answer to the question which has been raised with respect to which biological species are inactivated by hydroxyl radicals. However, there is the following observation and that is that as a general rule, those nerve cells which have the lowest

metabolic rate per unit volume of cytoplasm are the ones
which are knocked out first, which is in analogy to the inactivation of the enzyme which has the lowest turnover rate.
Vice versa, those nerve cells are usually best preserved
which as we know from all sorts of turnover studies have
the highest metabolic efficiency. So this would be in agreement
with the assumption that whatever radicals are formed do
inactivate biological species.

With respect to enzyme activity, which usually is expressed
as specific activity, i.e., per unit weight protein, the
cell reacts to the cumulative peroxidative damage, with a
loss of cytoplasmic bulk, retaining relatively normal ratios
of its various chemical components.

Now Dr. Miquel pointed out that the accurate measurements
on cells affected by lipid peroxidation do show a reduction
in RNA. Basically, this is similar to what we see, but when
you come down to measuring these concentrations in a homogenate
the results may not reflect the cytoplasmic loss.

Dr. Rider: Could you clarify what cells you're speaking
of when you say those were fast in metabolic turnover and
those that were slow in metabolic turnover. I'd like to
try and correlate it with the clinical picture.

Dr. Zeman: Cells with a high metabolic rate of activity
are generally those which have to maintain a very large surface
area because most of the energy is used up on the surface
of the nerve cell. If we measure the surface area of a cell
and this is done by measuring the dendritic apparatus because
it contains 95 percent of the cell surface, and relate this
to the volume of the perikaryon, that is the perinuclear
cytoplasm where 95 percent of the metabolic machinery is
housed, then we find a very good correlation of the coefficient
between surface area and perikaryon volume on the one hand
and the turnover rate of amino acid and RNA precursors on
the other. As a general rule, all large-bodied nerve cells,
such as motor cells, Purkinje cells, large pyramidal cells,
have a high metabolic coefficient, whereas small cells with
little cytoplasm which are generically referred to as granule
cells have a very low metabolic coefficient and these are
the cells which are preferentially damaged and lost in these
diseases.

Dr. Rider: I don't quite understand it because the
disease of course is manifested by lack of motor ability;
you're losing your Betz cells in the brain and so forth.
Now I'm not familiar with the granule cells, but certainly
in this disease, Wolf, those cells that are clinically implicated are the ones with the high metabolic rate.

Dr. Zeman: That is not quite so. We know that motor function can be lost, even so the primary motor neurons are fully preserved, because the motor system is not independent, only in our textbooks it is so. In reality, motor function can be lost by a lack of either facilitating or inhibitory influences at many different levels of the first and second motor neuron. This is a neurophysiological fact, but from the morphological aspect it is quite typical that the small nerve cells in the second and fourth cortical layer are lost at a time when the large nerve cells in the third, fifth and sixth layers are still preserved and this would certainly produce motor dysfunction. The loss of small neurons is particularly evident in the cerebellar cortex where we have something like 400 billion granule cells, most of which are destroyed. In contrast, a significant number of Purkinje cells, these are very large-bodied cells with a high metabolic activity, are preserved.

Dr. Miquel: In relation to this distribution of free radical injury of brain, I want to mention that Dr. Brizzee from the Delta Regional Primate Center has been involved in a very careful study of the lipofuscin distribution in the monkey brain and I have sent him recently six old mice from our colony that are 30 months old, very, very old. He has started to look at the distribution of the lipofuscin and to correlate it with that in the monkey brain. We are also planning to get involved in the topography of lipofuscin in the human brain and we may use the brains from the Institute of Neuropathology of Berlin, which has a tremendous collection of very old human brains because the population of Berlin is very old. The young people have left, so they have lots of brains from healthy old people, who died of old age. Brizzee is very interested in looking at the lipofuscin distribution of the human brain. I think it will be worthwhile to do similarly careful studies on the topography of lipofuscin in Batten's disease, because we may get some hints about the pathogenesis. In the mouse brain we see tremendous degeneration in the nucleus hypoglossus. We don't know why, but I wonder if anything is known about which areas deteriorate the most in Batten's disease. You know in the human brain the basal ganglia are very affected, you know, Parkinson's disease and also we see axonal dystrophy even in old normal mice, same as in human aging, some areas that for some reason deteriorate very fast. So I wonder if the distribution of this injury in Batten's disease is similar to normal aging.

Dr. Zeman: I believe we have to make a distinction between the accumulation of lipopigment and the loss or lethal damage of a cell due to the formation of lipopigment. Those cells in the human brain which disappear most readily in Batten's disease are not necessarily those which show the

371

heaviest accumulation of lipopigments. In fact, the largest
amounts of lipopigments are found in those cells which have
the capability to survive and I believe they survive because
of their enormous synthetic potential; that is to say, for
every mole of inactivated enzyme, membrane and nucleic acid
moiety another mole is very easily generated, whereas in
other cells, this loss is not compensated for to the same
extent by a lesser synthetic activity or capability and therefore the cell degenerates. Now, if we develop coefficients
of the density of endoplasmic reticulum, mitochondria and
the Golgi system, then we find that those cells which are
showing a very high coefficient are the ones which also harbor
large quantities of the pigment but are vital, whereas the
other cells which show very low coefficients have disappeared
at the same time.

Furthermore, and this is perhaps the explanation, a
cell which is subject to cytoplasmic damage of any type does
not necessarily keel over and die. It has an adaptive mechanism,
a relatively simple one; namely, it will reduce its surface
activity. So, for instance, a Purkinje cell which under
normal conditions in the physiological state has about 6,000
dendritic spines which represent an enormous surface area
for the cell, when subject to the accumulation of lipopigments,
it may wind up with no more than 100 dendritic spines and
the remainder of this expansive protoplasmatic system is
completely lost. The perikaryon will remain and that is
chock full with pigment.

Dr. Schonbaum: May I return for the moment to a discussion
of the hydroxyl radical. Dr. Fridovich had mentioned that
one way of intercepting hydroxyl radicals goes through the
benzoate system or ethanol in the course of which other radicals
are being formed. Nonetheless, at least in the benzoate
system the radical is less reactive and perhaps it serves
the useful purpose to dissipate the potential hydroxyl
radical in this manner. There is a partial contradiction
because if we do have reaction of hydroxyl radicals in an
extended cage, then the benzoate under those conditions will
not be effective or will not be a better trap than anything
else. But nonetheless, let's accept for a while the hypothesis
that such radicals are formed and that perhaps we should
do something to get rid of them. Now, I don't know at what
level the benzoate can be taken up by the mammalian organisms
without cell damage, but it would seem that perhaps other
aromatic or heterocyclic, carboxylic acids would not be less
effective than benzoate in trapping such radicals. Were
that the case and were such radicals formed, do you think,
and I tread on very dangerous grounds right now, because
I'm totally unfamiliar with this area, but would you consider,
perhaps as a therapy, use of high doses of nicotinic acid--
we know that nicotinic acid can be tolerated at massive doses--
gram quantities, in fact--do you see any virtue in attempting

such trials on a clinical basis in view of the fact that
nicotinic acid, apart from perhaps some minor side effects,
would be relatively non-toxic?

Dr. Zeman: You suggest to use nicotinic acid as a scavenger for hydroxyl radicals?

Dr. Schonbaum: Well, we have considered here a hypothesis.
The point is what are we going to do about it? In a sense
we say, well, is it an extended cage, is it a side reaction,
is it a diffusable one? We have talked yesterday about the
levels of glutathione which we didn't have any answer because
glutathione itself would be, of course, a trap for things
like that, but if we feel that something of this nature needs
to be taken care of and we need something which can be used
on a clinical basis, where one would prefer to use a substance
which is known to be as non-toxic as possible.

Dr. Zeman: The answer to your question is yes, we have
no good explanation for the biochemical aspects of this disease.
The hypothesis still is that there is damage by the products
of peroxidative reactants such as the hydroxyl radical and
we have tried to take care of this particular aspect by giving
our patients methionine as a radical scavenger. Perhaps what
you are suggesting is that there are different affinities
for different hydroxy and hydroperoxy radicals, for scission
fragments of aliphatic chains, and that a variety of radical
scavengers would do more than high doses of a single one.

Dr. Schonbaum: Well, we're grasping here at straws
you understand, it's totally hypothetical and we have at
the moment no evidence that there are hydroxyl radicals,
but we say if something like that does happen, if there is
a marginal chance that it could be intercepted in any way,
that it is not totally localized, not caged in effect, because
if it is totally in a cage, well before it can diffuse from
the cage, nothing can intercept it by the very definition
of the cage. But from the somewhat theoretical discussion
which we had before, one is wondering whether some practical
result would come, by attempting to use potential scavengers
which in themselves are physiologically acceptable.

Dr. Zeman: Just one question. Do you have data, or
would you stipulate that nicotinic acid and glutathione are
more efficient than methionine on a per weight basis?

Dr. Schonbaum: No certainly I have no data that nicotinic acid is more efficient. I have some understanding,
I believe, that nicotinic acid is relatively non-toxic; as
far as glutathione is concerned, I am quite sure it should
be far more effective than nicotinic acid in dissipating any

radicals whatsoever. But since we don't know what the level
is, or where we are trying to introduce high concentrations
of the scavengers, and since we cannot introduce glutathione
into the cells by increasing glutathione level, it is not
taken up, I don't know how effectively the methionine is
taken up by the cells, what intracellular concentrations
of methionine you can reach. The idea being that perhaps
using less effective scavenger, such as nicotinic acid, but
one which is readily permeable, that you might reach the
effective levels of the scavenger which are greater than
those which on an absolute basis would be more reactive.

Dr. Zeman: Right.

Dr. Fridovich: I'd just like to comment. It's kind
of amusing perhaps, but benzoic acid is actually rather non-
toxic. I have myself on occasion taken 5 to 10 grams in laboratory exercises so that we can isolate hippuric acid from
the urine. But I really, in a serious vein, I would really
not like to be the cause of the use of something like this.
The data that we have for in vitro systems, I consider is
fairly good, but it's an enormous step to be taken from a
reaction mixture with a pure enzyme etc. to what is perhaps
happening inside the cell, and it would certainly be premature
to be attempting to administer things which might function
as scavengers of hydroxyl radical in vivo. So, I don't want
to be responsible for that.

Dr. Rider: When we speak of nicotinic acid, I think
what's available is the nicotinamide, you know, niacin. I
don't think you can get the nicotinic acid.

Dr. Schonbaum: Yes, we can get nicotinic acid quite
readily.

Dr. Fridovich: I think the confusion here arises from
the fact that the ordinary vitamin form is the nicotinamide,
but the nicotinic acid is certainly available as Dr. Schonbaum says in large quantities. There is a difference, I
think, in the administration of the two. If large amounts
and I probably am getting them confused, but I believe if
large amounts of the nicotinamide are involved there are
certain rashes and things like this that would come up which
don't come up with nicotinic acid.

Dr. Miquel: We are obtaining excellent data on the
increase of the life span of drosophila and of mice with
a non-toxic antioxidant. I am amazed that it is not already
on the market here, because it is being used all over Europe.
I have the scientific literature on that. First I would
like to give you the formula of this drug and then I'll show

you some electromicrographs on its effects.

Dr. Rider: Are you talking about centrophenoxine?

Dr. Miquel: No. Thiazolidine carboxylic acid. It is a derivative of cysteine, and I can take at least 2-3 grams per day.

Dr. Zeman: Dr. Miquel will now present data on a water-soluble antioxidant, which may qualify as a therapeutic agent, as a chain-breaking principle for lipid oxidation.

Dr. Miquel: We know that tocopherol may have a very important role, but cysteine and other SH derivatives also play very important roles in preventing injury produced by free radicals. A few years ago I read in a review article by Bender on the Pharmacology of Aging that thiazolidine carboxylic acid is being used in experimental studies on rats in Roumania. The author claimed that rats lived longer when they were fed a diet containing the compound. Subsequently I suggested to some friends in the pharmaceutical industry that this chemical really showed potential. Now there is a lot of scientific literature on this compound, which shows that it protects liver cells against environmental injury. It is well tolerated by man, even at doses of 2 grams a day. In view of this data, I did some testing of the sodium salt, of thiazolidine carboxylic acid in drosophila, and I found the best increases in life span so far, among the 20 odd anti-oxidants that I have used. In fact, it produced a 22% increase in the mean and maximal longevity of the fruit fly. So in view of this data we set up aging experiments in 8-month-old retired C_{57} breeder mice. This is an excellent strain for aging studies. Some 200 mice were fed vitamin E, 3 parts per 1000 in the food. Their brains really look very well preserved, but the bad side of the treatment is that the animals, after about one year on this diet start losing weight. Also I got some early mortality in this experiment. I just saw by chance an advertisement for vitamin E as the best reducing agent for weight control, so I can now support that claim. The thyroid of these animals seems to be too well preserved, so I think we may stimulate the thyroid, although the toxicity is not very high. Nevertheless there is something there to worry about.

Dr. Rider: That's a very high dose of vitamin E.

Dr. Miquel: 3 per 1000 is a very high dose, but Tappel used the same dose in one of his experiments, and he didn't see any toxicity. Tappel claimed there was a reduction of lipopigments in testes, heart, and several other organs, but not in brain, as determined by spectrophotofluorometry, but with the light microscope we see a very marked decrease of pigment in brain cells. I think we have to worry a little bit about not going overboard on the dose. A few grams a day for humans is safe for the time being--I wouldn't go above that. But I would complement vitamin E with these other compounds for example one which combines tocopherol with centrophenoxine. Instead of using tocopherol acetate, and loading the body with acetate that is not doing anything, and instead of using the diethylaminoethanol, which is a non-functional part of centrophenoxine, we have combined the chlorophenoxyacetate with tocopherol producing a liposoluble antioxidant that has the activity of tocopherol plus whatever the centrophenoxine may do, because the active component really is in this part of the molecule. We are also able to obtain the magnesium salt of thiazolidine carboxylic acid; normally the sodium salt is used, but the sodium is not doing any good either. On the other hand, the magnesium may play a very important role in glia involved with fighting lipid peroxides in brain. I think it is worth looking into what magnesium may do to protect brain against lipid peroxidation.

We are feeding mice, with an equivalent age of about 55 years for a human subject, chlorophenoxy acetate tocopherol, and the same amount, namely 0.07%, of magnesium thiazolidine carboxylate. The animals are doing extremely well, they preserved their body weight better than the controls; I have tested them with some techniques we are developing to check neuromuscular coordination; we put the mice on a string and they just hold onto it and we measure for how long they can do it. We have also done some preliminary experiments with gas chromatography of the urine. The mice treated with these drugs show a pattern that is much closer to the young than the untreated controls. And, finally, with the electron microscope, we find a marked decrease in lipopigments, as compared with controls.

Dr. Zeman: Dr. Miquel, the theme of your presentation, it seems to me, would be that the situation in Batten's disease might be analogous to physiologic aging, perhaps being telescoped as regards time. If I understand the regimen correctly which you propose here, you give a combination of radical scavengers and antioxidants, which brings us back to the question of radical damage in these tissues.

Dr. Miquel: There is a further point in this combination. According to the old papers on centrophenoxine, or chlorophenoxyacetate or diethylaminoethanol from France, this drug is supposed to stimulate the pentose pathway, a point actually proven by appropriate enzyme determinations. This might be an unspecific stimulation of the metabolism of a cell to fight off any kind of injury. So this treatment has three different

components. A liposoluble antioxidant, a watersoluble antioxidant, and the unspecific metabolic stimulant. I don't
believe it is the elixir of youth, but it's as good a combination as we can figure out at the present time.

Dr. Zeman: Inasmuch as Batten's disease appears to be
particularly damaging to the brain tissue, and inasmuch as
we know that the oxidative reactions are probably going on
at a much higher rate in liver, I wonder whether Dr. Rahimtula
could tell us a little bit about his liver work, with respect
to peroxidation. Perhaps you can give us also a thumbnail
sketch as to the protective mechanisms that you have uncovered
in liver.

Dr. Rider: Dr. Miquel, could I ask you where is this
compound available? You say it's available in Europe, but
can we get it in the United States?

Dr. Miquel: Yes, it is available in the United States

Dr. Rider: I'm intrigued with the thiazolidine carboxylic
acid, because that's been used in humans.

Dr. Miquel: Yes, it's already cleared for human use.
No problem. No toxicity whatsoever.

Dr. Rahimtula: Let me say a few words about lipid peroxidation in the liver and some of the protective mechanisms
that might be operating. The peroxidation has primarily been
studied in the endoplasmic reticulum by several workers.
The usual way is by ferrous iron-mediated reactions and the
iron is kept in the ferrous state either enzymically through
the flavoprotein NADPH-cytochrome P450 reductase, or nonenzymical-
ly through ascorbate. Ascorbate would reduce ferric to ferrous.
Under these conditions you can get extensive lipid peroxidation, usually phosphatidyl serine is metabolized, and up to
15% of the lipid can be degraded. What usually happens is
that you get a radical formed and then you get a conjugation
with a double bond. You get a 232 or 234 peak when you get
the conjugated diene and the hydroperoxide formed. After
some time you get chain fission that gives rise to aldehydes,
ketones, and polymerization and other cross-linked products,
and what one usually measures as malonaldehyde is a breakdown
product, way down at the bottom, which is formed with a yield
of only 4-5%.

Once a lipid peroxide is formed, there are several ways
of breaking it. In the cytosol you have glutathione peroxidase,
which uses NADPH and it breaks down lipid peroxides to just
one product which is the corresponding alcohol. Hydroperoxide
can also be broken down in microsomes and in mitochondria.

In microsomes and mitochondria you have what is called a semi-dehydroascorbate reductase system which uses NADH and ascorbate. In tissues like adrenal where a high level of ascorbate is present, this enzyme may play quite an important role.

The other finding we have made is that cytochrome P450 in the liver can function as a very powerful peroxidase. In this system, oxygen uptake and malonaldehyde production are very similar, and they seem to go along together. The rate of oxygen uptake is about 150 nM. Eventually, malonaldehyde formation plateaus, because most of the cytochrome P450 is destroyed. We have also used cumene hydroperoxide as the initiator to start up this reaction. You can do this in a model system by using purified cytochrome P450, and either eggyolk lecithin, or extracted lipids from microsomes or arachidonate or lineolate and you can study the uptake of oxygen. If you use an unsaturated fatty acid that is slightly oxidized, like you just opened a vial of arachidonic acid and you put it in with P450, after a small lag period, you will get a massive oxygen uptake. So you don't even need a trigger; presumably there is a level of peroxide that is built up, and after that the reaction goes. There are two types of inhibitors which operate on this cytochrome P450 system. Type I binds to cytochrome P450 and so inhibits some of its function and Type II denatures it, for example, aniline or tetramethyl-p-phenylenediamine, which act as antioxidants. And they seem to inhibit lipid peroxidation to a more or less similar extent, both the microsomal one or the reconstituted one using cytochrome P450 and lecithin. These studies were performed on whole liver cells; the advantage in using liver cells is that there might be a protective mechanism that operates within the cell which you might not see using microsomes. We used two basically different approaches. One is to use the ADP-iron catalyzed peroxidation, and the other one is the cumene hydroperoxide catalyzing action; now these two reactions are mediated quite independently. The P450-dependent reaction is the one that uses cumene hydroperoxide, and the flavoprotein one uses NADPH and ADP-iron. The peroxide catalyzed reaction is very much faster, and is also attenuated very quickly, within 10 to 20 minutes there is no further malonaldehyde formation. Vice versa, the flavoprotein catalyzed reaction will go on for maybe 20, 30 minutes and then plateau off.

Now as far as protective mechanisms go, what could be the factor that would protect against further increase? One could look at NADPH levels during peroxidation or at glutathione levels during peroxidation. And the last thing is since some of these reactions are catalyzed by iron, you can look at the iron levels. We have found that during lipid peroxidation the NADPH level does not change significantly. You can measure

this fluorometrically, and find that for up to half an hour
or an hour, you don't get very significant levels of NADPH,
not much change. So if you get a plateau of lipid peroxidation it is not due to a change in NADPH. The flavoprotein
is not destroyed either; you can measure that, and it's more
or less constant. Now there is some change in the glutathione
levels, but what we really looked at is to see if iron levels
were affected. Once you add iron to the cells if you complex
it with the ADP to enter into the cell, it probably remains
there for some time, and then gets bound to apoferritin, and
gives you ferritin.

Although peroxide concentration increases with malonaldehyde production, the latter shows a lag period and that small
lag period can be removed by adding diethylmaleate, which
conjugates with glutathione. Thus glutathione acts as a very
good protective agent in the cell, and if you add peroxide
externally, all the glutathione is used up immediately, and
the moment the peroxide level goes above that of glutathione,
then you get lipid peroxidation, but not until then.

When you do lipid peroxidation, iron becomes bound to
the protein fraction. This you can demonstrate by washing
the cells, then lyse them, and precipitate most protein by
heating. If you add TCA and then look at the iron in the pre-
cipitated protein, you find that a considerable amount of
iron is bound, the one that you added externally. We feel
that this might be a cause that would attenuate lipid peroxidation. The other implication is that some of the enzymes
are solubilized by lipid peroxidation, like this flavoprotein,
and one feels that if you solubilize certain enzymes, like
the flavoprotein, it could travel up to the lysosomes or up
to the mitochondria, and then peroxidize lipids in the mitochondria and the lysosomes. In addition, the malonaldehyde
which is formed, about 90-95% remains with the cell and thus
could bring about peroxidative damage. Malonaldehyde is metabolized by mitochondria, and if you inhibit that particular reaction
by chloral, you find that about 50 to 60% more malonaldehyde
is formed. On the other hand, such peroxidative damage produced
by hydroperoxides might be prevented by cytochrome P450.

When you perform the ADP-iron peroxidation the cytochrome
P450 is not destroyed, it's not touched at all. But if you
do the cumene hydroperoxide catalyzed peroxidation, you get
a very drastic reduction in the P450 level, and that is responsible for stopping lipid peroxidation.

I'd like to say a few words about leukocytes, since all
of you are doing work on leukocytes. Most leukocytes, as
you know, are involved in phagocytosis and have bacteriocidal
action, and of course the enzyme that is responsible for producing

this hydrogen peroxide, is the so-called NADH or NADPH oxidase.
There is a controversy as to its location, some say it's granular, some people say it's in the cytosol. I'd like to present
some evidence from our lab that shows that it is an ectoenzyme
located on the plasma membrane. The evidence is as follows:
It is insensitive to cyanide, as is phagocytosis, and in the
presence of cyanide, oxygen uptake continues. The system
is stimulated by the addition of NADH or NADPH neither of
which penetrate the plasma membrane of the intact leukocyte.
So obviously anything that stimulates must act on the surface.
The third point is that p-chloromercurobenzoate (PCMB) also
inhibits this reaction and it is significant that PCMB does
not penetrate the plasma membrane. The other thing about
this reaction is that if you make the condition hypotonic
you can get oxygen uptake and hydrogen peroxide formation.
If you bring it back to isotonic conditions you will eliminate
the oxygen uptake completely and you can repeat this. You
can make it hypotonic and isotonic and you will get back from
uptake to non-uptake.

Another interesting aspect is that, if the leukocyte
enzyme is located on the plasma membrane, after invagination
during phagocytosis, the oxidase will be located on the inside
surface of the phagocytic vacuole. Now, I believe that very
little superoxide dismutase and catalase are in the plasma
membrane and once the oxidase is inside the phagosome, it
will be removed from superoxide dismutase and catalase and
therefore it can produce hydrogen peroxide and exert some
bacteriocidal action. Another aspect is that the granules
which contain myeloperoxidase fuse to the phagosome. This
means a release of myeloperoxidase into the phagosome where
it presumably takes part in bacteriocidal action, using iodide
or halide and hydrogen peroxide.

These reactions can be stimulated by adding something
like dichlorophenol. If added to the leukocyte system, uptake
of oxygen, formation of hydrogen peroxide and neutralization
of NADPH are greatly facilitated. You can see the complete
system will give you a good amount of oxygen uptake and NADHoxi-
dation. If you leave out either manganese or cyanide you
get a much reduced oxygen uptake and if you leave out dichlorophenol, or NADH, obviously you have very low oxygen uptake.

Dr. Fridovich: I merely need a point of information.
You mentioned the great increase in oxygen uptake by hypotoni-
city. Was the dichlorophenol present?

Dr. Rahimtula: That wasn't present. The dichlorophenol
is just another stimulant of peroxidation.

Dr. Rouser: Do you require lecithin for this system?

Dr. Rahimtula: Which one?

Dr. Rouser: The P450.

Dr. Rahimtula: I have used egg yolk lecithin but you could use any fatty acid.

Dr. Rouser: No, I mean is that a lipid requiring activity?

Dr. Rahimtula: For lipid peroxidation, yes.

Dr. Rouser: What I'm getting at is P450 and the reductase system, when they work together do they require phospholipid? So I'm asking can you leave phospholipid out and get this activity?

Dr. Rahimtula: I think it has been demonstrated recently in Dr. Kuhn's lab that the complex formed from cytochrome P450, the flavoprotein and the lipid is distinct and specific and you need all three components in combination to give you activity.

Dr. Fridovich: It should be commented also that it has been shown that polymorphs do exude or secrete superoxide into the surrounding medium in which they are activated, so that it would fit perfectly well with what you're saying about the NADPH or NADH oxidase being an ectoenzyme.   If it weren't, it wouldn't be possible for the superoxide to get out because it wouldn't survive, wouldn't run the gauntlet of the superoxide dismutase in the cell.   In terms of quantification, it's easily possible to account for 20 or 30% of the extra oxygen uptake in terms of the superoxide which can be intercepted in the outside medium.

Dr. Hoekstra: Along that line, would it be worth the effort to check superoxide production by Batten's leukocytes? I'm thinking particularly in terms of the supposed increased endogenous hydrogen peroxide level.   Any comment on that?

Dr. Fridovich: Not right offhand.

Dr. Rahimtula: If it is assumed that hydrogen peroxide production in Batten's disease is elevated, maybe this is a very good way of checking it.   Just make the leukocytes hypotonic and put NADH and NADPH in.   You would observe oxygen uptake. If you add catalase after the oxygen uptake has begun you can release some of the oxygen as recorded with an oxygen electrode.

Dr. Zeman: These are live cell suspensions on which you perform these determinations?

381

Dr. Rahimtula: Yes, this is pH 6.0, 50 mM phosphate buffer.

Dr. Zeman: With continuous recording by the oxygen electrode?

Dr. Rahimtula: That's right.

Dr. Zeman: Do you have any observations on activators or inhibitors which are biologically possible or usable in your system?

Dr. Rahimtula: For lipid peroxidation the most potent remedy found is tetramethyl-p-phenylenediamine (TMPD). You can oxidize it to Wooster's blue. It's very easy to make. In fact, we measure peroxidase activity by using TMPD and either an organic hydroperoxide or hydrogen peroxide and you measure the formation of Wooster blue at 610 nm.

Dr. Zeman: Apparently in your system the sensitivity is quite high if you use TMPD.

Dr. Rahimtula: We use it primarily to block peroxidation but also for assay of peroxidase.

Dr. Schonbaum: To put it in definitive terms, I don't recall what is the extinction coefficient of your dye.

Dr. Rahimtula: 20 or 21.

Dr. Schonbaum: Well, that is precisely the point I was making. You look at malachites or crystal violet you have on the order of 70 to 80,000 which means you should have a factor of 3 to 4 in your sensitivity gradient.

Dr. Zeman: I would like to return now to the question of activators of peroxidase activity. As you recall, Dr. Fridovich recognized that the data of Dr. Armstrong would be in agreement with the presence of an activator which may be absent in Batten's disease or at least decreased in activity. This observation raises several questions. What do we know in general about activators of peroxidases? Some aspects have certainly been discussed, especially the nitrogenous compounds. But in view of the fact that this does occur in a genetically determined heritable disease, we have to ask a more precise question, namely, what kind of analogy exists with respect to genetically controlled diseases where an activator is either not active or maybe missing on genetic grounds. It follows from this question that we have to develop some ideas as to the possible nature of such an activator. Dr. Fridovich, would you like to speculate a little bit?

Dr. Fridovich: I'm afraid that all I can do at this
point is speculate, because the observations which were reported
in the paper that I passed around yesterday are already published
a good number of years ago, 13 years ago or something like
that. I must admit that although I have since repeated most
of those observations quite recently so that I know they are
quite true, I haven't worked extensively on it in between,
nor to my knowledge has anybody else. I find it rather surprising that people in the peroxidase field have not pursued
this further. But the thing that stands out in my mind with
respect to the kinds of compounds that will work, is that
there was a great lack of specificity, so that one could use
ammonia, imidazole, dimethylamine, trimethylamine, pyridine,
etc., all these compounds. It was very clear that they all
worked in competition with each other, so that they all work
at the same site. It was further clear that none of them
activate by combining with the heme, because there was no
change in the absorption spectrum attributable to the heme.
So in conclusion then, there has to be a site distinct from
the active heme, so I'll call it an allosteric site, at which
these nitrogenous compounds can bind and the affinity was
fairly high because one could already see marked activation
at say a millimolar or a tenth-millimolar or even less concentration of the activators. So that almost any one of a
number of nitrogenous compounds could do, and I wouldn't have
any way of guessing, what the most active would be. Of course,
if Dr. Armstrong and his colleagues were able to show that
in fact a diffusible activator were present in the normal
and absent in only affected cells, it would be fairly easy
to isolate and then identify what it was, by using standard
techniques.

Dr. Schonbaum: Many of you wonder why nobody has pursued
that very intriguing observation by Dr. Fridovich. It's for
the same reason, I suppose, that he had run into and that
is to know precisely what can be done with it. That brings
perhaps into focus another observation, namely that this effect
is only seen, I believe, with o-dianisidine, but apparently
one does not obtain the reaction with guaiacol or substrates
of the phenolic type. The question therefore was that if
it is something which is specific to the enzyme in which you
have an allosteric modification of sorts, why does it express
itself with one substrate but not with another. We haven't
come to grips yet in trying to answer this question in definitive
mechanistic terms.

Dr. Fridovich: That's very true. A remarkable aspect
of it was that it didn't work with guaiacol but did work with
p-phenylenediamine or with o-dianisidine. I don't know why,
but of course that is kind of reminiscent of the kind of data
we've been hearing with respect to the peroxidase which is

383

supposed to be deficient in Batten's disease, that is, that deficiency is seen with one kind of substrate and not with the other. Maybe there is a relationship here.

Dr. Zeman: Let me return to the activator, and its place in the empirical treatment of these disorders. As Dr. Rider pointed out, we have tried a lot of things which are not in the book, and we are not afraid to try more. Essentially this is an incurable disease and anything which can be done to alleviate the lot of the patient or the problems which are generated for the parents, seems to provide us justification in this direction. Dr. Patel after reading your papers some time ago, came to me and asked me whether we should not treat these patients with imidazole, and I wondered whether this should be done and whether there are any data on the toxicity of imidazole. We have a very interesting situation in this respect, because patients with this particular disease excrete quantities of imidazole in the urine. It was on the strength of this observation that I told Dr. Patel, we would like to have a little more information, better data on this.

Dr. Fridovich: It's a fascinating observation about the excretion of imidazole. I hadn't heard that before.

Dr. Zeman: It does not occur in a large number of patients. I think the first to point this out was Dr. Bessman when he was still at Hopkins, and he did find it in one family. Then the idea was taken up by the Scandinavians who see a large number of these patients and if my memory doesn't play tricks, they found it in 4 out of 50 patients. So it is by no means a constant finding, but in comparison to the overall population it is significant. Significant also is that whenever this imidazoluria was found in the patient, it was also found to a lesser extent in the ascertained heterozygotes such as the parents.

Dr. Hoekstra: I wonder whether these patients excrete actually imidazole or rather histamine and similar substances that react like imidazole?

Dr. Zeman: It was some time ago that we checked out these reports and couldn't confirm the findings on any of our patients. Come to think of it, you're right, it was histidine and other imidazole reactive dipeptides.

Dr. Fridovich: It's the most common color test for imidazole coupling with diazosulfanylic acid, and it wouldn't distinguish between free imidazole or imidazole acetate or histamine or histidine, as long as the imidazole ring is there.

Dr. Hoekstra: I was just wondering about using histidine

relative to free imidazole, whether there would be less of
a problem. We fed a few chickens some imidazole, I can't
remember how much, but it didn't have any dramatic effect,
and I think we were somewhere between a tenth and five-tenths
percent of the diet, it was pretty high. I could, if you're
interested in that, I could send it to you, but I can't recall
it now.

Dr. Zeman: Well, would imidazole cross the blood-brain
barrier and hopefully get into cells, or do we know anything
about that?

Dr. Hoekstra: I don't know.

Dr. Zeman: Let me now try to summarize what has transpired here in these two half days. Somewhat embarrassingly,
it has turned out that one bit of evidence which we believed
had been reasonably well documented with respect to the pathogenesis, namely that this is a group of conditions in which
the connecting pathogenetic link is a molecular damage produced
by the peroxidation of unsaturated fatty acids by the intermediate formation of hydroperoxy radicals, may not be as com-
pelling as we had assumed. It was therefore suggested very
strongly that before we consider this a proven fact and continue
along this line of argument, that the peroxides which may
develop in the course of this presumed mechanism should be
more fully and specifically characterized.

This is particularly true with respect to the leukocytic
system, but may also be necessary with regards to the brain
tissue. Here lies really the greatest problem which we encounter
in our efforts to clarify the nature of this disease, because,
as it became clear during the past two days, peroxidative
reactions, chain-breaking mechanisms, and thus the detoxification
of peroxides, all require a very complex system of enzymes,
of activators and of cofactors, which is certainly not only
beyond the comprehension, but also beyond the imagination
of the average physician, and in particular the pathologists.
So what we must do, we must turn our attention to the chemical
characterization of the presumed peroxides. We must determine
the activity of the enzymes, not only in vitro but in the
tissue themselves, in order to obtain information as to the
availability of cofactors such as glutathione in particular,
and last, but not least, we must develop more reliable and
tighter systems for the measurement of these peroxidases,
procedures which give us reproducible results and which are
unequivocal with respect to the reaction product that is being
measured.

The major evidence which was presented in support of
a peroxidase deficiency was the data on the PPD-mediated peroxidase in leukocytes, and this concept probably has been

shot down. I'm not quite able to assess what is salvageable, but it appears that we must look very seriously into the possibilities to develop a system which is more in keeping with the theoretical considerations of Dr. Schonbaum or which, in practical terms, may combine with the system which Dr. P. J. O'Brien and his associates have developed.

In summary, then, we are really not much farther ahead at this time than we were last year, except that we have now a much clearer understanding of the mistakes which we have made in developing hypotheses, in developing concepts, and perhaps also in using the wrong technical procedures. On the other side of the coin, there seems to be acceptance of the possibility that this group of diseases is indeed due to the attack of the hydroperoxy radical upon biological species, and this should compel us to look at other possible mechanisms by which these hydroxyl radicals can form, as so lucidly pointed out by Dr. Fridovich. It is certainly worthwhile to consider his rather attractive hypothesis, namely that one of the barrels in the two-barrelled prevention of oxygen toxicity, could be faulty and that both barrels should be inspected for defects.

Notwithstanding our continued ignorance on the etiology of this group of diseases, I felt that there was considerable support and encouragement for continuing an empirical type of treatment which may actually take into account both the initiators of the peroxidation reaction as well as the chain-breaking mechanism, so that we should combine the pharmacological action of free radical scavengers with antioxidants. In view of the uncertainty of the primary initiator, it may very well be necessary to use an approach here which is widely used in the treatment of infectious diseases, of which the specific organism is not known, which is called broad-spectrum antibiotics. So we should have broad-spectrum radical scavengers and broad-spectrum antioxidants in order to cover the range of the unknowns.

Probably the most definitive result of this conference is the realization that Dr. Armstrong's data strongly suggests the suppression or absence of an activator in the enzyme preparations of patients affected with this syndrome, but present in the controls and in the heterozygotes. We have speculated on the nature of this activator, but it will take more than speculation; it will take hard work and sweat in order to come to grips with this particular problem. Also, and this shows at least the seriousness and the sincerity of our efforts, it now appears that some of the data which excited us last time may, following a more critical evaluation, no longer be so exciting. This relates to the interpretation which now seems to gain hold, at least in the mind of Dr. Armstrong, namely that the number of enzyme molecules which

he measures in his system may not change as a function of
the genetic endowment, but that there might be perhaps other
physicochemical factors which afford a change in the ratio
between the soluble and the insoluble phase of this enzyme.
So we have many more questions to answer now than we had
before we came together here, but with the exception of the
strong and convincing evidence of the activator, we do not
have more answers. Thank you very much for coming here.

INDEX

ADP-iron peroxidation, 378-379

Acidic lipid polymers
  as components of ceroid and
  lipofuscin, 124, 332

Activity of peroxidized enzymes,
  163

Aging in Drosophila, 150-155
  effect of vitamin E on, 154-155

Alkoxy radicals, 46

Alkyl peroxides, 353

Amaurotic idiocy
  definition, 2-3
  historical development, 15-16

γ-Aminobutyric acid
  as anticonvulsant, 114
  deficiency in Batten's
  disease, 102-103

δ-Aminolevulinic acid synthetase
  in Batten's disease, 140-141,
  147-149
  in heme synthesis, 136-138

2,3-AMP phosphohydrolase
  activity in lipopigments, 124,
  369

Arachidonic acid
  precursor of prostaglandins, 298
  rate of synthesis, 236

Batten's disease (Batten-Vogt Syndrome;
  neuronal ceroid-lipofuscinosis)
  abnormalities in ganglioside
  pattern, 298
  deficiency of PPD-mediated
  peroxidase, 255-265
  definition, 2-4, 18-19, 221-223
  diagnosis by rectal biopsy, 206
  dog model for, 207-208
  ethanolamine plasmalogen, 298
  genetic heterogeneity of, 182
  hypertension in, 117

imidazoluria in, 384
prevention of, 286-288

Biochemical genetics
  theory of, in Batten's disease,
  104-106

Bone marrow transplant, 197
  as treatment for Batten's disease, 193

Butylated hydroxytoluene
  as antioxidant, 48-50

Carbonyls
  as products of lipid peroxidation
  43-45, 82-85, 95-96

Catalase, 230, 257, 259
  activity in brain, 289
  activity in ducks, 344
  kinetics, 358
  specific substrates for, 344-345

Catalase deficiency, 343-344

Centrophenoxine, 50-51
  action on intralysosomal peroxidation, 240
  treatment of Batten's disease
  with, 295-296

Cerebrotendinous xanthomatosis, 235

Ceroid
  cation composition, 124
  definition and chemical properties, 121-126
  distribution of, 21
  formation in choline-deficient
  rats, 239
  in brain, 36
  in cirrhotic liver, 35
  in Drosophila, 38-40
  neutral lipid composition, 122
  polar lipid composition, 123
  stability, 30-31

Chicken encephalomalacia
  produced by unsaturated fatty
  acids, 90-94

389

Chlorophenoxy acetate-tocopherol
  extension of lifespan by, 376

Conjugated aldehydes, 44-45

Cross-linking
  of enzymes, 233
  of cholesterol, 235
  by malonaldehyde, 234

Curvilinear bodies, 127

Cytochrome C system, 350

Enzyme activity
  lipid requirements for, 342

Enzyme deficiency
  theory of, 112-113

Enzyme stabilization, 333

Ethanolamine plasmalogen
  (phosphatidal ethanolamine)
  loss of, in Batten's disease,
  298
  loss of, in lipid peroxidation,
  299

Fabry's disease, 195, 254
  treatment by kidney transplant, 200-201

Fatty acid turnover, 246-251
  in Batten's disease, 70-71, 74-77,
  247-248
  in Tay-Sachs disease, 69-73

Fingerprint bodies, 127

Fluorescent lipopigments
  conjugated aldehydes in, 44-45
  formation of, 42-44
  in brain explants, 252
  in tissue culture, 252-253

Free radicals
  chain reaction, 162
  in membrane peroxidation, 160-161

Gangliosides
  abnormalities in Batten's disease, 78-79, 164-165, 298

in SSPE, 77

Gaucher's disease, 195

Genetic replacement therapy by
  virus, 296-297

Glucose-6-phosphate dehydrogenase
  deficiency, 238-239

Glutamic decarboxylase deficiency,
  115-116

Glutathione, 227-230
  concentration in brain, 339-340

Glutathione peroxidase, 225-227
  absence in selenium deficiency,
  244-245
  activity in brain tissue in Batten's disease, 284-286, 322
  substrate specificity, 287-388

Haltia-Santavuori type
  definition, 3-4
  pathogenesis, 19
  ultrastructure of pigment, 128

Heme biosynthesis, 138

Homochronism, 278

Homotypism, 278

Horseradish peroxidase, 280-283
  treatment of Batten's disease
  with, 329-330

Hydroperoxides, 226

Hydrogen abstraction, 226

Hydrogen peroxide
  as substrate for peroxidase, 336-
  337

Hydroxylamine
  antioxidant effect, 52-53

Hypervitaminosis A, 133

390